# Lederman's
# Internal Medicine and
# Critical Care Pocketguide

## 6th Edition

Robert J. Lederman, MD, FACC, FAHA

Senior Investigator, Cardiovascular and Pulmonary Branch
National Heart, Lung, and Blood Institute
National Institutes of Health
Bethesda, MD

# Lederman's
# Internal Medicine and
# Critical Care Pocketguide

bibliohop

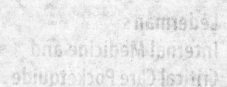

Robert Lederman, MD, FACP, FWA

Senior Investigator, Cardiovascular and Pulmonary Branch
National Heart, Lung and Blood Institute
National Institutes of Health
Bethesda, MD

Lederman's Internal Medicine and Critical Care Pocketguide (6th edition)
is published by

ANTIMICROBIAL THERAPY, INC.
*Publisher of the Sanford Guides*
P.O. Box 276, 11771 Lee Highway
Sperryville, VA 22740 USA
Tel +1 540 987 9480 Fax +1 540 987 9486
info@sanfordguide.com
www.sanfordguide.com

Printed in the United States of America
ISBN 978-1-930808-98-0

**IMPORTANT NOTE TO READER**

Every effort is made to ensure the accuracy of the content of this guide. Current full prescribing information available in the package insert for each drug referenced in this guide should be consulted before prescribing any product. The author and publisher are not responsible for errors or omissions or for any consequences from application of information in this guide and make no warranty, express or implied, with respect to the currency, accuracy or completeness of the contents of this guide. Application of information found in this guide in a particular situation remains the professional responsibility of the practitioner.

This book was authored by Robert J. Lederman in his private capacity. The views expressed in the book do not necessarily represent the views of the NIH, DHHS, or the United States.

Additional copies may be ordered from your bookstore or at www.sanfordguide.com.

**Lederman's Internal Medicine & Critical Care mobile apps**
may be purchased separately from the Apple App Store or Google Play.

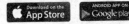

# Contents

Editorial Board.........................................................................xi

A Note from the Author..........................................................xii

Dedication..............................................................................xiii

Abbreviations........................................................................xiv

Handy Formulas.........................................................................1
    Acid-Base Rules of Thumb..............................................1
    Acid-Base Map...............................................................1
    Other Renal Equations....................................................2
    Pharmacology Equations.................................................3
    Anthropometric Equations..............................................4
    Hemodynamic Equations.................................................4
    Pulmonary Equations......................................................5
    Hemodynamic Values.......................................................6
    SI Lab Value Converter....................................................7
    Medical Statistics...........................................................7
    Pediatric Vital Signs.......................................................9
    Groovy Web Sites............................................................9

Code Algorithms.....................................................................10
    Basic Life Support for Professionals..............................10
    Adult Cardiac Arrest.....................................................11
    Bradycardia..................................................................14
    Tachycardia..................................................................15
    Immediate care after cardiac arrest..............................16

Cardiology.............................................................................19
    Hemodynamics–Cardiac Cycle.......................................19
    Jugular Venous Pulsations.............................................20
    Systolic Murmurs..........................................................20
    Echo/MRI/Nuclear Anatomy...........................................23
    Coronary Artery Anatomy..............................................24
    ECG Lead-Anatomy Relationship....................................25
    ECG ST elevation (STE) patterns....................................26
    ECG: Hypertrophy.........................................................28
    ECG: BBB, Fascicle Block & IWMI....................................29
    ECG: Wide-QRS Tachycardia...........................................31
    Torsades & Long QT syndromes......................................33
    Risk scores in atrial fibrillation: stroke & bleeding.........35
    Probability of Coronary Disease.....................................36
    Exercise Stress Testing..................................................37
    Emergency Cardiac Pacing Technique.............................39
    Intra-Aortic Balloon Pump.............................................40
    Hypertensive Emergencies.............................................42
    Perioperative Cardiovascular Risk.................................44
    Acute Coronary Syndromes & MI.....................................48

    Valve Formulae ........................................................ 54
    Valve Disease Severity ............................................. 55

**Critical Care** .............................................................**58**
    Shock ........................................................................ 58
    Sepsis ....................................................................... 60
    Anaphylaxis ............................................................. 62
    APACHE II Score ..................................................... 64
    Pulmonary Artery Catheters ................................. 65
    Using Mechanical Ventilators ................................ 68
    Ventilator Emergencies ......................................... 74
    Weaning from Mechanical Ventilation .................. 75
    Targeted temperature management ...................... 77

**Endocrinology** ........................................................**79**
    Thyroid Function in Critical Illness ........................ 79
    Myxedema Coma ..................................................... 80
    Thyroid Storm ......................................................... 82
    Hyperglycemia ........................................................ 84
    Adrenal Crisis .......................................................... 88

**Gastroenterology** ..................................................**90**
    Upper GI Hemorrhage ............................................ 90
    Acute Lower GI Bleeding ....................................... 94
    Acute Infectious Diarrhea ..................................... 95
    Clostrodium Difficile Colitis .................................. 97
    Viral Hepatitis Serologies ...................................... 99
    Serum-Ascites Albumin Gradient .......................... 100
    Spontaneous Bacterial Peritonitis ........................ 100
    Surgical Risk in Liver Disease ................................ 101
    Hepatorenal syndrome .......................................... 104
    Acute Pancreatitis .................................................. 105
    Nutrition: Enteral & Parenteral ............................ 107

**Hematology** ............................................................**113**
    Anemia Differential Diagnosis ............................... 113
    Hemolytic Anemia ................................................. 113
    Iron-Deficiency Anemia ......................................... 116
    Macrocytic Anemia ................................................ 118
    Thrombocytopenia ................................................. 120
    Heparin-Induced Thrombocytopenia ..................... 121
    Transfusion of Blood Products .............................. 125
    Transfusion Reactions ........................................... 126
    Coagulation Tests .................................................. 128

**Infectious Disease** .................................................**131**
    New fever in the ICU ............................................. 131
    Modified Duke Criteria for Endocarditis .............. 135
    Surgery for Infective Endocarditis ........................ 136
    Bacterial Endocarditis Prophylaxis ....................... 136
    Life-threatening Infective Rashes ......................... 138
    Bacterial Meningitis in Adults .............................. 139

# Contents

Community Acquired Pneumonia ........................... 141
Pharyngeal swab technique ................................. 145
Infections after Transplantation........................... 146

**Neurology** .......................................................**149**
Common Stroke Syndromes................................ 149
Stroke mimics .................................................... 150
Unusual Causes of Stroke .................................. 151
NIH Stroke Scale ................................................ 152
Modified Rankin Score ....................................... 153
Acute Ischemic Stroke ....................................... 154
ABCD2 Stroke Risk after TIA ............................. 158
Coma common reversible causes........................ 159
Status Epilepticus .............................................. 163
Alcohol Withdrawal Syndromes.......................... 166
Cerebrospinal Fluid Data ................................... 168
Muscle Innervation ............................................ 169
Spinal & Peripheral Nerves................................ 170
Visual Acuity Screen .......................................... 174
Folstein Mini-Mental State.................................. 175
Glasgow Coma Scale .......................................... 176
Neurologic Prognosis After Cardiac Arrest.......... 177
Brain Death Exam .............................................. 178

**Pulmonary** ......................................................**181**
Chest Anatomy - Radiographs ............................ 181
Chest Anatomy - CT ........................................... 184
Bronchoscopic Anatomy ..................................... 185
Fleishner Score: Incidental Pulmonary Nodules... 186
Pulmonary Function Testing................................ 186
Predicted Peak Expiratory Flow (L/min) .............. 189
Pulmonary thromboembolism (PE) ..................... 190
Pleural Fluid Analysis ......................................... 193
Pulmonary Hypertension .................................... 195
Preoperative Pulmonary Evaluation .................... 197

**Renal** ..............................................................**201**
Gaps and Deltas ................................................ 201
Metabolic Acidosis ............................................. 203
Lactic Acidosis .................................................. 204
Renal Tubular Acidosis ...................................... 206
Metabolic Alkalosis ............................................ 207
Hyponatremia .................................................... 209
Syndrome of Inappropriate Antidiuretic Hormone
(SIADH) ............................................................ 211
Hypernatremia ................................................... 212
Hypokalemia ..................................................... 214
Hyperkalemia .................................................... 216
Hypomagnesemia .............................................. 217
Hypocalcemia .................................................... 219

    Hypercalcemia.........................................................220
    Hypophosphatemia..................................................222
    FENa............................................................................223
    FE-Urea......................................................................224
    Tumor Lysis Syndrome...........................................224

**Rheumatology**..........................................................**225**
    Autoantibody Tests.................................................225
    Vasculitis....................................................................227
    Systemic Lupus Erythematosus: ARA Criteria.....229
    Synovial Fluid Analysis...........................................231
    Arthritis & Fever......................................................232

**Toxicology**.................................................................**234**
    General Management..............................................234
    Common Toxic Syndromes.....................................237
    Tricyclic antidepressant toxicity...........................238
    Beta-adrenergic blocker & calcium-channel blocker
    toxicity.......................................................................240
    Neuroleptic Malignant Syndrome.........................241
    Serotonin Syndromes.............................................242
    Ethylene Glycol & Methanol Toxicity....................243
    Acetaminophen (APAP) Toxicity............................245
    Salicylate Toxicity...................................................247
    Cyanide Poisoning...................................................249
    Methemoglobinemia, acquired.............................251
    Nerve Agents............................................................252

**Groovy Drugs**............................................................**255**
    Cytochrome P450 (CYP) interactions....................256
    Abciximab..................................................................258
    Acetylcysteine (Mucomyst, Acetadote)...............258
    Adenosine (Adenocard, Adenoscan).....................258
    Alteplase (tPA; Activase).........................................259
    Aminophylline...........................................................259
    Amiodarone (Cordarone).......................................260
    Anticholinesterases.................................................262
    Anticoagulants.........................................................263
    Argatroban................................................................264
    Atracurium (Tracrium)............................................265
    Atropine.....................................................................265
    Beta-Adrenergic Blockers.......................................266
    Bicarbonate...............................................................268
    Bivalirudin (Angiomax)............................................269
    Bumetanide (Bumex)...............................................269
    Calcium......................................................................270
    Calcium channel blockers.......................................270
    Charcoal, activated..................................................271
    Chlorothiazide (Diuril)............................................271
    Cisatracurium (Nimbex)..........................................271

Clevidipine (Cleviprex)............................................ 272
Clonidine (Catapres).............................................. 272
Corticosteroids.................................................... 273
Dabigatran (Pradaxa)............................................. 273
Dantrolene......................................................... 274
Desmopressin (ddAVP, Stimate)................................. 274
Dexmedotomidine (Precedex)................................... 275
Digoxin............................................................. 276
Digoxin Immune Fab (Digifab)................................... 277
Diltiazem IV....................................................... 278
Diuretics, Loop.................................................... 279
Dobutamine........................................................ 279
Dopamine.......................................................... 280
Enoxaparin (Lovenox)............................................ 281
Epinephrine (Adrenalin).......................................... 281
Eptifibatide (Integrilin).......................................... 282
Esmolol (Brevibloc)............................................... 282
Ethanol............................................................ 283
Etomidate (Amidate).............................................. 284
Fibrinolytic Agents................................................ 284
Flumazenil (Romazicon).......................................... 289
Fomepizole (Antizol)............................................. 290
Fondaparinux (Arixtra)........................................... 291
Fosphenytoin (Cerebyx IV)....................................... 292
Furosemide (Lasix)............................................... 292
Glucagon.......................................................... 292
Glycoprotein $II_bIII_a$ Inhibitors............................... 293
Haloperidol (Haldol).............................................. 295
Heparin (UFH)..................................................... 296
Heparin (LMWH)................................................... 298
Hydralazine (Apresoline)......................................... 300
Hydroxocobalamin (Cyanokit)................................... 301
Hypoglycemic Agents............................................ 301
Insulin............................................................. 304
Ibutilide (Corvert)................................................ 306
Idarucizumab (Praxbind)......................................... 307
Iron Intravenous.................................................. 308
Iron sucrose (Venofer)........................................... 309
Isoproterenol (Isuprel).......................................... 310
Kayexalate........................................................ 310
Ketamine (Ketalar)............................................... 310
Labetalol.......................................................... 311
Levetiracetem (Keppra).......................................... 312
Levothyroxine (T4)............................................... 313
Lidocaine.......................................................... 313
Liothyronine (T3)................................................. 314
Lipid or fat emulsion (Intralipid)................................ 315
Magnesium........................................................ 315
Mannitol........................................................... 316

Methylene Blue .................................................. 316
Methylnaltrexone (Relistor) ............................... 317
Midazolam (Versed) ........................................... 317
Milrinone (Primacor) .......................................... 318
Naloxone (Narcan) ............................................. 319
Neostigmine ....................................................... 319
Neuromuscular blockers .................................... 320
Nicardipine IV (Cardene) ................................... 323
Nimodipine ........................................................ 324
Nitrite ................................................................ 324
Nitroglycerin ...................................................... 325
Nitroprusside (Nipride) ...................................... 325
Norepinephrine (Levophed) ............................... 327
Novel Oral Anticoagulants (NOACs) .................. 328
Octreotide (Sandostatin) ................................... 331
Ondansetron (Zofran) ........................................ 331
Opiate Analgesics .............................................. 332
Pamidronate (Aredia) ........................................ 333
Pancuronium ..................................................... 334
Pentobarbital (Nembutal) .................................. 334
Phenobarbital sodium ....................................... 334
Phentolamine (Regitine) .................................... 335
Phenylephrine (Neo-Synephrine) ...................... 336
Phenytoin (Dilantin) .......................................... 336
Phosphorus ....................................................... 338
Physostigmine ................................................... 339
Platelet $P2Y_{12}$ Inhibitors .................................. 339
Pralidoxime (2-PAM) .......................................... 340
Procainamide ..................................................... 341
Propofol (Diprivan) ............................................ 343
Propylene Glycol Diluent ................................... 344
Protamine ........................................................... 344
Prothrombin (4-factor PCC, Kcentra) ................ 345
Pulmonary Vasodilators ..................................... 346
Rasburicase (Elitek) ........................................... 350
Remifentanil (Ultiva) ......................................... 351
Sodium (Kayexalate) .......................................... 351
Vasopressin ........................................................ 352
Verapamil ........................................................... 354
Warfarin (Coumadin) ......................................... 354
Zoledronic Acid (Zometa) .................................. 357

**Index** ............................................................... 359

# Editorial Board

# A Note from the Author

This guide is intended as a "head of the bed" reference for a variety of internal medicine emergencies. While the 6th edition has been expanded and updated, we have continued to include only a selection of life-threatening or less-common clinical problems.

To use this book effectively, please take a few minutes to familiarize yourself with its structure and contents.

Many users have sent in comments; we are grateful for their input. If you find an error or wish to make a suggestion, please let us know (e-mail: info@sanfordguide.com).

# Dedication

This book is dedicated to my son Adam and my wife Laura with all my love, and to the memory of my father Ezjel.

As before, this book also is dedicated to the memory of James S. Winshall, and to his insistence on excellence.

# Abbreviations

↓: decrease, low
↑: increase, high
Δ: change

Ab: antibody
ABG: arterial blood gas
ACE: angiotensin converting enzyme
ACLS: advanced cardiac life support
ACS: acute coronary syndrome
ADH: antidiuretic hormone
AF or A-fib: atrial fibrillation
Ag: antigen
AI: aortic insufficiency
ALT: alanine aminotransferase
AML: acute myelogenous leukemia
Amp: ampule
ANA: antinuclear antibody
aPTT: activated partial thromboplastin time
ARDS: adult respiratory distress syndrome
ARF: acute renal failure
AS: aortic stenosis
ASD: atrial septal defect
AST: aspartate aminotransferase
ATN: acute tubular necrosis
AV: atrioventricular
AVB: atrioventricular block
AVM: arteriovenous malformation
AWMI: anterior wall myocardial infarction

BBB: bundle branch block

BLS: basic life support
BMT: bone marrow transplant
BP: Blood pressure

Ca: calcium
CABG: coronary artery bypass graft
CAD: coronary artery disease
CAPD: continuous ambulatory peritoneal dialysis
CAVH/D: continuous arteriovenous hemofiltration/dialysis
CCS: Canadian angina class
CHF: congestive heart failure
CLL: chronic lymphocytic leukemia
CMV: cytomegalovirus
CNS: central nervous system
CO: carbon monoxide
COPD: chronic obstructive pulmonary disease
CPR: cardiopulmonary resuscitation
Cr: creatinine
CrCL: creatinine clearance
CSF: cerebrospinal fluid
CT: computed tomography
CTA: CT angiography
CXR: chest radiograph

d: day
D5W: dextrose 5% in water
D50: dextrose 50% in water
DA: dopamine
DC: discontinue
DBP: diastolic BP

DIC: disseminated intravascular coagulation
DKA: diabetic ketoacidosis
dL: deciliter
DVT: deep vein thrombosis
DM: diabetes mellitus
Dx: diagnosis
Dz: disease

EBV: Epstein-Barr virus
ECG: electrocardiogram
EEG: electroencephalogram
*e.g.*: for example
eGFR: estimated glomerular filtration rate
EP: electrophysiologic testing
ERCP: endoscopic retrograde cholangio-pancreatography
ESRD: end-stage renal disease
EtOH: ethanol

FENa: fractional excretion of sodium
$FEV_1$: forced expiratory volume in 1 second
$FiO_2$: inspired oxygen fraction
FFP: fresh frozen plasma
FVC: forced vital capacity

G6PD: glucose-6-phosphate dehydrogenase
GFR: glomerular filtration rate
GI: gastrointestinal
gm: gram
GP $II_bIII_a$: Glycoprotein $II_bIII_a$
gtts: drops
GVHD: graft vs. host disease

h or hr: hour
Hb: hemoglobin
HBsAb/Ag: hepatitis B surface Ab, Antigen
HBV: hepatitis B virus
HCV: hepatitis C virus
$HCO_3$: bicarbonate
HELLP: hemolytic anemia, elevated liver enzymes and low platelets
HIT: heparin-induced thrombocytopenia
H&P: history & physical exam
HR: heart rate
HSV: herpes simplex virus
HTN: hypertension
HUS: hemolytic-uremic syndrome

IABP: intraaortic balloon counterpulsation pump
ICD: implantable cardiac defibrillator
IE: infective endocarditis
IM: intramuscular
IMV: intermittent mandatory ventilation
IU: international units
IV: intravenous
IVC: inferior vena cava
IVDU: intravenous drug user
IVIG: intravenous immunoglobulin
IVP: intravenous push
IWMI: inferior wall myocardial infarction

JVP: jugular vein pressure

K: potassium

L: left, liter
LA: left atrium

LAO: left anterior oblique

LBBB: left bundle branch block

LDH: lactate dehydrogenase

LMWH: low molecular weight heparin

LN: lymph node

LV: left ventricle

LVEDP: left ventricular end-diastolic pressure

LVH: left ventricular hypertrophy

MAOI: monoamine oxidase inhibitor

MetHb: methemoglobin

Mg: magnesium

MI: myocardial infarction

min: minutes

MS: mitral stenosis

$M_VO_2$: myocardial oxygen consumption

MVP: mitral valve prolapse

Na: sodium

n/a: not available

NE: norepinephrine

Nml: normal

n/r: not recommended

NS: normal (0.9%) saline

NSAID: nonsteroidal antiinflammatory drug

NSR: normal sinus rhythm

NSTEMI: non-ST elevation myocardial infarction

NTG: nitroglycerin

N/V/D: nausea, vomiting, diarrhea

$O_2$sat: arterial oxygen saturation

PA: pulmonary artery, posteroanterior

PAD: PA diastolic pressure, Peripheral artery disease

$P_aCO_2$: arterial partial pressure of carbon dioxide

PAgram: pulmonary arteriogram

$P_aO_2$: arterial partial pressure of oxygen

$P_AO_2$: alveolar partial pressure of oxygen

PCA: procainamide

PCI: percutaneous coronary intervention

PCN: penicillin

PCP: *Pneumocystis carinii* pneumonia

PCR: polymerase chain reaction

PCWP: pulmonary capillary wedge pressure

PDA: patent ductus arteriosus

PE: pulmonary embolism

PEEP: positive end-expiratory pressure

PFT: pulmonary function test

PGp: P-glycoprotein

PMN: polymorphonuclear leukocyte

PNGT: via nasogastric tube

PO: orally

PRBC: packed RBCs

PSA: prostate specific antigen

PSVT: paroxysmal supra-ventricular tachycardia

Pt: patient

PT: prothrombin time

PTCA: percutaneous transluminal coronary angioplasty

PTU: propylthiouracil

PUD: peptic ulcer disease
PVR: pulmonary vascular resistance

R: right
RA: right atrium
RAO: right anterior oblique
RBBB: right bundle branch block
RBC: red blood cell
RCT: randomized controlled trial
R/O: rule out
RSV: respiratory syncytial virus
RTA: renal tubular acidosis
RV: right ventricle
RVEDP: right ventricular end-diastolic pressure
Rx: therapy

SA: sinoatrial
SAH: subarachnoid hemorrhage
$S_aO_2$: arterial oxygen saturation
SBP: systolic blood pressure; spontaneous bacterial peritonitis
SC: subcutaneous
SIADH: syndrome of inappropriate ADH secretion
SLE: systemic lupus erythematosus
SNRT: sinus node recovery time
s/p: status post
STEMI: ST elevation myocardial infarction
SVC: superior vena cava
SVR: systemic vascular resistance

SVT: supraventricular tachycardia
Sx: symptoms

$T_{1/2}$: half-life
TB: tuberculosis
TCA: tricyclic antidepressant
Td: tetanus-diphtheria vaccine
TIA: transient ischemic attack
tid: three times daily
TEE: transesophageal echocardiography
TN: true negative
Tn: troponin
TP: true positive
TPN: total parenteral nutrition
TTKG: trans-tubular potassium gradient
TTP: thrombotic thrombocytopenia purpura

U: Unit
UGI: upper gastrointestinal
US: ultrasound

VC: vital capacity
$V_D$: volume of distribution, or dead-space volume
VF: ventricular fibrillation
V/Q: ventilation/perfusion
VSD: ventricular septal defect
VT: ventricular tachycardia
vWF: von Willebrand factor
VZV: varicella-zoster virus

WBC: white blood cell
WPW: Wolff-Parkinson-White syndrome

XRT: radiation therapy

# Handy Formulas

## Acid-Base Rules of Thumb

| | | Acidosis | Alkalosis |
|---|---|---|---|
| Respiratory | Acute | $\Delta$ pH = − 0.008 x $\Delta$ PaCO$_2$<br>$\Delta$ [HCO$_3^-$] = 0.1 x $\Delta$ PaCO$_2$ (± 3) | $\Delta$ pH = 0.008 x $\Delta$ PaCO$_2$<br>$\Delta$ [HCO$_3^-$] = − 0.2 x $\Delta$ PaCO$_2$ (usually not to less than 18 mEq/L) |
| | Chronic | P$_a$CO$_2$ = 2.4 x [HCO$_3^-$] - 22<br>$\Delta$ [HCO$_3^-$] = 0.35 x $\Delta$ PaCO$_2$ (± 4) | $\Delta$ [HCO$_3^-$] = − 0.4 x $\Delta$ PaCO$_2$ (usually not to less than 18 mEq/L) |
| Metabolic | | P$_a$CO$_2$ = 1.5 x [HCO$_3^-$] + 8 ± 2<br>P$_a$CO$_2$ ≅ last two digits of pH<br>$\Delta$ P$_a$CO$_2$ = 1.2 x $\Delta$ [HCO$_3^-$] | P$_a$CO$_2$ = 0.9 x [HCO$_3^-$] + 9 ± 2<br>$\Delta$ P$_a$CO$_2$ = 0.6 x $\Delta$ [HCO$_3^-$] |

## Acid-Base Map[1]

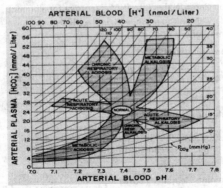

[1] Reprinted with permission from Brenner BM, Rector FC. *Brenner and Rector's The Kidney*. 6th ed. Figure 21-9. Philadelphia: Elsevier, 2000.

# *Other Renal Equations*

mmol/L = mg/dL x 10 ÷ molecular weight

mEq/L = mmol/L x valence

mOsm/kg = mmol/L x n (where *n* is number of dissociable particles per molecule)

Calculated Osmolarity = $2 \times Na(mEq/L) + \frac{BUN\ (mg/dL)}{2.8}$

$+ \frac{Glucose\ (mg/dL)}{18} + \frac{EtOH\ (mg/dL)}{4.6} + \frac{Isopropanol\ (mg/dL)}{6}$

$+ \frac{methanol}{3.2} + \frac{ethylene\ glycol}{6.2}$ (Normal 275-290 mOsm/kg)

Osmolar gap = Measured − calculated osmolarity
(normal < 10 mOsm/kg)

Anion Gap = [Na] − [Cl] − [$HCO_3$] (correct for albumin)

Urinary anion gap = [Na] + [K] − Cl − [$HCO_3$]
(may ignore $HCO_3$ if pH < 6.5)

Free water deficit (L) =

$$0.4 \times lean\ body\ wt \times \left\{ \frac{plasma\ [Na+]}{140} - 1 \right\}$$

Creatinine Clearance = $\frac{UCr \times V}{PCr}$ =

$$\frac{[Urine\ creatinine\ (mg/dL)] \times [Urine\ volume\ (ml/d)]}{[Plasma\ creatinine\ (mg/dL)] \times 1440\ min/d}$$

Creatinine Clearance (eGFR) $\approx \dfrac{140 - Age\ (yrs)}{Serum\ creatinine\ (mg/dL) \times 7.}$

x weight (kg) (x 0.85 if a woman)

Creatinine Clearance (eGFR, mL/min/1.73m²; Abbreviated MDRD formula[2]) = 186 x [Cr mg/dL]$^{-1.154}$ x Age (yr)$^{-0.203}$ x [.742 if female] x [1.210 if African-American]

Fractional Excretion of Sodium (FENa) =

$$\frac{[Urine\ Na]\ x\ [Plasma\ Cr]}{[Urine\ Cr]\ x\ [Plasma\ Na]}$$

Trans-tubular K$^+$ gradient (TTKG) = $(U_K \times P_{Osm}) \div (P_K \times U_{Osm})$

**Rules of thumb:**

Estimated 24-hr urinary protein excretion (g/day) ≈ spot urine prot/creat ratio

Potassium and pH: [K$^+$] increases 0.6 mEq/L for each pH drop of 0.1

Sodium and glucose: [Na$^+$] decreased 1.6 mEq/L per 100 mg/dl ↑ in glucose

Calcium and albumin: [Ca$^{++}$] decreases 0.8 mg/dl for each 1.0 g/dl ↓ in albumin

# *Pharmacology Equations*

Elimination constant: $K_{el} = \ln \frac{[peak]}{[trough]} \div (Time_{peak} - Time_{trough})$

Clearance: $Cl = V_d \times K_{el}$

Half-life: $T_{\frac{1}{2}} = 0.693 \div K_{el} = 0.693 \times V_d \div Cl$

Dosing interval = $\frac{1}{K_{el}} \times \ln\left(\frac{[desired\ peak]}{[desired\ trough]}\right)$ + infusion time

Loading dose = $V_d \times$ [target peak]

[2] K/DOQI clinical practice guidelines for chronic kidney disease: evaluation, classification, and stratification. *Am J Kidney Dis.* 2002;39 (2 Suppl 1): S1-266.

# *Anthropometric Equations*

Ideal body weight (male)[3] = 50 kg + (2.3 kg per inch over 5 feet)

Ideal body weight (female)[3] = 45 kg + (2.3 kg per inch over 5 feet)

Ideal body weight (male)[4] = 48 kg + (1.1 kg/cm per cm over 150 cm)

Ideal body weight (female)[4] = 45 kg + (0.9 kg/cm per cm over 150 cm)

Body mass index (BMI) $= mass (kg) / [height (m)]^2$ (Normal 18.5–25)

$$= mass (lb) \times 703 / [height (in)]^2$$

Body surface area (BSA) in $m^2 = \sqrt{\dfrac{height\ (cm) \times weight\ (kg)}{3600}}$

# *Hemodynamic Equations*

Blood pressure:

$$MAP = \frac{Systolic\ BP + (2 \times Diastolic\ BP)}{3} = DBP + \frac{SBP - DBP}{3}$$

Fick Cardiac Output:

$$CO = \frac{O_2\ Consumption}{(Arterial - Venous)O_2\ Content}$$

$$= \frac{10 \times V_{O_2}\ (ml/min/m^2)}{Hb\ (gm/dL) \times 1.36 \times (Arterial\ O_2\ Sat\% - Venous\ O_2\ Sat\%)}$$

Cardiac Index: $CI = \dfrac{CO}{BSA}$ (Normal 2.5–4.2 L/min/m$^2$)

Stroke Volume: $SV = \dfrac{CO}{HR}$

---

[3] Devine BJ. Gentamicin therapy. *Drug Intell Clin Pharm* 1974;8:650-655

[4] Hamwi/Hammond (1964): Add or subtract 10% for heavy or light frame.

Pulmonary vascular resistance (PVR, dyne/sec/cm$^5$) =

$$\frac{80 \times [\text{Mean PA Pressure} - \text{mean PCWP}]}{\text{Cardiac output (L/min)}}$$

Systemic vascular resistance (SVR, dyne/sec/cm$^5$) =

$$\frac{80 \times [\text{MAP (mmHg)} - \text{RA pressure (mmHg)}]}{\text{Cardiac output (L/min)}}$$

Oxygen consumption: $VO_2/BSA = K + 0.483 \times HR$
(mL/min/M$^2$),
where K=99.7 (men), 85.9 (women)
or $VO_2 \approx 125$ mL/kg/min

# *Pulmonary Equations*

Tidal Volume: $V_T = (V_{dead\ space} + V_{alveolar\ space}) = V_D + V_A$

Minute Ventilation: $V_E = \dfrac{0.863 \times V_{CO_2}(ml/min)}{P_aCO_2 \times (1 - V_D/V_T)}$ (Normal 0.2-0.3)

Bohr Dead Space: $\dfrac{V_D}{V_T} = \dfrac{P_ACO_2 - P_{expired}CO_2}{P_ACO_2}$ (Normal 0.2-0.3)

Physiologic Dead Space: $\dfrac{V_D}{V_T} = \dfrac{P_aCO_2 - P_{expired}CO_2}{P_aCO_2}$

Static Compliance = $\dfrac{V_T}{P_{plateau} - P_{end\ expiration}}$ (Normal > 60 mL/cmH$_2$O)

Surface Tension LaPlace Law: Pressure = $\dfrac{2 \times \text{Tension}}{\text{Radius}}$

Alveolar O$_2$ estimate:
$P_AO_2 = FiO_2 \times [\text{pAtmospheric} - \text{pH}_2O] - \dfrac{pCO_2}{\text{Resp Quotient}}$

$\quad = FiO_2 \times [760 - 47 \text{ mmHg}] - \dfrac{pCO_2}{0.8}$

Alveolar – arterial $O_2$ gradient = $P_AO_2 - P_aO_2 \approx 2.5 + 0.21 \times$ Age (yr) upright

$P_aO_2$ upright $\approx 104.2 - 0.27 \times$ Age (yr)

$P_aO_2$ supine $\approx 103.5 - 0.42 \times$ Age (yr)

$$P_aCO_2 = K \times \frac{CO_2 \text{ Production}}{\text{Alveolar Ventilation}} = 0.863 \times \frac{VCO_2}{VA}$$

Shunt Fraction: $\dfrac{Q_s}{Q_t} = \dfrac{(A - aDO_2) \times 0.0031}{(A - aDO_2) \times 0.0031 + C_aO_2 - C_vO_2}$

$C_aO_2$ = Arterial $O_2$ content
$C_vO_2$ = Mixed venous $O_2$ content (from PA catheter)
$C_xO_2$ = [1.39 x Hb (g/dl) x ($O_2$sat %)] + [0.0031 x $P_xO_2$]
A-a$DO_2$ = Alveolar – arterial oxygen difference (mmHg)

# *Hemodynamic Values*[5]

| Pressure Parameter (mmHg) | Normal |
|---|---|
| Right atrium (RA), mean | 0-8 |
| "a"-wave | 2-10 |
| "v"-wave | 2-10 |
| Right ventricle (RV) | |
| systolic | 15-30 |
| diastolic | 0-8 |
| Pulmonary artery (PA), mean | 9-16 |
| systolic | 15-30 |
| diastolic | 3-12 |
| PA wedge, mean | 1-10 |
| "a"-wave | 3-15 |
| "v"-wave | 3-12 |

| Parameter | Normal Value |
|---|---|
| Cardiac output | 4.0-6.0 L/min |
| Cardiac index | 2.6-4.2 L/min/m² |
| Systemic vascular resistance (SVR) | 1130 ± 178 dyne/sec/cm⁻⁵ |
| Pulmonary vascular resistance (PVR) | 67 ± 23 dyne/sec/cm⁻⁵ |
| $O_2$ consumption | 110-150 mL/min/m² |
| Arterial-venous $O_2$ difference (AVD$O_2$) | 3.0-4.5 mL/dL |

[5] Lambert CR *et al.* Pressure measurement and determination of vascular resistance. In: *Diagnostic and Therapeutic Cardiac Catheterization*, 3rd ed. Pepine CJ (ed). Baltimore: Williams & Wilkins 1998.

# SI Lab Value Converter[6]

| Lab Value | US Unit | SI Unit | Factor* | Lab Value | US Unit | SI Unit | Factor* |
|---|---|---|---|---|---|---|---|
| **Chemistry** | | | | **Blood Gas** | | | |
| ALT, AST | U/L | μkat/L | 0.0167 | PaCO$_2$ | mmHg | kPa | 0.133 |
| Alk phos | U/L | μkat/L | 0.0167 | PaO$_2$ | mmHg | kPa | 0.133 |
| Amylase | U/L | nkat/L | 0.0167 | **Toxicology & Drug Monitoring** | | | |
| Bilirubin | mg/dl | μmol/L | 17.1 | Acetaminophen | mcg/ml | μmol/L | 6.62 |
| BUN | mg/dl | mmol/L | 0.357 | Amikacin | mcg/ml | μmol/L | 1.71 |
| Calcium | mg/dl | mmol/L | 0.25 | Carbamazepine | mcg/ml | μmol/L | 4.23 |
| Cholesterol | mg/dl | mmol/L | 0.0259 | Digoxin | ng/ml | nmol/L | 1.28 |
| Cortisol | mcg/dl | mmol/L | 27.6 | Gentamicin | mcg/ml | μmol/L | 2.09 |
| Cr Kinase | U/L | μkat/L | 0.0167 | Phenytoin | mcg/ml | μmol/L | 3.96 |
| Creatinine | mg/dl | μmol/L | 88.4 | Salicylate | mg/L | mmol/L | .00724 |
| Glucose | mg/dl | mmol/L | 0.0555 | Theophylline | mcg/ml | μmol/L | 5.55 |
| LDH | U/L | μkat/L | 0.0167 | Tobramycin | mcg/ml | μmol/L | 2.14 |
| Lipase | U/dl | μkat/L | 0.167 | Valproate | mcg/ml | μmol/L | 6.93 |
| Mg$^{++}$ | mEq/L | mmol/L | 0.5 | Vancomycin | mcg/ml | μmol/L | 0.690 |
| 5'-NT | U/L | μkat/L | 0.0167 | **Hematology** | | | |
| Phos | mg/dl | mmol/L | 0.322 | Folate | ng/ml | nmol/L | 2.27 |
| T$_4$ | mcg/dl | nmol/L | 12.9 | Hemoglobin | g/dl | mmol/L | 0.621 |
| T$_3$ | mcg/dl | nmol/L | 0.0154 | Iron, TIBC | mcg/dl | μmol/L | 0.179 |
| Uric acid | mg/dl | μmol/L | 59.5 | Vit B12 | pg/ml | pmol/L | 0.738 |

* Multiply by Factor to convert US unit to SI units

## Medical Statistics

| | Disease Present | Disease Absent |
|---|---|---|
| Test Positive | TP | FP |
| Test Negative | FN | TN |

---

[6] Adapted from Kratz, SI Lab Converter, *N Engl J Med* 1998; 339 (15): 1063-72

**Prevalence**
(prior probability) = (TP+FN)/(ALL) = All patients with disease/all pts

**Sensitivity** = TP / (TP + FN) = True positive/all diseased

**Specificity** = TN / (FP + TN) = True negative/all healthy

**False positive rate** = 1 - Specificity

**False negative rate** = 1 - Sensitivity

**Positive predictive value** = TP / (TP + FP) = True-positive/all positives

**Negative predictive value** = TN / (FN + TN) = True-negative/all negatives

**Accuracy** = (TP + TN) / (ALL) = True results/all patients

**Likelihood ratio**
(pos. results) = Sensitivity ÷ (1 - Specificity)

**Likelihood ratio**
(neg. results) = (1 – Sensitivity) ÷ Specificity

**Pre-test odds ratio** = Pre-test probability ÷ (1 – Pre-test probability)

**Post-test odds ratio** = Pre-test odds ratio x Likelihood ratio

**Post-test probability** = Post-test odds ratio ÷ (Post-test odds ratio + 1)

| Likelihood ratio | Change from Pre-test to Post-test Probability[7] |
|---|---|
| > 10 or < 0.1 | Large, often conclusive |
| 5-10 or 0.1-0.2 | Moderate |
| 2-5 or 0.2-0.5 | Small; sometimes important |
| 0.5-2 | Rarely important |

---

[7] Jaeschke R, et al. Users' guides to the medical literature. III. How to use an article about a diagnostic test. B. What are the results and will they help me in caring for my patients?. *JAMA* 1994; 271: 703-707

# *Pediatric Vital Signs*[8]

| Age | Awake HR | Asleep HR | Respiratory Rate | Systolic BP | Diastolic BP |
|---|---|---|---|---|---|
| Birth (12h, < 1 kg) | | | | 39-59 | 16-36 |
| Birth (12h, 3 kg) | | | | 50-70 | 25-45 |
| Neonate (96 hr) | 100-180 | 80-60 | | 60-90 | 20-60 |
| Infant (6 mo) | 100-160 | 75-160 | 30-60 | 87-105 | 53-66 |
| Toddler (2 yr) | 80-110 | 60-90 | 24-40 | 95-108 | 53-66 |
| Preschooler | 70-110 | 60-90 | 22-34 | 96-110 | 55-69 |
| School-age child (7 yr) | 65-110 | 60-90 | 18-30 | 97-112 | 57-71 |
| Adolescent (15 yr) | 60-90 | 50-90 | 12-16 | 112-128 | 66-80 |

# *Groovy Web Sites*

| Topic | Link |
|---|---|
| Medical calculators | www.mdcalc.com |
| Surgical risk calculators | www.surgicalriskcalculator.com |
| Pubmed ID to get details on risk calculators | www.pmidcalc.org |
| Pubmed National Library of Medicine | pubmed.gov |
| Textbook: Up-to-date (Subscription) | www.uptodate.com |
| Drug Instructions for Use (FDA inserts) | dailymed.nlm.nih.gov |
| Long QT Drugs | crediblemeds.org |
| Agency for Toxic Substances & Dz Registry | www.atsdr.cdc.gov |
| Toxnet | toxnet.nlm.nih.gov |
| Bronchoscopy Training | bronchoscopy.org |
| Medical image viewers | Mac: www.osirix-viewer.com<br>Windows: microdicom.com<br>All: Weasis: dcm4che.atlassian.net/wiki/display/WEA |

---

[8] Cummins RO (ed). *Textbook of Advanced Cardiac Life Support*. Dallas: American Heart Association, 1994, page 1:65.

# Code Algorithms

## *Basic Life Support for Professionals*[1]

For unresponsive patients not breathing or not breathing normally.

Cardiac arrest in children & infants usually asphyxiation requiring ventilations + compressions. Consider foreign-body airway obstruction.

|  | Adults | Children | Infants |
|---|---|---|---|
| Upon recognition | Verify scene safety<br>Get help; Get AED; Activate EMS (via cellphone)<br>Start CPR: Compression, Airway, Breathing sequence | | |
| Possible opioid overdose | Administer naloxone intranasal 2 mg or IM 0.4 mg if available | | |
| Compression Rate | 100-120/min | | |
| Compression Depth | ≥ 5 cm & < 6 cm, allow complete recoil & don't lean on chest | $\geq \frac{1}{3}$ AP depth (~ 5 cm; 5-6 cm after puberty); allow complete recoil | $\geq \frac{1}{3}$ anteroposterior depth (~ 4 cm); allow complete recoil |
| Interruptions | Minimize, < 10s for breaths;<br>Rotate compressors q 2 min | | |
| Airway | Head tilt and chin lift; Possible spinal injury → jaw thrust; | | |
| Suspected spinal injury | Manual spine immobilization preferred at first | | |
| Untrained rescuers | Compressions-only is reasonable | | |
| Compression: Ventilation (No airway device) | 30:2 | 30:2 single rescuer;<br>15:2 two rescuers | |
| Compressions: Ventilation (Airway device) | 1 breath every 6 sec, lasting ~ 1 sec, asynchronous with chest compressions, visible chest rise | | |
| Defibrillation | AED/Defibrillator as soon as possible, minimize interruptions in compressions. Resume CPR immediately after each shock. | | |

Pulse checks allocated < 10 sec unless definite pulse identified.

[1] Atkins DL, *et al.* Pediatric BLS and CPR Quality: 2015 AHA Guidelines Update. *Circulation 2015; 132: S519-525.* Kleinman ME, et al. Adult BLS and CPR Quality: 2015 AHA Guidelines Update. *Circulation 2015; 132: S414-435.*

Place in (lateral recumbent) recovery position after clearly normal breathing and effective circulation restored.

Drowning victims (unresponsive) should receive rescue breathing

## Adult Cardiac Arrest[2]

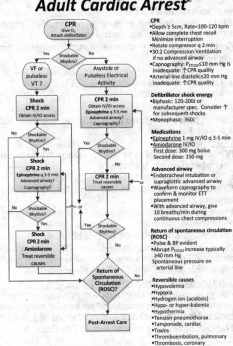

**CPR**
- Depth ≥ 5cm, Rate=100-120 bpm
- Allow complete chest recoil
- Minimize interruption
- Rotate compressor q 2 min
- 30:2 Compression:Ventilation if no advanced airway
- Capnography: $P_{ETCO_2} \le 10$ mm Hg is inadequate: ↑CPR quality
- Arterial-line diastolics≤20 mm Hg inadequate: ↑CPR quality

**Defibrillator shock energy**
- Biphasic: 120-200J or manufacturer spec. Consider ↑ for subsequent shocks
- Monophasic: 360J

**Medications**
- Epinephrine 1 mg IV/IO q 3-5 min
- Amiodarone IV/IO
  First dose: 300 mg bolus
  Second dose: 150 mg

**Advanced airway**
- Endotracheal intubation or supraglottic advanced airway
- Waveform capnography to confirm & monitor ETT placement
- With advanced airway, give 10 breaths/min during continuous chest compressions

**Return of spontaneous circulation (ROSC)**
- Pulse & BP evident
- Abrupt $P_{ETCO_2}$ increase typically ≥40 mm Hg
- Spontaneous pressure on arterial line

**Reversible causes**
- Hypovolemia
- Hypoxia
- Hydrogen ion (acidosis)
- Hypo- or hyper-kalemia
- Hypothermia
- Tension pneumothorax
- Tamponade, cardiac
- Toxins
- Thromboembolism, pulmonary
- Thrombosis, coronary

[2] Link MS, *et al.* Adult ACLS: 2015 AHA Guidelines Update. *Circulation* 2015; 132: S444-464.

## Additional comments on adult cardiac arrest[3]
### Ventilation, $CO_2$ detectors and oximetry

1 breath ever 6 sec during chest compressions
Use airway **suction** devices
**Colorimetric $CO_2$ detectors** may be misleading if contaminated with acidic gastric contents or drugs (*e.g.* epinephrine via ETT)
**$ETCO_2$** may be low in lung hypoperfusion (cardiac arrest) or severe airflow obstruction
Ominous **physiology prognosticators** (removed from guidelines):

- $P_{ETCO2}$ < 10 mmHg via ETT after 20 min;
- Central vein $O_2$ saturation < 30%
- Diastolic BP < 20 mmHg during CPR;

**Avoid hyperventilation**
**Don't pause compressions for ventilation with advanced airway**
### Drug Delivery
**IV Access: central line unnecessary if large-bore peripheral access is obtained**
IV access **should not delay** CPR & defibrillation
**Remember Intraosseous** and **endotracheal** delivery option
**Think ahead:** Prepare drugs before rhythm & pulse checks
**Flush** drugs with 10-20 mL IV fluid bolus.
Drugs **can** be **administered via ETT**: epinephrine, atropine, lidocaine, vasopressin, naloxone; Use 2-2.5 x usual dose diluted in 5-10 mL saline or dextrose
### Ultrasound/echocardiography during CPR
Potential value to identify hypovolemia, pneumothorax, pulmonary thromboembolism, pericardial tamponade, cardiac function, mechanical complications of acute MI
Tracheal ultrasound can confirm ETT position.

[3] Brooks SC, *et al.* Alternative Techniques and Ancillary Devices for CPR: 2015 AHA American Heart Association Guidelines Update. *Circulation* 2015; 132: S436-443.

## Ventricular Tachycardia or Ventricular Fibrillation

**Magnesium** IV is indicated only for Torsades related to prolonged QT (1-2 g in 10 mL)

Consider differential diagnosis: H's & T's on algorithm

Accelerated idioventricular rhythm: Do not treat if adequate perfusion.

## Asystole or Pulseless Electrical Activity

Pacing: No utility in arrest except selected events such as iatrogenic asystole

Consider differential diagnosis of reversible etiologies (H's & T's on algorithm)

## Extracorporeal CPR aka ECMO CPR aka ECPR

Routine use not recommended.

Possible value if rapidly implemented for selected cardiogenic shock, pulmonary thromboembolism, refractory VF, profound hypothermia, drug intoxication, or as a bridge to LVAD/transplant.

## Local anesthesia systemic toxicity

For example bupivacaine; may respond to lipid emulsion. *See* Lipid emulsion *on page 315.*

## Opiod life-threatening intoxication

Naloxone 2 mg intranasal or 0.4 mg IM. May repeat in 4 min.

## Pulmonary embolism:

*See* pulmonary thromboembolism *on page 190*

# Bradycardia[4]

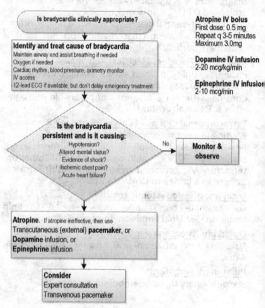

**Is bradycardia clinically appropriate?**

**Identify and treat cause of bradycardia**
Maintain airway and assist breathing if needed
Oxygen if needed
Cardiac rhythm, blood pressure, oximetry monitor
IV access
12-lead ECG if available, but don't delay emergency treatment

**Is the bradycardia persistent and is it causing:**
Hypotension?
Altered mental status?
Evidence of shock?
Ischemic chest pain?
Acute heart failure?

No → **Monitor & observe**

**Atropine.** If atropine ineffective, then use
**Transcutaneous (external) pacemaker,** or
**Dopamine** infusion, or
**Epinephrine** infusion

**Consider**
Expert consultation
Transvenous pacemaker

**Atropine IV bolus**
First dose: 0.5 mg
Repeat q 3-5 minutes
Maximum 3.0mg

**Dopamine IV infusion**
2-20 mcg/kg/min

**Epinephrine IV infusion**
2-10 mcg/min

---

[4] AHA, ACLS Provider Manual, Dallas: American Heart Association, 2016.

# Tachycardia[5]

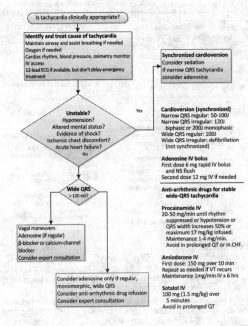

Is tachycardia clinically appropriate?

**Identify and treat cause of tachycardia**
Maintain airway and assist breathing if needed
Oxygen if needed
Cardiac rhythm, blood pressure, oximetry monitor
IV access
12-lead ECG if available, but don't delay emergency
treatment

**Synchronized cardioversion**
Consider sedation
If narrow QRS tachycardia
consider adenosine

**Unstable?**
Hypotension?
Altered mental status?
Evidence of shock?
Ischemic chest discomfort?
Acute heart failure?
No                          Yes

**Cardioversion (synchronized)**
Narrow QRS regular: 50-100J
Narrow QRS irregular: 120J
biphasic or 200J monophasic
Wide QRS regular: 100J
Wide QRS irregular: defibrillation
(not synchronized)

**Adenosine IV bolus**
First dose 6 mg rapid IV bolus
and NS flush
Second dose 12 mg IV if needed

**Anti-arrhythmic drugs for stable
wide-QRS tachycardia**

**Procainamide IV**
20-50 mg/min until rhythm
suppressed or hypotension or
QRS width increases 50% or
maximum 17 mg/kg infused.
Maintenance 1-4 mg/min.
Avoid in prolonged QT or in CHF.

**Wide QRS**
> 120 ms?

Vagal maneuvers
Adenosine (if regular)
β-blocker or calcium-channel
blocker
Consider expert consultation

**Amiodarone IV**
First dose: 150 mg over 10 min
Repeat as needed if VT recurs
Maintenance 1mg/min IV x 6 hrs

Consider adenosine only if regular,
monomorphic, wide QRS
Consider anti-arrhythmic drug infusion
Consider expert consultation

**Sotalol IV**
100 mg (1.5 mg/kg) over
5 minutes
Avoid in prolonged QT

---

[5] AHA, ACLS Provider Manual, Dallas: American Heart Association,
2016.

# Immediate care after cardiac arrest[6]

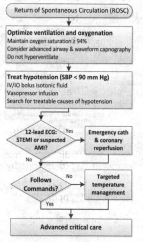

```
Return of Spontaneous Circulation (ROSC)
            │
            ▼
Optimize ventilation and oxygenation
Maintain oxygen saturation ≥ 94%
Consider advanced airway & waveform capnography
Do not hyperventilate
            │
            ▼
Treat hypotension (SBP < 90 mm Hg)
IV/IO bolus isotonic fluid
Vasopressor infusion
Search for treatable causes of hypotension
            │
            ▼
12-lead ECG:          Yes    Emergency cath
STEMI or suspected  ──────▶  & coronary
AMI?                          reperfusion
            │ No
            ▼
Follows             No    Targeted
Commands?         ──────▶  temperature
                            management
            │ Yes
            ▼
Advanced critical care
```

**Ventilation & Oxygenation**
Do not hyperventilate.
Start 10 breaths/min.
Titrate to $P_{ETCO2}$ ~ 35-40 mm Hg.
Down-titrate $F_{IO2}$ to $S_{pO2}$ ≥ 94%

**IV bolus fluid**
1-2L NS or LR

**Epinephrine IV infusion**
0.1-0.5 mcg/kg/min
(7-35 mcg/min for 70 kg adult)

**Dopamine IV infusion**
5-10 mcg/kg/min

**Norepinephrine IV infusion**
0.1-0.5 mcg/kg/min
(7-35 mcg/min for 70 kg adult)

**Reversible causes**
- Hypovolemia
- Hypoxia
- Hydrogen ion (acidosis)
- Hypo/hyperkalemia
- Hypothermia
- Tension pneumothorax
- Tamponade, cardiac
- Toxins
- Thromboembolism, pulmonary
- Thrombosis, coronary

## Ventilation:
• <u>Capnography</u> to confirm airway;
• <u>ETT</u> if comatose;
• <u>Chest X-ray</u>: confirm airway, detect pneumonitis, edema, pneumonia, etc;
• <u>Oxygenation</u>: Use pulse-ox or ABG; Start with highest $FiO_2$ and downtitrate to keep $P_aO_2$ ~ 100 mmHg and $S_pO_2$ ≥ 94%; calculate $P_aO_2/FiO_2$ index of acute lung injury;
• <u>Mechanical ventilation</u>: Tidal Volume 6-8 mL/kg; Physiological range $P_aCO_2$ is desirable ($P_{ET}CO_2$ ~ 35-40 mmHg and $P_aCO_2$ ~ 40-45 mmHg), unless permissive hypercapnia needed (acute lung injury, high airway

---

[6] AHA, ACLS Provider Manual, Dallas: American Heart Association, 2016.

pressure) or temporizing hypocapnia (cerebral edema, mindful of risk of cerebral vasoconstriction)

**Hemodynamics:**
- Monitor frequently using <u>NIBP or arterial line</u>; maintain SBP ≥ 90, MAP ≥ 65;
- Treat <u>hypotension</u>: with fluid bolus and vasopressors as indicated

**Cardiovascular:**
- Monitor and treat <u>rhythm</u>;
- <u>No prophylactic</u> antiarrhythmics;
- Treat reversible causes such as electrolytes and ischemia;
  - 12-lead <u>ECG</u> and troponin to assess ACS and QT interval;
- Treat <u>ACS</u> with aspirin, heparin, transfer for catheterization or fibrinolysis;
- <u>Echocardiogram</u> to detect myocardial stunning, regional wall motion abnormality, cardiomyopathy, structural heart disease;
- Treat myocardial <u>stunning</u> with fluid optimization, dobutamine, mechanical circulatory support

**Neurological:**
- <u>Serial neuro exam</u>: define coma, brain injury & prognosis;
- Test <u>response</u> to commands & stimuli;
- Pupillary light and corneal <u>reflexes</u> & spontaneous eye movement;
- <u>Gag</u>, cough, spontaneous breaths;
- <u>EEG</u> monitor if comatose to exclude and treat seizures;
- <u>Targeted temperature management</u> if comatose; Higher T preferred in risk of bleeding; Lower T preferred for seizures and cerebral edema. Duration ≥ 24 hr, perhaps as long as coma persists. Avoid fever if possible.
- Consider non-enhanced <u>CT</u>: exclude primary intracranial process;
- <u>Sedation and muscle relaxants</u>: control shivering, agitation, and ventilator dyssychrony

**Metabolic:**
- Serial <u>lactate</u>: confirm adequate perfusion;
- Monitor & replace <u>potassium</u> to > 3.5 mEq/L;
- Monitor <u>urine output</u>, maintain euvolemia, renal replacement therapy if necessary;
- <u>Glycemic control</u> with permissive targets;
- <u>Avoid hypotonic fluids</u> which risk cerebral edema

# Cardiology

## *Hemodynamics—Cardiac Cycle*[1]

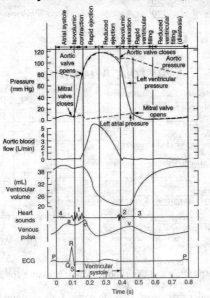

[1] Reprinted with permission from Berne & Levy. *Cardiovascular Physiology*, 6th ed. St. Louis: Mosby, 1986; figure 3-13.

# *Jugular Venous Pulsations*[2]

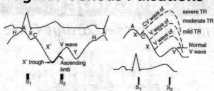

# *Systolic Murmurs*[3]

| Maneuver | Response | Sens (%) | Spec (%) | PPV (%) | NPV (%) |
|---|---|---|---|---|---|
| **Right-sided murmurs** | | | | | |
| Inspiration | Increase | 100 | 88 | 67 | 100 |
| Expiration | Decrease | 100 | 88 | 67 | 100 |
| Müller maneuver | Increase | 15 | 92 | 33 | 81 |
| **Hypertrophic cardiomyopathy** | | | | | |
| Valsalva | Increase | 65 | 96 | 81 | 92 |
| Squatting to Standing | Increase | 95 | 84 | 59 | 98 |
| Standing to Squatting | Decrease | 95 | 85 | 61 | 99 |
| Leg elevation | Decrease | 85 | 91 | 71 | 96 |
| Handgrip | Decrease | 85 | 75 | 46 | 95 |
| **Mitral regurgitation & ventricular septal defect** | | | | | |
| Handgrip | Increase | 68 | 92 | 84 | 81 |
| Transient arterial occl | Increase | 78 | 100 | 100 | 87 |
| Amyl nitrite inhalation | Decrease | 80 | 90 | 84 | 87 |

Sens=Sensitivity;   Spec=specificity;   PPV=Positive predictive value;
NPV=Negative predictive value

- Aortic stenosis diagnosed by exclusion
- Inspiration and Expiration: Patient breathes following listener's arm signal
- Müller maneuver: Occlude nares; Suck manometer (-)40-50 mmHg x 10 sec
- Valsalva: Exhale into manometer +40 mmHg x 20 sec. Listen at end of strain phase.

---

[2]   Reproduced with permission from Constant J. *Bedside Cardiology*, 3/e. Boston: Little, Brown, 1985; pp. 95, 105.
[3]   Lembo NJ, *et al.* Bedside diagnosis of systolic murmurs. *N Engl J Med.* 1988;318:1572-1578  Adapted with permission.

- Squatting to standing: Squat 30 sec then rapidly stand. Listen first 15-20 sec standing.
- Standing to squatting: Avoid Valsalva. Listen immediately after squatting.
- Passive leg elevation: Patient supine, elevate 45 degrees. Listen 15-20 sec later.
- Isometric handgrip: Hand dynamometer, listen after one minute max contraction.
- Transient arterial occlusion: Sphygmomanometer cuffs on both arms inflated 20-40 mm above systolic. Listen 20 sec later.
- Amyl nitrite: 0.3 mL ampule broken, 3 rapid deep breaths. Listen 15-30 sec later.

## Patterns of systolic heart murmurs[4]

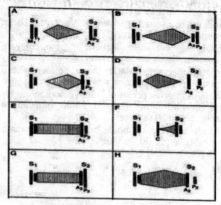

A: **Systolic ejection murmur.** Early peak

B: **Severe aortic stenosis.** Late peak, ↓ $A_2$ intensity

C: **Pulmonary valve stenosis.** Late peaking murmur extends through $A_2$. $P_2$ is delayed.

D: **Atrial septal defect.** Wide, fixed $S_2$ splitting.

E: **Mitral regurgitation.** Holosystolic through $A_2$.

F: **Mitral valve prolapse.** Late systolic murmur after midsystolic click.

G: **Tricuspid regurgitation** due to pulmonary hypertension. Holosystolic murmur begins with $S_1$. $P_2$ is loud.

H: **Ventricular septal defect.** Loud, holosystolic murmur with midsystolic accentuation and slightly delayed $P_2$.

[4] Alpert MA. Systolic murmurs. In: *Clinical Methods*. HK Walker (ed). Boston: Butterworth-Heineman, 1991. Adapted with permission.

# Echo/MRI/Nuclear Anatomy[5]

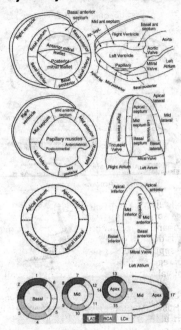

---

[5] Adapted from Cerqueira MD, *et al.* Standardized myocardial segmentation and nomenclature for tomographic imaging of the heart. *Circulation.* 2002;105:539-542

# Coronary Artery Anatomy[6]

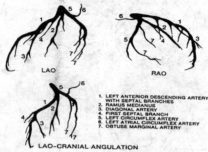

LEFT CORONARY ARTERY

LAO        RAO

LAO-CRANIAL ANGULATION

1. LEFT ANTERIOR DESCENDING ARTERY
   WITH SEPTAL BRANCHES
2. RAMUS MEDIANUS
3. DIAGONAL ARTERY
4. FIRST SEPTAL BRANCH
5. LEFT CIRCUMFLEX ARTERY
6. LEFT ATRIAL CIRCUMFLEX ARTERY
7. OBTUSE MARGINAL ARTERY

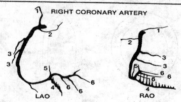

RIGHT CORONARY ARTERY

LAO        RAO

1. CONUS ARTERY
2. S-A NODE ARTERY
3. ACUTE MARGINAL ARTERY
4. POSTERIOR DESCENDING ARTERY WITH SEPTAL BRANCHES
5. A-V NODE ARTERY
6. POSTERIOR LEFT VENTRICULAR ARTERY

---
[6] Reproduced with permission from Grossman WG. *Cardiac Catheterization and Angiography*, 4th ed. Philadelphia: Lea and Febiger, 1991.

# ECG Lead-Anatomy Relationship[7]

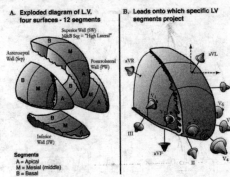

A. Exploded diagram of L.V. four surfaces - 12 segments

Superior Wall (SW)
M&B Seg = "High Lateral"

Anteroseptal Wall (Sep)

Posterolateral Wall (PW)

Inferior Wall (IW)

Segments
A = Apical
M = Mesial (middle)
B = Basal

B. Leads onto which specific LV segments project

[7] Reproduced with permission, Boineau JP. The ECG in multiple myocardial infarction and the progression of ischemic heart disease : new criteria for diagnosis of concealed MI. St. Louis: CardioRhythms.com; 2004.

# *ECG ST elevation (STE) patterns*[8]

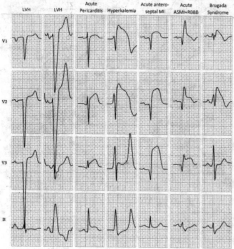

[8] Adapted from Wang K, et al. ST-segment elevation in conditions other than acute myocardial infarction. *N Engl J Med 2003; 349: 2128-2135.*

**Normal or benign patterns of STE:** stable over time: (1) <u>Male pattern</u>: upward concavity, STE ≤ 0.3 mV in precordial leads; (2) "<u>Early repolarization</u>": young black men, upward concavity, notched J point especially $V_4$, concordant large T waves.

**Left ventricular hypertrophy (LVH) :** STE initial upward concave "smiley" (LVH) rather than flat/convex "frown" (AMI). Asymmetrical T wave inversion, unlike symmetric T wave inversion of ischemia.

**Left bundle branch block (LBBB) and acute myocardial infarction:** (*See p 29*)

**Acute pericarditis:** Diffuse STE, upward concavity, with PR-depression. PR-elevation in lead $aV_R$. Unlike acute MI, T-waves invert only after STE normalizes. Unlike benign early repolarization, ST/T ratio ≥ 0.25[9].

**Hyperkalemia:** "Pseudoinfarction" widened QRS, tall-peaked T waves, reduced or absent P waves. STE may be downward-sloping.

**Myocardial infarction, Acute STEMI:** Upward convex or flat STE resembles "frown." <u>Anterior</u> $V_3$-$V_4$; Septal $V_2$-$V_3$; ASMI $V_{1/2}$-$V_{4/5}$: LAD; <u>Lateral</u> I, $V_5$/$V_6$: LCx, or apical LAD; <u>Inferior</u>: II, III, $aV_F$, dominant RCA or LCx; <u>Posterior</u>: ST depression downsloping and R > S in R precordial leads, also STE in leads $V_7$-$V_8$

**STE resembling STEMI:** <u>Prinzmetal</u> Angina (transient STE); <u>Pulmonary embolism</u> (RV strain pattern), <u>Stress</u> (Takotsubo) <u>cardiomyopathy</u>, large <u>stroke</u> (with deep precordial TW inversion), <u>LV aneurysm</u> (chronic STE), profound <u>hypothermia</u> (Osborne "J" wave: extra deflection between QRS and T)

**Brugada syndrome pattern**[10]: RBBB+ coved STE ≥ 0.2 mV in $V_1$-$V_3$. RSR' pattern rather than normal rsR'. ECG pattern may fluctuate or be concealed without sodium blocker. Syndrome includes VT, VF, family history, structurally normal heart, normal $QT_c$.

**Diffuse STE:** Lasting minutes after **cardioversion**; persistent in **pericarditis**

---

[9] Ginzton LE, et al. The differential diagnosis of acute pericarditis from the normal variant. *Circulation* 1982; 65: 1004-1009.

[10] Antzelevitch C, et al. Brugada syndrome: report of the second consensus conference. *Circulation* 2005; 111: 659-670.

# ECG: Hypertrophy[11]

## Left Ventricular Hypertrophy
• Romhilt-Estes criteria:

| | | |
|---|---|---|
| Limb lead R or S amplitude > 2.0 mV or S in V$_1$ or V$_2$ > 3.0 mV or R in V$_5$ or V$_6$ > 3.0 mV | 3 points | **Total Points:** 4: LVH likely 5: LVH present |
| ST segment abnormality: Without digitalis | 2 points | |
| With digitalis | 1 point | |
| Left atrial enlargement | 3 points | Sensitivity 40-50% |
| Left axis deviation > -30° | 2 points | Specificity 80-90% |
| QRS duration > 0.09 sec | 1 point | |
| Intrinsicoid deflection V$_5$ and V$_6$ > 0.05 sec | 1 point | |

• **Cornell criteria[12]:** R (aV$_L$) + S (V$_3$) ≥ 2.8 mV (men), ≥ 2.0 mV (women). Sensitivity 42%, specificity 96%
• **Other:** R in aV$_L$ > 1.1 mV (97% specific)

## Right ventricular hypertrophy (any of the following)
• Right axis deviation > 90° without anterior/inferior MI, left posterior fascicle block, or RBBB (99% specific)
• R > S in V$_1$ **and** R in V$_1$ > 0.5 mV (90% specific; highest sensitivity at 44%)
• S in V$_5$ or V$_6$ ≥ 0.7 mV (95% spec)
• S1Q3 pattern (93% specific)
• P-pulmonale (97% specific)
**Note:** Sensitivity and specificity generally higher in absence of LVH

## Causes of dominant R in V1 and V2
• Normal variant • RVH • Posterior or lateral infarction • WPW • LV diastolic overload • Hypertrophic cardiomyopathy • Duchenne's muscular dystrophy

---

[11] Romhilt DW, et al. A critical appraisal of the electrocardiographic criteria for the diagnosis of left ventricular hypertrophy. *Circulation* 1969; 40: 185-195.

[12] Casale PN, et al. Improved sex-specific criteria of left ventricular hypertrophy for clinical and computer interpretation of electrocardiograms: validation with autopsy findings. *Circulation* 1987; 75: 565-572.

# ECG: BBB, Fascicle Block & IWMI[13]

## Left bundle branch block
- QRS > 120 msec
- Absent septal Q (abnormal septal activation R → L)
- Slurred R wave leads I & V6 (slow R → L activation)
- Notched R in I and V6 (prominent delay late in QRS)
- Unpredictable A-P, inferosuperior activation patterns:
  - frontal axis may be normal or leftward
  - right-precordial R waves may be present or absent
- Absent Q waves in LBBB obscure myocardial scar
- ST- and T-wave vector opposite to QRS vector
- **Incomplete LBBB:** • QRS 100-120 msec • loss of septal Q wave • slurred/notched QRS in I and V6

## LBBB and acute MI [14]
- ST-segment elevation ≥ 1 mm **concordant** with QRS complex – highly sensitive and specific for acute MI under appropriate clinical circumstances (*e.g.*, chest pain)
- ST-segment depression ≥ 1 mm in lead V1, V2 or V3 – highly specific but less sensitive (36-78%) for MI
- ST-segment elevation ≥ 5 mm discordant with QRS complex – suggestive of MI but confirmatory data needed

## Right bundle branch block
- QRS > 120 msec
- Normal septal activation
- Terminal portion of QRS vector rightward and anterior
  - V1: initial R from normal septal activation; subsequent S from LV activation; terminal R' from delayed RV activation

---

[13] Warner RA, *et al.* Improved electrocardiographic criteria for the diagnosis of left anterior hemiblock. *Am J Cardiol* 1983; 51: 723-726.

[14] Sgarbossa EB, *et al.* Electrocardiographic diagnosis of evolving acute myocardial infarction in the presence of left bundle-branch block. *N Engl J Med* 1996; 334: 481-487.

- I, $V_5$, $V_6$: initial Q from normal septal activation, R from normal LV activation, prolonged shallow S wave from delayed RV activation
- T wave vector opposite the **terminal** portion of QRS
- Early activation intact (including Q wave of myocardial scar)
- **Incomplete RBBB:** • QRS 100-120 msec • morphology criteria of RBBB (RsR' pattern in $V_1$, prolonged shallow S wave in lateral leads)

**Left anterior fascicular block (LAFB)**
- Vectorcardiogram: frontal plane forces counter-clockwise, initially inferior and terminally superior; therefore $_aV_L$ peaks before $_aV_R$
- ECG: **(1)** QRS complexes in $_aV_R$ and $_aV_L$ each end in an R wave **and (2)** peak of the terminal R wave in $_aV_R$ occurs later than the peak of terminal R wave in $_aV_L$
- Scalar criteria: • QRS axis -45° to -90° • QRS < 120 msec • small Q in lead I
  • small R in II, III, $_aV_F$ • late intrinsicoid deflection in $_aV_L$ (> 45 msec)

**Left posterior fascicular block (LPFB)**
- Vectorcardiogram: QR complex in II, III, $_aV_F$ from initial superior and final inferior force
- Scalar criteria: • QRS axis > +90° • initial R in I, $_aV_L$+ small Q in II, III, $_aV_F$ • QRS < 120 msec • late intrinsicoid deflection in $_aV_F$ (> 45 msec) • absence of pulmonary disease, vertical heart position, RVH, W-P-W

**Inferior wall MI (sensitivity & specificity > 90%)**
- Vectorcardiogram: initial frontal forces clockwise and superior
- Clockwise rotation of frontal plane (lead II peaks before lead III) **and**
- Q waves > 30 msec in lead II **or** regression of initial inferior forces from lead III to lead II (initial portion of QRS is more negative in lead II than in lead III)
- Right coronary culprit: ST elevation lead III > lead II & ST depression in lead I and lead $_aV_L$
- Left circumflex culprit: ST elevation lead II > lead III & isoelectric or elevated ST in lead $_aV_L$

**Inferior wall MI + left anterior fascicular block (requires both)**
- $_aV_R$ and $_aV_L$ both end in R waves; terminal R of $_aV_L$ before $_aV_R$; and
- Q of any magnitude in lead II
- VCG: initial superior and clockwise; terminal superior and counterclockwise

# ECG: Wide-QRS Tachycardia

**Inexact features suggestive of ventricular tachycardia (VT)**
**Tachycardia: Wide-QRS**
- Extreme left axis deviation
- QRS duration > 140 msec (RBBB morphology) or > 160 msec (LBBB morph)
- "Capture" (narrow complex) and "fusion" (hybrid narrow-wide complex) beats
- Net area under QRS negative both in leads I and II

**Brugada criteria (99% sensitive, 97% specific)[15]**
- Rhythm is **ventricular tachycardia** if **any** of the following is present (in stepwise fashion):
  **(1)** RS absent in **all** precordial leads (may include QS, QR, monophasic R)
  **(2)** R-S interval > 100 msec (onset of R to nadir of S) in any precordial leads
  **(3)** Evidence of atrioventricular (A-V) dissociation

---

[15] Brugada P, et al. A new approach to the differential diagnosis of a regular tachycardia with a wide QRS complex. *Circulation* 1991; 83: 1649-1659; Eckardt L, et al. Approach to wide complex tachycardias in patients without structural heart disease. *Heart* 2006; 92: 704-711.
Note: these patients were not taking antiarrhythmic drugs.
Diagrams adapted with permission from Tom Evans, MD.

**(4)** Morphology criteria for VT in **both** leads $V_{1-2}$ and $V_6$: • RBBB-like QRS (predominantly positive in $V_1$)

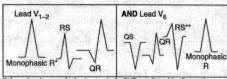

Other classic morphologies typical of VT not listed by Brugada are:
* RBBB: RSR' with R>R'
** RBBB: R/S<1 more suggestive of VT than R/S>1
*** LBBB: QS in $V_{1-2}$

• LBBB - like QRS (predominantly negative in lead $V_1$)

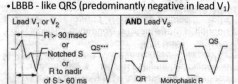

Other classic morphologies typical of VT not listed by Brugada are:
*RBBB: RSR' with R > R'
**RBBB: R/S < 1 more suggestive of VT than R/S > 1
***LBBB: QS in $V_{1-2}$

- If **all** of above criteria are absent, 99% likelihood that rhythm is **supraventricular**

**Pearls**
- In **structural heart disease** and reduced LV systolic function, a wide complex tachycardia is VT in 95% of cases
- Clinical appearance (*i.e.* whether patient is symptomatic or hemodynamically stable) is poor predictor of ventricular vs. supraventricular tachycardia

• If there is uncertainty about whether an arrhythmia is VT or SVT and patient does not require immediate electrical cardioversion, IV amiodarone or procainamide are the drugs of choice to terminate arrhythmia. **Avoid verapamil and diltiazem.** Adenosine may be tried, but **(1)** response may not reliably determine VT vs. SVT and **(2)** there is a small (1%) but definite risk of ventricular fibrillation (VF).

# Torsades & Long QT syndromes[16]

**Drugs clearly or probably associated with Torsades de Pointes[17]**

• **Anti-arrhythmic:** amiodarone, disopyramide, dofetilide, dronedarone, flecainide, ibutilide, procainamide, quinidine, sotalol; • **Cardiovascular Other:** bepridil, diuretic-induced electrolyte disorder, indapamide, isradipine, moexipril/hctz, nicardipine, ranolazine; • **Anti-cancer:** arsenic trioxide, lapatinib, nilotinib, sunitinib, tamoxifen; • **Anti-emetic / GI:** cisapride, dolasetron, granisetron, ondansetron; • **Anti-infective:** atazanavir, azithromycin, chloroquine, clarithromycin, erythromycin, foscarnet, gatifloxacin, gemifloxacin, halofantrine, levofloxacin, moxifloxacin, ofloxacin, pentamidine, sparfloxacin, telithromycin, voriconazole; • **Psychiatric:** chloral hydrate, chlorpromazine, clozapine, droperidol, escitalopram, haloperidol, imipramine, lithium, paliperidone, pimozide, quetiapine, risperidone, selective serotonin reuptake inhibitors, thioridazine, tizanidine, tricyclic antidepressants, venlafaxine, ziprasidone; • **Other:** alfuzosin, amantadine, felbamate, fosphenytoin, methadone, octreotide, oxytocin, propofol, tacrolimus, vardenafil

---

[16] Roden DM. Long-QT syndrome. *N Engl J Med* 2008; 358: 169-176. Drew BJ, et al. Prevention of torsade de pointes in hospital settings. *J Am Coll Cardiol* 2010; 55: 934-947.
[17] See database at www.crediblemeds.org

**Other risk factors and precipitants**
• QT$_c$ > 500 mS; • QT-prolonging drugs; • Concurrent 2 or more QT-prolonging drugs; • Structural heart disease; • Drug-induced CYP3A4 inhibition of associated drugs; • Female; • "Stimulant" conditions including endogenous or exogenous catecholamines; • QT-prolonging electrolyte abnormalities: hypokalemia, hypomagnesemia, including from diuretics; • Bradycardia, or pauses induced by frequent PVCs; • Starvation; • Anorexia nervosa; • Liquid protein diet; • Intracranial disease: subarachnoid hemorrhage, stroke or head trauma • autonomic manipulation from surgery (vagotomy, carotid endarterectomy)

**Treatment of Torsades de Pointes (TdP):**
• DC cardioversion if sustained; • Magnesium IV; • Correct electrolyte abnormality; • Withdraw precipitating drugs; • Overdrive suppression with pacing; • **Warning:** Amiodarone is useful in PMVT but potentially harmful in LQTS or TdP

**Hereditary repolarization syndromes: LQTS & Brugada**
TdP or sudden death often precipitated by metabolic (electrolyte, catecholamine) alteration, medication, or bradycardia. Genetic LQTS may be rare, but gene variants may predispose to drug-induced LQTS.

Brugada: coved ST elevation leads V1-V3 (*see page 27*) associated with VT, syncope, family history, nocturnal agonal respiration.

LQTS and Brugada syndromes are channelopathies having variable clinical penetrance. Some are autosomal dominant, others recessive and include congenital deafness. A short QT syndrome also is recognized.

Risk in LQTS: Highest after arrest or spontaneous TdP; High after prior syncope or QT$_c$ > 500 ms; Low (5-year risk of arrest ~ 0.5%) if Qt$_c$ ≤ 440-500 ms.

Prophylactic therapy in LQTS: Beta-blockers for medium- or high-risk LQTS. Some advocate beta blockers in all. ICD in highest risk or persistently symptomatic. Role of surgical sympathectomy and pacing (for bradycardia) is controversial.

Management of Brugada syndrome: Risk increased in ST elevation, higher in symptomatic. Sodium blockers and EP testing used in diagnostic evaluation. ICDs used widely, adjunctive pharmacotherapy controversial.

Expert consultation is recommended.

## *Risk scores in a-fib: stroke & bleeding*

### HAS-BLED risk of bleeding[18]

| Risk | Points |
|---|---|
| Hypertension uncontrolled > 60 mmHg | 1 |
| Abnormal liver or renal function, 1 pt each | 1-2 |
| Stroke | 1 |
| Bleeding history or anemia | 1 |
| Labile INR, in-range < 60% of time | 1 |
| Elderly > 65 years | 1 |
| Drugs (antiplatelet or NSAID) or Alcohol, 1 pt each | 1-2 |

| Score | Bleeds per 100 patient-years |
|---|---|
| 0 | 1.13 |
| 1 | 1.02 |
| 2 | 1.88 |
| 3 | 3.74 |
| 4 | 8.70 |
| 5-9 | Inadequate data |

### $CHADS_2$ and $CHA_2DS_2$-VASc stroke risk in atrial Fibrillation[19]

| $CHADS_2$ Criterion | Score |
|---|---|
| Congestive heart failure ever | 1 |
| Hypertension | 1 |
| Age ≥ 75 years | 1 |
| Diabetes mellitus | 1 |
| Stroke, TIA, thromboembolism in past | 2 |
| Max | 6 |

| Score | Adj Stroke Risk %/yr |
|---|---|
| 0 | 1.9 |
| 1 | 2.8 |
| 2 | 4.0 |
| 3 | 5.9 |
| 4 | 8.5 |
| 5 | 12.5 |
| 6 | 18.2 |

[18] Pisters R, *et al.* A novel user-friendly score (HAS-BLED) to assess 1-year risk of major bleeding in patients with atrial fibrillation. *Chest* 2010; 138: 1093-1100.

[19] Gage BF, *et al.* Validation of clinical classification schemes for predicting stroke. *JAMA* 2001; 285: 2864-2870. Lip GY, et al. Refining clinical risk stratification for predicting stroke and thromboembolism in atrial fibrillation using a novel risk factor-based approach. *Chest* 2010; 137: 263-272. January CT, et al. AHA/ACC/HRS guideline for the mgmt of patients with atrial fibrillation. *J Am Coll Cardiol* 2014; 64: e1-76.

| CHA₂DS₂-VASc Criterion | Score |
|---|---|
| Congestive heart failure ever | 1 |
| Hypertension | 1 |
| Age ≥75 yr | 2 |
| Diabetes mellitus | 1 |
| Stroke, TIA, thromboembolism in past | 2 |
| Vascular dz (prior MI, PAD, or aorta plaque) | 1 |
| Age 65-74 yr | 1 |
| Female sex | 1 |
| Max | 9 |

| Score | Adj Stroke Risk %/yr |
|---|---|
| 0 | 0 |
| 1 | 1.3 |
| 2 | 2.2 |
| 3 | 3.2 |
| 4 | 4.0 |
| 5 | 6.7 |
| 6 | 9.8 |
| 7 | 9.6 |
| 8 | 6.7 |
| 9 | 15.2 |

| Score | Recommended therapy |
|---|---|
| 0 | Reasonable to omit atithrombotic therapy in non-valvular afib |
| 1 | No antithrombic therapy or oral anticoagulant or aspirin |
| 2 | Oral anticoagulant. Concurrent clopidogrel without aspirin if needed after stent revascularization. |

# Probability of Coronary Disease[20]

### Likelihood of significant coronary disease based on history

| Age | Asymptomatic | Non-Anginal | Atypical Angina | Typical Angina |
|---|---|---|---|---|
| **Men** | | | | |
| 60-69 | .12 | .28 | .67 | .94 |
| 50-59 | .10 | .22 | .59 | .92 |
| 40-49 | .06 | .14 | .46 | .87 |
| 30-39 | .02 | .05 | .22 | .70 |
| **Women** | | | | |
| 60-69 | .08 | .19 | .54 | .91 |
| 50-59 | .03 | .08 | .32 | .79 |
| 40-49 | .01 | .03 | .13 | .55 |
| 30-39 | .00 | .01 | .04 | .26 |

[20] Diamond GA, et al. Analysis of probability as an aid in the clinical diagnosis of coronary-artery disease. *N Engl J Med 1979; 300: 1350-1358.* Adapted with permission of *The New England Journal of Medicine*, copyright 1979, Massachusetts Medical Society.

## Post-exercise test probability (%) of significant CAD

| Age | Asymptomatic | | Non-Anginal | | Atypical Angina | | Typical Angina | |
|-----|------|------|------|------|------|------|------|------|
| Sex | M | F | M | F | M | F | M | F |
| **ST depression > 2.5 mm** | | | | | | | | |
| 30-39 | 43±25 | 11±9 | 68±22 | 24±20 | 92±8 | 63±25 | 99±1 | 93±7 |
| 40-49 | 69±21 | 28±21 | 87±12 | 53±26 | 97±3 | 86±13 | 100±.4 | 98±2 |
| 50-59 | 81±16 | 56±25 | 91±8 | 78±17 | 98±2 | 95±5 | 100±.2 | 99±.7 |
| 60-69 | 85±13 | 76±18 | 94±6 | 90±9 | 99±1 | 98±2 | 100±.2 | 100±.3 |
| **ST depression 2-2.5 mm** | | | | | | | | |
| 30-39 | 18±10 | 3±2 | 38±17 | 8±6 | 76±13 | 33±17 | 96±3 | 79±13 |
| 40-49 | 39±17 | 10±7 | 65±16 | 24±14 | 91±6 | 63±17 | 98±1 | 93±5 |
| 50-59 | 54±17 | 27±14 | 75±13 | 50±18 | 94±4 | 84±9 | 99±.5 | 98±2 |
| 60-69 | 61±16 | 47±17 | 81±11 | 72±14 | 96±3 | 93±5 | 100±.4 | 99±.6 |
| **ST depression 1.5-2.0 mm** | | | | | | | | |
| 30-39 | 8±5 | 1±1 | 19±11 | 3±2.5 | 55±18 | 16±10 | 91±6 | 59±19 |
| 40-49 | 20±11 | 4±3 | 41±17 | 11±7.2 | 78±12 | 39±18 | 97±2 | 84±10 |
| 50-59 | 31±15 | 12±8 | 53±18 | 28±14 | 86±9 | 67±16 | 98±1 | 94±4 |
| 60-69 | 37±16 | 25±13 | 62±17 | 49±18 | 90±7 | 83±10 | 99±1 | 98±2 |
| **ST depression 1.0-1.5** | | | | | | | | |
| 30-39 | 4±1 | 0.6±.2 | 10±2 | 2±.7 | 38±5 | 9±3 | 83±3 | 42±9 |
| 40-49 | 11±2 | 2±.5 | 26±4 | 6±2 | 64±4 | 25±6 | 94±1 | 72±6 |
| 50-59 | 19±2.6 | 7±1 | 37±5 | 16±3 | 75±3 | 50±5 | 96±.7 | 89±2 |
| 60-69 | 23±3 | 15±2 | 45±5 | 33±5 | 81±3 | 72±4 | 97±.5 | 95±1 |
| **ST depression 0.5-1.0** | | | | | | | | |
| 30-39 | 2±.6 | 0.3±.1 | 5±2 | 0.7±.4 | 21±6 | 4±2 | 68±7 | 24±8 |
| 40-49 | 5±2 | 1±.3 | 13±4 | 3±1 | 44±8 | 12±4 | 86±4 | 53±10 |
| 50-59 | 9±3 | 3±1 | 20±5 | 8±2 | 57±8 | 31±7 | 91±3 | 78±6 |
| 60-69 | 11±3 | 7±2 | 26±6 | 17±5 | 65±7 | 52±8 | 94±2 | 90±3 |

# Exercise Stress Testing

**Limitations in detecting coronary artery disease (CAD)**

• Limited value in certain common situations: • **Women:** high false-positive rate (ST segment response); positive tests add little to predictive value of history alone • **Beta-blockers:** limit max work (heart rate x blood pressure) → sensitivity decreased • **Digitalis:** depresses ST segments, usually ≤ 0.1 mV. Further exertional ST-depression usually reflects ischemia.

Consider stopping digoxin > one week before test
• Conduction abnormalities (BBB, pre-excitation): ST segments uninterpretable (except lateral precordial leads in RBBB) • **Pressure overload (LVH, aortic stenosis):** subendocardial ischemia and ST depression even in absence of CAD (true-positive test for ischemia; false-positive for epicardial coronary obstruction) • **Metabolic abnormalities:** anemia, hypoxia, hypokalemia and hyperventilation
• The patient has to be **able to exercise**
• **Uncertainty** about whether a positive tests reflects an anatomic abnormality
• ST-segment **depression** suggests presence of but **does not localize** ischemia
• **Myocardial imaging** (nuclear scintigraphy, echocardiography, MRI) modestly increases sensivity and specificity for CAD, are best applied when CAD likelihood is intermediate and resting ECG abnormal.
• **Pharmacologic stimulation** (reg/adenosine, dipyridamole, dobutamine) when unable to exercise but functional implications less clear. Adenosine agonists contraindicated in bronchospasm or high-grade A-V block; theophylline & caffeine decrease effectiveness

## The Duke Treadmill Prognostic Score[21]

Treadmill angina index: 0 = none;   1 = non-limiting angina;   2 = angina stops test

Score = (Exercise duration in min) — (5 x max ST-deviation in mm) — (4 x treadmill angina index)

| Risk of death (score) | Inpatients | | Outpatients | |
|---|---|---|---|---|
| | Patients | 4-yr Survival | Patients | 4-yr survival |
| Low (≥ +5) | 470 (34%) | 98 % | 379 (62%) | 99 % |
| Mod (-10 to +4) | 795 (57%) | 92 % | 211 (34%) | 95 % |
| High (< -10) | 129 (9%) | 71 % | 23 (4%) | 79 % |

---

[21] Mark DB, et al. Prognostic value of a treadmill exercise score in outpatients with suspected CAD. *N Engl J Med* 1991; 325: 849-853.

# *Emergency Cardiac Pacing Technique*

**Transcutaneous (noninvasive) pacing method**
(1) Attach electrodes to dry skin anterior & posterior to cardiac apex; (2) Set 70-100 bpm; (3) Confirm capture pace-spike followed by consistent ST-T-wave. Do not confuse with stimulation of skeletal muscles! (4) Confirm BP and pulse. (5) **Brady-asystolic arrest:** Set initial output to maximum; confirm capture, then decrease output slowly until threshold determined.
**Conscious patient:** Set output to minimum and increase until capture. (6) Set output at 20% above capture threshold; (7) Sedatives and analgesia as needed. (8) Transvenous pacing if cause not immediately reversible.

**Transvenous pacing wires: "Pace-capture" technique:**
• If fluoroscope unavailable, use balloon flotation for ventricle and J-wire for atrium.
• **"Pace-capture" technique:** Monitor ECG.
(1) Connect pacing catheter to generator. Set rate 70-100 bpm, maximum output, minimum sensitivity (demand mode). (2) Advance catheter until ventricular capture. (3) Deflate balloon and test thresholds (below).

**Failed capture:** check for: stimulus artifact on ECG, battery, connections, placement; consider myocardial unresponsiveness (*e.g.* acidosis).

**Threshold testing**
**Pacing (stimulation) threshold:** minimum energy for successful capture. (1) Set rate 10-20 bpm higher than intrinsic heart rate. (2) Set to maximum output and confirm capture. (3) Decrease output (mA) until capture fails: the *stimulation threshold*. (4) Operate at output 2-3 times stimulation threshold.
**Sensing (inhibition) threshold:** voltage at which pacing is inhibited (when intrinsic heart rate is adequate). Proper sensing distinguishes normal QRS from T, avoids R-on-T pacing.

- **Technique:** (1) Set rate to 10-20 bpm below intrinsic heart rate (assuming hemodynamically acceptable). Gradually decrease pacemaker rate. (2) Start at highest sensitivity (lowest mV setting or "demand"), which inhibits pacing. Then gradually increase sensing millivoltage until inappropriate pacing occurs, at the *sensing threshold*, usually 0.5-2 mV. (3) Set sensitivity to approximately half of the sensing threshold for safety margin. Assure pacing is not inhibited by artifacts like T waves.
- **Terminology:** "Demand mode" = highest sensitivity: minimal energy will inhibit pacer, *e.g.* unwanted stimuli such as muscle movement or T waves.
"Asynchronous mode" = lowest sensitivity: pacemaker will fire even though it detects considerable energy, *e.g.* from the QRS complex.

# Intra-Aortic Balloon Pump

### Indications
- **Myocardial ischemia:** refractory unstable angina or postinfarction angina; refractory polymorphic VT; support for PCI
- **Cardiogenic shock:** pump failure; acute mitral regurgitation or acute ventricular septal rupture (as a bridge to definitive treatment)
- **Pre- and Postoperative:** myocardial depression and weaning from bypass

### Contraindications
- Aortic valve insufficiency > mild-moderate; • Severe obstructive aortic or iliofemoral artery disease; • Aortic dissection, aortic aneurysm

### Operating the intra-aortic balloon pump (IABP)
- **Balloon deflation:** nadir of end-diastolic pressure should occur just before arterial upstroke (aortic valve opening) begins • Late deflation: ventricle contracts against inflated balloon • Premature deflation: suboptimal afterload reduction

- **Balloon inflation:** should occur just after dicrotic notch • **Early inflation:** ventricle contracts against inflated balloon • **Late inflation:** excessive diastolic hypotension and suboptimal augmentation of coronary flow
- **Anticoagulation** is optional as long as pump is not in "standby"
- During CPR the IABP should be turned off or set to "standby" mode

**Timing examples[22]: Arterial pressure waveforms with 1:2 counterpulsation**

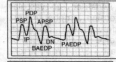

**Correct timing.** Balloon aortic end-diastolic pressure (BAEDP) is lower than aortic end-diastolic pressure (PAEDP). Assisted peak systolic pressure (APSP) is lower than native peak systolic pressure (PSP). IP=inflation point.

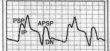

**Early inflation.** Inflation point (IP) occurs before aortic valve closure, before dicrotic notch (DN).

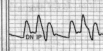

**Late inflation.** IP occurs after DN with shortening of diastolic augmentation time and small augmented waveform.

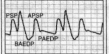

**Early deflation.** BAEDP occurs early and equilibrates rapidly with nonaugmented PAEDP; augmented peak systolic pressure (APSP) is improperly higher than nonaugmented PSP.

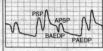

**Late deflation.** BAEDP exceeds PAEDP (should be lower).

[22] Sorrentino M, Feldman T. Techniques for IABP timing, use, and discontinuance. *J Critical Illness* 1992; 7(4): 597-604; with permission of Cliggott Publishing.

# Hypertensive Emergencies[23]

## Diagnosis
- Defined by end-organ damage, *e.g.* encephalopathy, renal dysfunction, CHF, cardiac ischemia, decreased placental perfusion
- DBP usually > 120 mmHg but BP can be as low as 160/100 in previously normotensive patient (*e.g.* pregnant woman, drug reaction in young adult)
- "Hypertensive urgency": elevated BP without end-organ damage; usually appropriate to treat as outpatient with oral medications

**Etiology:** • Chronic HTN • Renal or renovascular disease • Drug ingestion (cocaine, amphetamines) • Non-adherence or withdrawal (esp. clonidine, β-blocker) • Pheochromocytoma • Scleroderma or other collagen-vascular disease • S/p carotid artery or neurosurgery • Head or spinal cord injury • Guillain-Barré syndrome

| Clinical Scenario | Goal of Treatment | 1st Line Rx [24] | Comments |
|---|---|---|---|
| Hypertensive encephalopathy | 20-25% reduction in MAP over 2-3 hr (but keep DBP > 100 mmHg) | SNP, CVP, labetalol, nicardipine | Treatment may worsen neuro fxn. Avoid clonidine, βB (CNS effects). |
| Ischemic stroke | If BP > 220/120 lower 15-25% in first day (*See* stroke hypertension *on page 157*) | Labetalol, nicardipine | SNP and NTG may increase ICP. Goal BP 185/110 if fibrinolytics. |
| Intracerebral hemorrhage | Gradually reach 160/80, MAP < 110, CPP > 60 with ICP monitor, or pre-stroke level | Labetalol, SNP, nicardipine | Monitor for worsening neuro function after lowering BP |

*(Continued)*

---

[23] Marik PE, et al. Hypertensive crises. *Chest 2007; 131: 1949-1962.*
[24] For specific drug dosages and administration guidelines *see Groovy Drugs*

| Clinical Scenario | Goal of Treatment | 1st Line Rx [25] | Comments |
|---|---|---|---|
| Subarachnoid hemorrhage | Same as intracerebral hemorrhage | Nimodipine 60 mg PO/PNGT q 4 hr (to prevent spasm) ± labetalol | Avoid SNP and NTG (increase ICP) |
| Pulmonary edema | DBP ≤ 100 mmHg or resolution of symptoms | SNP plus NTG plus diuretic | Avoid (-) inotropes in LV dysfunction. Search for myocardial ischemia. In CAD or PAD, seek RAS. |
| Myocardial infarction or unstable angina | DBP ≤ 100 mmHg or resolution of symptoms | NTG, β-B. Add SNP if DBP remains elevated | |
| Aortic dissection | SBP 100-120 or MAP 80 mmHg (watch urine output) | SNP or CVP plus βB or labetalol | Decrease dP/dT. Avoid vasodilator monotherapy. |
| Sympathomimetic crisis (cocaine, amphet., pheochromocytoma, MAOI reaction, βB or clonidine withdrawal) | DBP ~ 100-105 (but ≤ 25% reduction in presenting BP) over 2-6 hr | Phentolamine (1st) then βB or labetalol. Benzodiazepine for cocaine-like drugs. Alternative: NTG ± Ca blocker. | Avoid βB or labetalol alone (unopposed α stimulation). Restart βB or clonidine if withdrawing. |
| Pregnancy (eclampsia) | DBP 90-105 or MAP ≤ 126 mmHg | Hydralazine[26], labetalol, nifedipine | PO: methyldopa. Avoid SNP, ACE-I. |
| Post-operative | Pre-op BP | SNP, labetalol, diuretic | Treat pain, ↑ volume, & ↓ O₂ |
| Acute renal insufficiency | DBP ~ 100-105 (but ≤ 25% reduction in presenting BP) | Ca channel blockers, CVP | Avoid diuretics. Maintain renal blood flow. |

*SNP = sodium nitroprusside   βB = β-blocker;   CVP = clevidipine;*
*NTG = nitroglycerin;   ICP = intracranial pressure*

---

[25] For specific drug dosages and administration guidelines
see *Groovy Drugs*
[26] Magee LA, *et al.* Hydralazine for treatment of severe hypertension in pregnancy. *BMJ 2003; 327:* 955-960.

# Perioperative Cardiovascular Risk[27]

## Risk classification schemes
## Surgery risk: European Society of Cardiology (ESC) Risk Classification of Surgery

| Low risk < 1% | Intermediate 1-5% | High risk > 5% |
|---|---|---|
| Superficial surgery | Intraperitoneal: splectomy, hiatal hernia, cholecystectomy | Aortic & major vascular surgery |
| Breast | | Open limb revascularization, amputation, or thromboembolectomy |
| Dental | | |
| Endocrine: thyroid & parathyroid | Carotid endarterectomy symptomatic | Lung resection |
| Eye | Endovascular AAA or TAA | Esophagectomy |
| Reconstructive | | Exploratory laparotomy |
| Carotid endarterectomy asymptomatic | Peripheral artery angioplasty | Gastric surgery |
| Dialysis access | Neurological or orthopedic: major hip or spine | Repair of bowel perforation |
| Gastric bypass | | Small bowel or colon resection |
| Gynecologic minor | Urology or gynecology major | • Enterostomy |
| Orthopedic minor (meniscectomy) | Renal transplant | Liver resection |
| Urology minor (transurethral prostate resection) | Intra-thoracic: non-major | Duodeno-pancreatic or biliary surgery |
| | | Adrenal resection |

## American Society of Anesthesiologists (ASA) class
Class I completely healthy;
Class II mild systemic disease;
Class III severe systemic disease that is not incapacitating;
Class IV incapacitating disease that is a constant threat to life;
Class V moribund, not expected to live 24 hr, with or without surgery

---

[27] Fleisher LA, et al. 2014 ACC/AHA guideline on perioperative cardiovascular evaluation and management of patients undergoing noncardiac surgery. J Am Coll Cardiol 2014; 64: e77-137. Kristensen SD, et al. 2014 ESC/ESA Guidelines on non-cardiac surgery: cardiovascular assessment and management. Eur Heart J 2014; 35: 2383-2431. Patel AY, et al. Cardiac Risk of Noncardiac Surgery. J Am Coll Cardiol 2015; 66: 2140-2148. Devereaux PJ, et al. Cardiac Complications in Patients Undergoing Major Noncardiac Surgery. N Engl J Med 2015; 373: 2258-2269.

**Clinical Risk: Lee Revised cardiac risk index (RCRI)**[28]
High-risk surgery (Intrathoracic, intra-abdominal, or
  vascular surgery above groin)
Ischemic heart disease (angina or prior MI)
Congestive heart failure
Stroke or TIA
Diabetes requiring insulin
Serum creatinine > 2.0 mg/dL

**Clinical Risk: American College of Surgery NSQIP**
  **risk calculator**
(http://www.surgicalriskcalculator.com/miorcardiacarrest)

**Functional "testing" from history**
Can you walk up two flights of stairs? (= 4 mets)

**Risk-oriented operative management (flowchart)**
• Consider the **risk of surgery** (table above) and its
  urgency
• Consider **patient risk**: age, ASA classification (table
  above), functional capacity, risk estimation models
  (Lee RCRI and ACS NSQIP tables above).
• **Emergency surgery** proceeds with risk stratification
  & perioperative surveillance
• **Low risk surgery** or patient: proceed without
  further testing
• Preoperative **cardiac (stress) testing** only for
  moderate or high risk, poor or unknown functional
  capacity, and when results will alter management.
• **Unstable heart disease** (ACS, acute heart failure,
  significant cardiac arrhythmia, symptomatic heart
  disease, recent MI < 30 d with residual myocardial
  ischemia): stabilize the patient including delay of
  surgery and cath if necessary. Team review of timing,
  surgical and anesthesia options, revascularization,
  antiplatelet therapy. For example, extensive ischemic burden may prompt cath & revascularization or a
  less extensive surgery or a noninvasive approach.

---

[28] Lee TH, et al. Derivation and prospective validation of a simple
index for prediction of cardiac risk of major noncardiac surgery.
*Circulation* 1999; 100: 1043-1049.

- **Revascularization** before surgery is controversial because it may paradoxically ↑ operative risk. Generally used as indicated apart from non-cardiac surgery, and less desirable unless CCS3+ angina or extensive ischemia. Delay surgery 2 wk after balloon angioplasty, 4 wk after bare metal stents, and 6-12 mo after drug-eluting stents.
- **Beta-blockers:** continue if in use, unclear benefit and possible harm unless RCRI ≥ 3 or intermediate-high risk preoperative testing. Initiate days-weeks preoperatively and slowly titrate to HR 60-70 and SBP > 100. β1-selective may be better.
- **Statins:** reasonable to initiate before vascular surgery or if otherwise indicated.
- Dual **antiplatelet** (aspirin + P2Y$_{12}$ blocker) and stents: withdrawal is hazardous and requires expert consultation. Continue if possible as indicated by stent status. Discontinue clopidogrel/prasugrel/ticagrelor 5/7/3 d before surgery.
- **Nitroglycerin**, α-adrenergic blockers have no benefit intraoperatively.
- **ACE inhibitors or ARBs:** continue if in use, restart postoperatively if withheld.
- Maintain normal temperature unless intentional hypothermic organ preservation
- Assure meticulous **postoperative** pain control, BP, volume management, normoxia, glycemic control, *etc.*

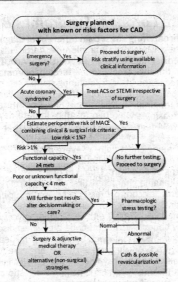

# Acute Coronary Syndromes & MI[29]

**Life-threatening chest pain differential diagnosis**
• Acute myocardial infarction; • Aortic dissection; • Mediastinitis/esophageal rupture; • Acute pulmonary thromboembolism; • Tension pneumothorax; • Myocarditis

**Principal presentations of UA/NSTEMI**
• Rest angina; • New onset angina (to CCS 3); • Increasing angina (to CCS 3);

**High risk features of suspected ACS that should trigger EMS**
• Continuing chest pain; • Severe dyspnea; • Syncope or presyncope; • Palpitation

**Patterns of discomfort/pain in ACS**

**Typical angina characteristics:** • Poorly-localized chest or arm discomfort associated reproducibly with physical exertion or emotional upset, relieved promptly (< 5 min) with rest and nitroglycerin. Note many patients do not describe their chest discomfort as "pain." Sole jaw, neck, ear, throat, back, epigastric discomfort or dyspnea may be angina-equivalent ("atypical angina") symptoms. Other **atypical symptoms** include • Epigastric pain; • Indigestion; • Nausea; • Vomiting; • Diaphoresis; • Profound fatigue; • Stabbing or • pleuritic pain; • Increasing dyspnea

[29] Amsterdam EA, *et al.* 2014 AHA/ACC Guideline for the Management of Patients with Non-ST-Elevation Acute Coronary Syndromes. *J Am Coll Cardiol* 2014; 64: e139-228. O'Gara PT, *et al.* 2013 ACCF/AHA guideline for the management of ST-elevation MI. *J Am Coll Cardiol* 2013; 61: e78-140. Steg PG, *et al.* ESC Guidelines for the management of acute MI in patients presenting with ST-segment elevation. *Eur Heart J* 2012; 33: 2569-2619. Hamm CW, *et al.* ESC Guidelines for the management of acute coronary syndromes in patients presenting without persistent ST-segment elevation. *Eur Heart J* 2011; 32: 2999-3054.

**Pain not characteristic of myocardial ischemia:**
• Mid- or lower-abdominal pain; • Localized 1-0 q fingertip pain at costochondral border or LV apex; • Pain reproduced with palpation or movement of arms or chest wall; • Pain lasting a few seconds or less; • Pain radiating to lower extremity

### Prognostication

*TIMI-Risk Score for UA/NSTEMI*[30]
(markers of 14 d risk of death, MI or urgent revascularization): • Age ≥ 65; • 3 CAD risk factors; • CAD with > 50% stenosis; • ST ↑ on initial ECG; • 2 angina episodes in preceding 24hr; • ASA in past 7d; • ↑ serum cardiac markers

| # of Markers | 0/1 | 2 | 3 | 4 | 5 | 6/7 |
|---|---|---|---|---|---|---|
| 14 d risk | 5% | 8% | 13% | 20% | 26% | 41% |

*GRACE risk model: http://www.gracescore.org/WebSite*

*Adverse Prognosticators From PURSUIT* [31]
• Age > 60; • Male; • Prior CCS 3 angina; • HR > 100-120; • SBP < 80-100; • CHF signs; • ST depression

### Syndrome-specific emergency treatment

**All patients**
• 12-lead ECG; leads $V_3R$, $V_4R$, $V_5R$ in inferior wall MI; leads $V_7$-$V_9$ in suspected circumflex territory MI and/or non-diagnostic ECG. Extent & magnitude of ST depression confers worse prognosis.
• Repeat ECGs q 15 min if non-diagnostic & high suspicion ACS and persistent symptoms
• Serial troponins immediately, after 3-6 hr, and subsequently if high suspicion persists
• Echocardiography evaluates regional & global LV function & adds specificity to diagnosis

---

[30] Antman EM, *et al.* The TIMI risk score for unstable angina/non-ST elevation MI: A method for prognostication and therapeutic decision making. *JAMA* 2000; 284: 835-842.
[31] PURSUIT Investigators. Inhibition of platelet glycoprotein IIb/IIIa with eptifibatide in patients with acute coronary syndromes. *N Engl J Med* 1998; 339: 436-443.

*Low risk:*
- Consider non-invasive stress test if normal serial ECG & troponins
- Consider CTA if no prior CAD, and ECG and troponin are inconclusive

### Non-ST-Elevation Acute Myocardial Infarction (NSTEMI)

*(1) Adjunctive **anti-ischemic** and heart failure treatments:*

- Nitroglycerin SL/IV, if not hypotensive and has not taken sildenafil/vardenafil < 24 hr, tadalafil < 48 hr. Avoid in inferior wall MI with right ventricular involvement
- β-adrenergic blockers: (1) assure no contraindications (signs of heart failure, low-output, risk of heart block, bronchospasm) & low risk of shock (age > 70, HR > 110, SBP < 120, late presentation). Avoid agents with intrinsic sympathomimetic activity. Initiate oral therapy within 24 hr especially in LV dysfunction, but avoid IV if risk of shock.
- Non-dihydropyridine calcium blockers: recommended if β-blockers unsuitable or in addition to β-blockers, if no risk of heart block. Helpful in coronary spasm.
- Morphine analgesia is reasonable if other antiischemics fail, NSAIDS should be avoided
- Oxygen if $SaO_2$ < 90%, respiratory distress, or features of hypoxia
- ACE inhibitors in left LVEF < 0.40, CHF, diabetes, hypertension, stable chronic kidney disease. Avoid IV. Use ARB if ACEI intolerant.
- If LVEF < 0.40 or DM or systolic heart failure, aldosterone blocker after MI without significant renal dysfunction or hyperkalemia
- Statin should be initiated at high doses
- **Note:** Fibrinolytic therapy is contraindicated in NSTEMI

*(2) Adjunctive **anti-platelet** treatments:*
- Aspirin 160-325 mg chewed po/pr, not enteric-coated

- P2Y$_{12}$ platelet inhibitor (clopidogrel 300-600 mg load + 75 mg daily; or ticagrelor 180 mg load + 90 mg bid; or prasugrel 60 mg load + daily dose) added to aspirin for up to 12 mo.
- If troponin+ and early-invasive strategy, consider IV GPII$_b$III$_a$ inhibitor (tirofiban or eptifibatide)

*(3) Adjunctive anti-coagulant treatments (follow institutional practices) for duration of hospital or until PCI is performed*

- Enoxaparin 1 mg/kg SQ q 12 h (qd if CrCL < 30 mL/min/m$^2$). IV load 30mg selected pts. OR
- Bivalirudin 0.10 mg/kg load + (if early invasive) 0.25 mg/kg/hr
- Fondaparinux 2.5 mg SQ qd. If PCI additional UFH or bivalirudin is required.
- UFH IV load 60 unit/kg max 4000 unit, infuse 12 unit/kg/hr max 1000 unit/hr to maintain therapeutic aPTT for 48 hr or PCI.

*(4) Choose Invasive or Ischemia-guided (conservative) strategy:*

**Initial invasive** = Urgent catheterization + revascularization of suspected culprit lesions, before discharge irrespective of non-invasive testing

- <u>Immediate invasive within 2 hr</u>: • Refractory angina; • heart failure or • mitral regurgitation; • hemodynamic instability; • recurrent angina at rest or minimal effort despite pharmacologic treatment; • sustained VT/VF
- <u>Early-invasive within 24 hr</u>: • GRACE risk score > 140; • Rise in Troponin; • New ST ↓
- <u>Delayed invasive within 72 hr</u>: • Diabetes; • Renal insufficiency; • Postinfarction angina; • PCI within 6 mo; • Prior CABG; • GRACE risk score 109-140 or TIMI score ≥ 2

**Ischemia-guided** strategy = initial pharmacologic stabilization

- Attractive if • Low-risk score TIMI 0-1 or GRACE < 109; • Low-risk Tn-negative women; • Patient or clinician preference

- Crossover to invasive strategy if • refractory angina at rest or minimal exertion, or • ischemia on noninvasive testing or dynamic ECG ischemia, or • high risk TIMI or GRACE score

## ST-Elevation Acute Myocardial Infarction (STEMI):

### ECG criteria

- New ST ↑ at J-point in at least 2 contiguous leads ≥ 2 mm (0.2 mV) in men or ≥ 1.5 mm in women in leads V2-V3 and/or ≥ 1 mm in other contiguous chest leads or limb leads. *See ECG ST elevation patterns on page 26*
- New LBBB is a presumed STEMI equivalent.

### Out of hospital cardiac arrest

- Therapeutic hypothermia if comatose and STEMI with VF/VT undergoing primary PCI
- Primary PCI should be offered after resuscitated out-of-hospital cardiac arrest and STEMI

### Primary PCI

- Perform in STEMI with • symptoms < 12 hr duration;
  - contraindications to fibrinolytics;
- Perform in • cardiogenic shock; • acute severe heart failure; irrespective of time from onset
- Reasonable 12-24 hr after symptom onset if evidence of ongoing ischemia
- Non-culprit artery PCI may be acceptable staged or immediate, even if hemodynamically stable[32]

### Adjunctive therapy for primary PCI

- ASA 162-325, continue indefinitely, AND
- Loading dose P2Y$_{12}$ inhibitor as soon as possible: clopidogrel 600 mg, prasugrel 60 mg, or ticagrelor 180 mg and continued at maintence dose for 1 yr. Assure low-dose ASA when used with ticagrelor.

---

[32] Levine GN, et al. 2015 ACC/AHA/SCAI Focused Update on Primary Percutaneous Coronary Intervention for Patients With ST-Elevation Myocardial Infarction. *Circulation.* 2016;133:1135-1147.

Anticoagulants for primary PCI
- Unfractionated heparin (UFH) 50-70 unit/kg with- and 70-100 unit/kg without- GPII$_b$III$_a$ inhibitor. OR
- Bivalirudin 0.75 mg/kg bolus then 1.75 mg/kg/h irrespective of UFH. Re-bolus 0.3mg/kg if needed. Reduce to 1 mg/kg/h if CrCL < 30 mL/min. Bivalirudin monotherapy may be preferred if bleeding risk is high.
- Fondaparinux is NOT recommended
- IV GPII$_b$III$_a$ inhibitor in conjunction with UFH or bivalirudin

Fibrinolytic therapy: when there is a delay > 120 min to a PCI-capable center
- Perform in STEMI with ischemic symptoms < 12 hr; • STEMI with ongoing ischemia for 12-24 hr and large myocardial risk area or hemodynamic instability; • Posterior myocardial infarction manifest as ST ↑ in lead aVR
- Do not use fibrinolytic therapy for ST ↓ except true posterior MI
- Administer within 30 min of arrival
- <u>Contraindications</u> and dosing: *see* fibrinolytics on *page 284*.
- <u>Agents</u>: Tenecteplase TNK-tPA, Reteplase rPA, Alteplase tPA weight-based dose, AND
- <u>Aspirin</u> 162-325 mg loading dose, continue indefinitely, at 81 mg if desired, AND
- <u>Clopidogrel</u> 300 mg age < 75; 75 mg age > 75 y. Continue 14 d-12 mo, AND
- <u>Anticoagulation</u> options: • UFH to achieve aPTT 1.5-2.0 elevation for 48 hr or until PCI; • Enoxaparin IV bolus then SQ 15 min later for duration admission up to 8 d; • Fondapariinux IV then SQ daily if CrCL > 30 mL/min for duration of admission up to 8 d or PCI
- <u>Transfer</u> to PCI facility for • shock or instability; • reperfusion failure; • consider immediate transfer irrespective of reperfusion to allow early remedy of reperfusion failure

Cardiogenic Shock:
- Emergency PCI or CABG for cardiogenic shock after STEMI irrespective of time delay.
- Fibrinolytics if otherwise unsuitable for PCI or CABG
- Intraaortic balloon pump or other mechanical circulatory support useful if unstable
- Seek mechanical complications (rupture, mitral valve regurgitation, *etc.*)

Convalescence:
- Initiate oral β-blockers if not contraindicated. Reevaluate eligibility later in course.
- ACEI within 24 hr if anterior MI, heart failure, EF < 0.40. ARB if ACEI intolerant.
- Aldosterone if EF < 0.40 and ACEI and β-blocker and (diabetes or symptomatic)
- High intensity statins
- Implanted defibrillator: Indicated if VT/VF after first inpatient 48 hr. May be indicated in moderate-severe LV dysfunction > 6wk post MI after expert consultation.
- Address comorbidities: • tobacco; • obesity; • lipids; • hypertension; • diabetes; • heart failure; • rhythm disorder; • sexual health; • mental health; • diet; • physical fitness and activity.

# *Valve Formulae*

## Gorlin Valve Stenosis Estimates[33]

Aortic Valve Area(cm$^2$)

$$= \frac{Cardiac\ Output\,(L/min)}{HR\,(bpm)\times Flow\ Time\,(s)\times k\times \sqrt{Mean\ Gradient\,(mmHg)}}$$

For aortic valve: Flow Time = Systolic Ejection Period, k = 44.3
For mitral valve: Flow Time = Diastolic Filling Period, k = 37.7

---

[33] Gorlin R, *et al.* Hydraulic formula for calculation of the area of the stenotic mitral valve, other cardiac valves, and central circulatory shunts. *Am Heart J* 1951; 41: 1-29.

## Hakki Simplified Valve Area-Gradient Relationship[34]

$$\text{Valve Area}(cm^2) \approx \frac{\text{Cardiac Output (L/min)}}{\sqrt{\text{Mean Gradient (mmHg)}}}$$

## Continuity Equation for Echo Aortic Valve Area Estimate

Valve Area (cm$^2$) =

$$\frac{\underline{\text{(Velocity at LVOT) x (Cross-sectional of LVOT)}}}{\text{(Velocity at Aortic Valve}}$$

### Pressure half-time method for mitral valve stenosis area

Mitral valve area (cm$^2$) = 220 ÷ Pressure half-time (ms)

# *Valve Disease Severity*[35]

### Aortic valve stenosis

| Severity | Mild | Moderate | Severe[§,¶] |
|---|---|---|---|
| Area | > 1.5 cm$^2$ | 1.0-1.5 cm$^2$ | < 1.0 cm$^2$ or < 0.6 cm$^2$/m$^2$ BSA |
| Mean gradient | < 25 mmHg | 25-40 mmHg | > 40 mmHg |
| Jet velocity | < 3.0 m/s | 3.0-4.0 m/s | > 4.0 m/s |
| Dimensionless index* | — | — | < 0.25 |
| Prosthetic valve EOA‡ patient mismatch[36] | > 0.85 cm$^2$/m$^2$ | 0.65-0.85 cm$^2$/m$^2$ | <0.65 cm$^2$/m$^2$ |

*\* Dimensionless Index = velocity-time integral (VTI) of aortic valve / VTI of LV outflow tract. ‡ EOA=Effective orifice area. § Area may be higher in mixed AS+AR. ¶Severe low-gradient AS may require provocation if low-flow, or "paradoxical" if stroke volume<35mL/m$^2$.*
Symptoms portend ominous prognosis if untreated.

---

[34] Hakki AH, *et al*. A simplified valve formula for the calculation of stenotic cardiac valve areas. *Circulation 1981; 63: 1050-1055.*

[35] Nishimura RA, *et al*. 2014 AHA/ACC guideline for the management of patients with valvular heart disease. *J Am Coll Cardiol 2014; 63: e57-185.*

[36] Pibarot P, *et al*. Prosthetic heart valves: selection of the optimal prosthesis and long-term management. *Circulation 2009; 119: 1034-1048.*

## Aortic valve regurgitation

| Severity | Mild | Moderate | Severe |
|---|---|---|---|
| Angiography | 1+ | 2+ | 3-4+ |
| Color Doppler jet if central | < 0.25 x LVOT | | > 0.65 x LVOT |
| Doppler vena contract width | < 0.3 cm | 0.3-0.60 cm | ≥0.60 cm |
| Regurgitant volume/beat | < 30 mL | 30-59 mL | ≥ 60 mL |
| Regurgitant fraction | < 0.30 | 0.30-0.49 | ≥ 0.50 |
| Regurgitant orifice area | < 0.10 cm$^2$ | 0.10-0.29 cm$^2$ | ≥ 0.30 cm$^2$ |
| Other | | | LV enlarged |

## Mitral valve stenosis

| Severity | Mild | Moderate | Severe |
|---|---|---|---|
| Area | > 1.5 cm$^2$ | 1.0-1.5 cm$^2$ | < 1.0 cm$^2$ |
| Mean gradient | < 5 mmHg | 5-10 mmHg | > 10 mmHg |
| Pulmonary Artery Pressure | < 30 mmHg | 30-50 mmHg | > 50 mmHg |
| Prosthetic valve EOA patient mismatch[36] | >1.2 cm$^2$/m$^2$ | 0.9-1.2 cm$^2$/m$^2$ | <0.9 cm$^2$/m$^2$ |

Consider balloon valvuloplasty if favorable echo valvuloplasty score *(see below)* and (1) PASP > 50 or (2) Poor exercise tolerance, or exercise PASP > 60, or exercise PAWP > 25, or new atrial fibrillation.

## MGH echo valvuloplasty score[37]:

| Grade | Leaflet Mobility | Subvalvular thickening | Leaflet Thickening | Calcification |
|---|---|---|---|---|
| 1 | Only leaflet tips restricted | Minimal below leaflets | Near-normal 4-5mm | Single area of echo brightness |
| 2 | Normal mid & base mobility | Extending to proximal 1/3 of chordae | Margins 5-8mm | Scattered brightness at leaflet margins only |
| 3 | Basal diastolic movement | Extending to distal 1/3 of chordae | Entire leaflet 5-8mm | Brightness into leaflet midportion |
| 4 | Minimal forward leaflet movement in diastole | Extensive through papillary muscles | Thickening throughout > 8-10 mm | Extensive brightness throughout leaflet |

Sum of scores on all categories ≤ 8 and no severe mitral regurgitation suggests suitable for balloon valvuloplasty. Higher scores: higher risk of failure, complications, and recurrence.

---

[37] Wilkins GT, *et al.* Percutaneous balloon dilatation of the mitral valve. *Br Heart J 1988; 60: 299-308.*

## Mitral valve regurgitation

| Severity | Mild | Moderate | Severe |
|---|---|---|---|
| Angiography | 1+ | 2+ | 3-4+ |
| Doppler vena contracta width | < 0.3 cm | 0.3-0.69 cm | ≥0.70 cm |
| Regurgitant volume/beat | < 30 mL | 30-59 mL | ≥ 60 mL |
| Regurgitant fraction | < 0.30 | 0.30-0.49 | ≥ 0.50 |
| Regurgitant orifice area | < 0.20 cm$^2$ | 0.20-0.39 cm$^2$ | ≥ 0.40 cm$^2$ |
| Other | | | LA or LV enlarged |

## Tricuspid valve

Severe tricuspid stenosis: area < 1.0 cm$^2$
Severe tricuspid regurgitation: Doppler vena contracta width ≥ 0.70 cm and systolic flow reversal in hepatic veins

# Critical Care

## Shock[1]

### Hemodynamic Profiles in Shock

| Classification | PCWP | CO | SVR | Comments |
|---|---|---|---|---|
| **Cardiogenic** | | | | |
| Myocardial dysfunction | ↑ | ↓ | ↑ | Hemodynamic goals: • PCWP 15-18; • MAP ≥ 70 mmHg; • CI ≥ 2.2; • SVR 1000-1200 |
| Acute MR | ↑ | ↓ (forward) | ↑ | |
| Acute VSD | ↑ | ↓ | ↑ | O₂ "step-up" at RV. |
| RV infarction | ↔/↓ | ↓ | ↑ | RA pressure >> PCWP |
| Pericardial Tamponade | ↑ | ↓ | ↑ | RAP=RVEDP=PAD=PCWP Pulsus paradoxicus increased |
| **Distributive** | | | | |
| Sepsis (early) | ↔/↓ | Usually ↑ | ↓ | CO may ↓ due to sepsis-mediated LV dysfunction, especially in later phases (mixed cardiogenic-septic physiology) |
| Anaphylaxis, liver disease, spinal shock, adrenal insufficiency | ↔/↓ | ↑ | ↓ | Epinephrine for anaphylaxis after treating underlying cause; pure α agonists in spinal shock |
| **Hypovolemic** | | | | |
| Hemorrhage, dehydration | ↓ | ↓ | ↑ | Invasive monitoring needed only if co-existing LV dysfunction |

### Choice of drugs in shock[2]

| Hemodynamics | Initial Treatment | Comments |
|---|---|---|
| PCWP (or CVP) ↓ | Aggressive volume expansion | Volume >> pressors; reevaluate once PCWP ≥ 18 or CVP ≥ 12 |
| CO ↓, SVR ↑ | Dobutamine | Alternatives include milrinone or dopamine plus nitroprusside |
| CO ↓, SVR ↔ or ↓ | Dopamine vs norepinephrine | |
| SVR ↓, CO ↑ | High dose dopamine or norepinephrine | Add epinephrine or phenylephrine for refractory hypotension |

---

[1] Vincent JL, *et al.* Circulatory shock. *N Engl J Med* 2013; 369: 1726-1734.
[2] Beale RJ, *et al.* Vasopressor and inotropic support in septic shock. *Crit Care Med* 2004; 32: S455-465.

## Relative action of vasopressors

| Drug | Receptor | HR | Inotropy | SVR | Comments |
|------|----------|-----|----------|-----|----------|
| Dopamine, *Low dose* | DA | 0 | 0 | ↔↓ | Renal & splanchnic vasodilator. Unlikely clinical benefit. |
| Dopamine, *High dose* | $\beta_1 \rightarrow \alpha_1$ | ↑ | ↑↑ | ↑↑ | Versatile vasopressor, not better than norepinephrine |
| Dobutamine | $\beta_1, \beta_2 > \alpha_1$ | ↔↑ | ↑↑ | ↓↓ | Inotrope & vasodilator; may lower BP |
| Norepine-phrine | $\alpha_1, \alpha_2, \beta_1$ | ↔↑ | ↑↑ | ↑↑↑ | For hypotension refractory to dopamine; initial choice in sepsis |
| Epinephrine | $\alpha_1, \alpha_2$ $\beta_1, \beta_2$ | ↑↑ | ↑↑↑ | ↑↑↑ | For refractory cardiac failure (*e.g.* post CABG) or anaphylaxis. More arrhythmia than norepi. |
| Phenylephrine | $\alpha_1$ | 0 | 0 | ↑↑↑ | For refractory hypotension, esp. vasculogenic |
| Isoproterenol | $\beta_1, \beta_2$ | ↑↑↑ | ↑↑ | ↔↓ | Primarily increases HR. May cause reflex hypotension. |
| Vasopressin | V1a | 0 | 0 | ↑↑ | Despite acidosis. Use only with adequate cardiac output. |
| Milrinone | PDIII inhibitor | ↑ | ↑↑ | ↓↓ | May reinforce dobutamine. Useful in downregulated or blocked β-adrenergic receptors. |
| Glucagon[‡] | ↑cAMP | ↑↔ | ↑ | ↔ | Counteracts β-blocker or calcium-blocker overdose |

[‡] *Off-label application supported by low-quality evidence.*

# Sepsis

**Severe sepsis (tissue hypoperfusion or organ dysfunction)[3]:**
- Sepsis-induced hypotension; • Lactate > upper limits of normal; • Oliguria < 0.5 mL/kg/hr x 2 hrs, despite adequate volume infusion; • Acute lung injury with $P_aO_2/FiO_2 < 250$ (no pneumonia) or < 200 (pneumonia); • Creatinine >2.0 mg/dL; • Bilirubin > 2 mg/dL; • Platelets < 100k/mm[3]; • Coagulopathy (INR>1.5)

**Controversy**
- Aggressive CVP catheter-guided therapy had shown high mortality benefit. Wide adoption of early aggressive volume resuscitation subsequently undermined benefit of protocolized "early goal directed therapy," with control arms receiving ~ 4L IV fluid in 1st 6-8 hr[4].

**Goal: normalize perfusion including lactate.**
**Resuscitate even before ICU arrival.**

- Crystalloid <u>volume</u> (30mL/kg) preferred over colloid & albumin[5] and over vasopressors.
- <u>Vasopressors</u> if fluids insufficient to maintain adequate BP, *i.e.* MAP > 65 mmHg.
- Norepinephrine is preferred agent; may add epinephrine, vasopressin. • Dopamine not recommended for renal protection. • Phenylephrine reserved for tachyarrhythmia from other agents. • Vasopressin doses > 0.03-0.04 unit/m reserved for salvage. • Dobutamine inotropic trial may be added in myocardial dysfunction.

---

[3] Dellinger RP, *et al.* Surviving Sepsis Campaign: international guidelines for management of severe sepsis and septic shock. *Intensive Care Med* 2013; 39: 165-228.
[4] Mouncey PR, *et al.* Trial of early, goal-directed resuscitation for septic shock. N Engl J Med 2015; 372: 1301-1311.; Caironi P, *et al.* Albumin replacement in patients with severe sepsis or septic shock. *N Engl J Med* 2014; 370: 1412-1421; Yealy DM, et al. A randomized trial of protocol-based care for early septic shock. *N Engl J Med* 2014; 370: 1683-1693.
[5] Caironi P, et al. Albumin replacement in patients with severe sepsis or septic shock. N Engl J Med 2014; 370: 1412-1421.

- Glucocorticoids if no hemodynamic stability despite fluid and vasopressors: hydrocortisone IV 200 mg/d.
- Empiric antimicrobials early, after blood cultures. De-escalate as soon as possible. • Low procalcitonin may guide discontinuation of antimicrobials
- Aggressive search for infection source, mechanical intervention as required
- Blood transfusion for permissive targets Hb < 7.0 g/dL with target > 7 g/dL
- Platelet transfusion prophylactically for platelet ≤ 10 k if high risk, ≤ 20 k normal risk, ≤ 50 k if bleeding or invasive procedures.
- Bicarbonate NOT indicated for lactic acidosis pH > 7.15.

## Mechanical ventilation in sepsis with ARDS
(see page 70)

- Tidal volume (TV) target 6 mL/kg predicted body weight.
- Plateau ≤ 30 cm $H_2O$. Permissive hypercapnea to minimize TV & plateau pressure.
- Use PEEP to avoid alveolar collapse, higher rather than lower pressures
- Use recruitment maneuvers
- Prone positioning if feasible & refractory hypoxemia ($PaO_2/FIO2 < 100$ mmHg)
- Semi-recumbent position (head of bed to 45°), as feasible
- Routine weaning trials once stable, low vent pressures, low $FiO_2$ requirements
- Neuromuscular blockers risk prolonged blockade, should be reserved for ARDS, titrated to train-of-four peripheral nerve stimulation, limited in duration

# *Anaphylaxis*[6]

## Diagnostic criteria: One of three scenarios

- Acute onset reaction (within minutes to hours) involving skin and/or mucosae (pruritis, flushing, hives, angioedema) and at least one of respiratory compromise (dyspnea, bronchospasm, stridor, hypoxemia), reduced blood pressure, symptoms of end-organ dysfunction
- After exposure to a likely allergen, two or more of skin/mucosal involvement, respiratory compromise, reduced blood pressure, or associated symptoms, persistent gastrointestinal symptoms (vomiting, cramping abdominal pain, diarrhea)
- Reduced blood pressure after exposure to a known allergen

## Pearls

- Use epinephrine; physician hesitation can lead to death
- Do not rely on signs of shock for the diagnosis!
- Anaphylaxis diagnosis may be obscured by catheter angiography, surgery, or hemodialysis precipitants
- Anaphylaxis may occur without skin signs 10-20%
- Hypotension may be the sole manifestation of anaphylaxis 10-20%
- Anaphylaxis in patient with known asthma may appear to be "just" severe asthma
- Concurrent adrenergic blockers, ACE inhibitors may predispose or exacerbate anaphylaxis
- "Biphasic" anaphylaxis: occurs 1-23% after initial resuscitation, warrants careful observation and repeat treatment if necessary

## Differential diagnosis

- Rare but may resemble anaphylactoid: pheochromocytoma, carcinoid, VIPoma;

---

[6] Lieberman P, *et al.* The diagnosis and management of anaphylaxis practice parameter: 2010 update. *J Allergy Clin Immunol 2010; 126*: 477-480.

- Common but distinct: Profound myocardial ischemia or dysfunction, pulmonary thromboembolism, panic disorder, aspiration, vasodepressor phenomenon

**Triggers**

- Food (peanuts, tree nuts, sesame seed, fish, shellfish, cow's milk, soy, egg); • Latex; • Perioperative/Procedural: iodinated radiocontrast; thiopental; succinylcholine- or opioid-induced histamine release; Antimicrobials, *e.g.* β-lactams; protamine; blood transfusion; methylmethacrylate bone cement; • Coital; • Exercise or hereditary or acquired angioedema (C1 esterase deficiency); • Allergen immunotherapy; • Drugs and biological response modifiers: β-lactam antibiotics; aspirin and NSAIDs; omalizumab; • Insect sting (occasionally a marker of underlying mast cell disease); Idiopathic

**Emergency Management**

- Remove <u>precipitant</u> (*i.e.* stop medication infusion)
- <u>Airway</u> management
- <u>Epinephrine</u> IM 1:1000 or 1 mg/mL or 0.1%, dose 200-500 µg into anterolateral thigh (vastus lateralis, preferred over deltoid or SQ). Repeat q 5 min or as needed
- <u>Oxygen</u>
- Aggressive <u>volume</u> (10-20 mL/kg or 1-2L IV or IO, repeated),
- Assume <u>supine</u> posture, elevate legs to increase central vascular volume
- Urticaria: <u>H1 antihistamine</u>; • <u>H2 antihistamine</u> <u>and</u>; • <u>Glucocorticoid</u> for subacute management. Do not administer instead of epinephrine
- Prolonged <u>aggressive resuscitation</u> is suggested for cardiac arrest caused by anaphylaxis because of greater likelihood of favorable outcome. Include high-dose epinephrine (in contrast to ACLS recommendations)
- Treat <u>bronchospasm</u> with albuterol in addition to epinephrine

### Refractory Anaphylaxis
- Epinephrine infusion, other vasopressors. Epinephrine 1:10,000 or 0.01% or 0.1 mg/mL, infusion 2-10 µg/min IV
- Glucagon 1-5 mg IV then 5-15 µg/min may have value

### Convalescence
- <u>Lab tests</u>: timing is critical. Tryptase (peak 60-90 min after event), histamine (plasma, elevated only 30-60 min), urinary methyl histamine, carboxypeptidase.
- <u>Expert consultation</u> is recommended, including education about how to avoid and manage recurrence

# APACHE II Score[7]

**Acute Physiology Score (APS):** Sum variables 1-12 (use one each for 5 & 9), add to Age and Chronic Health Points below. *Use worst value from preceding 24 hr.*

| Physiologic Variable | 0 | 1 | 2 | 3 | 4 |
|---|---|---|---|---|---|
| 1 Temperature (°F) | $96^8$-$101^2$ | $101^3$-$102^1$<br>$93^2$-$96^7$ | $89^6$-$93^1$ | $102^2$-$105^7$<br>$86^0$-$89^5$ | $\geq 105^8$<br>$\leq 85^9$ |
| 2 Heart Rate *Ventricular response* | 70-109 | n/a | 110-139<br>55-69 | 140-179<br>40-54 | ≥ 180<br>≤ 39 |
| 3 Mean Art Pressure (2 x DBP + SBP)÷3 | 70-109 | n/a | 110-129<br>50-69 | 130-159 | ≥ 160<br>≤ 49 |
| 4 Resp Rate *On or off ventilator* | 12-24 | 25-34<br>10-11 | 6-9 | 35-49 | ≥ 50<br>≤ 5 |
| 5 Oxygenation: *Use 5a if $FiO_2 \geq 0.5$, or 5b if $FiO_2 < 0.5$*<br>*A-a gradient = $(713 \times FiO_2) - (1.25 \times PaCO_2) - PaO_2$* | | | | | |
| 5a: A-a gradient | < 200 | | 200-349 | 350-499 | ≥ 500 |
| 5b: $PaO_2$ | > 70 | 61-70 | | 55-60 | ≤ 54 |
| 6 Serum Na⁺ | 130-139 | 150-154 | 155-159<br>120-129 | 160-179<br>111-119 | ≥ 180<br>≤ 110 |
| 7 Serum K⁺ | 3.5-5.4 | 5.5-5.9<br>3.0-3.4 | 2.5-2.9 | 6.0-6.9 | ≥ 7.0<br>≤ 2.4 |
| 8 Serum Creatinine *Double if Acute RF* | 0.6-1.4 | n/a | 1.5-1.9<br>< 0.6 | 2.0-3.4 | ≥ 3.5 |

*(Continued)*

---

[7] Knaus WA, et al. APACHE II: a severity of disease classification system. Crit Care Med. 1985;13:818-829

| Physiologic Variable | | 0 | 1 | 2 | 3 | 4 |
|---|---|---|---|---|---|---|
| 9 | 9a: Arterial pH *Preferred* | 7.33-7.49 | 7.50-7.59 | 7.25-7.32 | 7.60-7.69 | ≥ 7.70 |
| | | | | | 7.15-7.24 | ≤ 7.14 |
| | 9b: Venous $HCO_3$ *Use only if no ABG* | 22-31.9 | 32-40.9 | 18-21.9 | 41-51.9 | ≥ 52 |
| | | | | | 15-17.9 | ≤ 14 |
| 10 | WBC | 3.0-14.9 | 15 -19.9 | 20-39.9 | n/a | ≥ 40 |
| | | | | 1.0-2.9 | | < 1.0 |
| 11 | Hematocrit | 30-45.9 | 46-49.9 | 50-59.9 | n/a | ≥ 60 |
| | | | | 20-29.9 | | < 20 |
| 12 | GCS *(see below)* | Score = 15 – GCS Score (Eye + Motor + Verbal) | | | | |

| Glasgow Coma Scale (GCS) | | Chronic Health Points | | Age Points | |
|---|---|---|---|---|---|
| **Eye Opening** | *Verbal* | Non-operative, or emergency post-op & any conditions below* | 5 | ≤ 44 | 0 |
| 4:Spontaneously | 5: Oriented and conversant; seems able to talk if intubated | | | 45-54 | 2 |
| 3:To command | | | | 55-64 | 3 |
| 2:To pain | | Elective operation & any conditions below* | 2 | 65-74 | 5 |
| 1:No response | | | | ≥ 75 | 6 |
| **Motor Response** | 4: Confused | *Cirrhosis with portal hypertension or encephalopathy; class IV angina; chronic hypoxia, hypercarbia or polycythemia; chronic dialysis; immunocompromised | | | |
| 6: Obeys commands | 3: Inappropriate speech; questionable ability to speak if intubated | | | | |
| 5: Localizes to pain | | | | | |
| 4: Withdraws to pain | | | | | |
| 3: Flexion to pain | | **Total APACHE II Score = Acute Physiology Score + Chronic Health Points + Age Points** | | | |
| 2: Extension to pain | 2: Incomprehensible | | | | |
| 1: No response | 1: No response | | | | |

# *Pulmonary Artery Catheters*[8]

**Utility:** Determine cause of **pulmonary edema** (cardiogenic vs. non-cardiogenic), **hypotension** (cardiac vs. volume status vs. vascular tone) or **oliguria** (cardiac function vs. volume status vs. renal disease), **PA hypertension** etiology & management; **Severe** or **discordant RV/LV** heart failure; No benefit and possible harm used routinely

**Risks:** LBBB risks complete heart block; Coagulopathy; PA rupture

---

[8] Figures copyright 1987 Lawrence Martin MD, with permission.

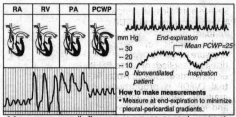

- Measure mean "*a*" wave pressure at end expiration (peak "*a*" wave follows ECG "*p*" wave by ~ 0.24 ms and *v*-wave follows ECG *T*-wave)
- PEEP Correction: Subtract ½ of PEEP (x 0.8 cm $H_2O$/mmHg), less in ARDS
- Caution if there is excessive catheter whip or marked respiratory variation

## Quality assurance for PAWP

- Catheter is calibrated, level and flushes easily;
- Correct position on CXR (AP: < 3-5 cm from midline; lateral: below LA); • Characteristic PA waveforms with balloon deflated; • PAWP < PADP; • Mean PAWP < mean PAP

## Interpretation of PAWP

- PAWP correlates with LV filling pressures (LVEDP) – *see exceptions below*
- "Physiologic" LVEDP is rate-dependent
  - Bradycardia increases LVEDP, tachycardia decreases LVEDP
- High LVEDP does not always correlate with radiographic pulmonary edema
  - No edema with chronically ↑ LVEDP (↑ lymph drainage, ↓ vasc. permeability)
  - Non-cardiogenic pulmonary edema (normal LVEDP) occurs with endothelial injury (*e.g.* ARDS) or low albumin states
- PAWP *underestimates* LVEDP (pre-load) in
  - Decreased LV compliance (MI, LVH, diastolic dysfunction, pericardial disease)

- Severe aortic insufficiency
- **PAWP *overestimates* LVEDP (pre-load)** in
  - High thoracic or pericardial pressure, *e.g.* obstructive lung disease, applied or auto-PEEP, or pericardial disease. **Note:** Actual LVEDP is proportional to gradient between intracardiac and *intrapericardial* pressure; Measured PAWP is proportional to gradient between intracardiac and *atmospheric* pressure

PA · V wave · Balloon inflated · Giant V Waves

  - Mitral regurgitation or stenosis
  - Non-"zone III" catheter position (PAWP > PAD), "over wedged" waveform (unnaturally smooth with marked respiratory variation)
  - Increased PA vascular tone (hypoxia, hypovolemia, dopamine)
  - "Catheter whip" in hyperdynamic states
  - Catheter tip obstruction (LA myxoma, thoracic tumors, mediastinal fibrosis)

| Specific findings on PA catheterization<br>*Also see jugular vein pulsations, page 20* | Cause |
|---|---|
| Giant "*v*" waves with obliteration of *a* waves (balloon inflated), and bifid PA waveform (ballon deflated) *See diagram* | • Acute mitral regurgitation<br>• LA enlargement or LV failure<br>• Acute ventriculoseptal defect |
| PA diastolic pressure exceeds PAWP by > 5-7 mmHg | • PA hypertension, embolism, hypoxic vasoconstriction, venooclusive disease)<br>• Pulmonary parenchymal disease<br>• Tachycardia |
| O₂sat "step-up" (> 10%) between RA and PA = L → R shunt | • Atrial or ventricular septal defect<br>• Patent ductus arteriosus |
| Elevated RA pressure with prominent *x* and *y* descents (*y* usually > *x*). RA pressure does not decrease with negative intrathoracic pressure (Kussmaul sign). | • RV infarction<br>• Restrictive/constrictive physiology |
| Elevated RA pressure with prominent *x* descent & diminished or absent *y* descent. RAP = RVEDP = PAD = mean PAWP. Absent Kussmaul sign. Pulsus paradox. | • Pericardial Tamponade |

## Common problems

| | |
|---|---|
| Reported mean, not end-expiratory pressures | • Inspiration is driven by transthoracic gradients; • End-expiration minimizes exterior-pleural gradient. |
| Catheter is persistently wedged | • Flush tip; • Make sure balloon is deflated; • Pullback to PA tracing, then inflate and re-advance |
| Catheter will not wedge | • Make sure that balloon is intact (air returns from balloon) and that tip is not over wedged; • Inflate balloon while in PA and advance; • Use fluoroscopy guidance; • Use PAD if shown to correspond with PAWP |
| Ventricular ectopy | • Suggests RV position or catheter "pretzeled:" withdraw to cavae or reposition; • Check electrolytes |

# Using Mechanical Ventilators[9]

## Modes of Mechanical Ventilation

| Mode | Advantages | Disadvantages |
|---|---|---|
| Assist-control (AC) | • Full tidal volume regardless of respiratory effort or drive • Can set minute volume | • Tachypnea causes resp alkalosis • Poor patient-vent synchrony → "breath-stacking" & auto-PEEP |
| Intermittent Mandatory Ventilation (IMV) | • Patient determines tidal volume for spontaneous breath • Possible ↓ resp alkalosis • Possible respiratory conditioning | • May ↑ work of breathing & resp. muscle fatigue • Resistance of respiratory circuit during spontaneous breath (unless also pressure support) |
| Pressure Support Ventilation (PSV) | • Patient determines volumes, rate & flow • Potentially ↓ peak inspiratory pressures (PIPs) | • Monitor to assure adequate tidal volumes & minute ventilation • Requires consistent respiratory effort |
| Pressure Control Ventilation (PCV) | • Easier control of inspire time & peak airway pressures • May be used with AC or IMV | • Assure adequate tidal volumes & minute ventilation • May increase risk of auto-PEEP |

(Continued)

[9] Schmidt GA, *et al.* Management of the Ventilated Patient. In: Hall JB, et al., editors. *Principles of Critical Care, 4e*: McGraw-Hill; 2015. Tobin MJ. Advances in mechanical ventilation. *N Engl J Med* 2001; 344: 1986-1996.

| Mode | Advantages | Disadvantages |
|------|-----------|---------------|
| Non-invasive Positive Pressure Ventilation (NIPPV) - *see page 73* | • Allows ventilation without intubation<br>• Easily taken on/off | • Requires careful patient selection and trained respiratory therapists<br>• No airway control |

## Initial ventilator settings and mechanics

| Parameter | Suggested Initial Settings / Normal | Comments |
|-----------|-------------------------------------|----------|
| $FiO_2$ | 100% | • May taper rapidly to level adequate to maintain $PaO_2/O_2$sat<br>• Keep < 60% to ↓ $O_2$ toxicity & lung injury |
| Respiratory Rate (RR) | 8-12/min | • Titrate to pH<br>• Consider 18-24/min for "therapeutic" hyperventilation (↓ respiratory effort in shock)<br>• Rate > 20/min may ↑ auto-PEEP |
| Mode | IMV or AC | • Consider PSV in neuromuscular disease if respiratory effort enough to trigger cycle |
| Tidal Volume ($V_T$) | 6 ml/kg ideal body weight | • Higher volumes increase alveolar overdistention ("barotrauma") and worsen ventilator lung injury |
| Inspiratory Flow Rate (IFR) | 60 L/min | • Set only on volume cycled ventilators<br>• IFR set too low may increase auto-PEEP by allowing insufficient exhalation time<br>• IFR set too high may increase PIPs |
| Inspiratory to Expiratory (I:E) Ratio | 1:3 | • Determined by IFR and respiratory rate during volume-cycled ventilation<br>• Can be specifically adjusted during PCV<br>• Increased I:E ratio (*e.g.* 1:4) may be useful in severe obstruction (↑ expiratory phase)<br>• Inverse ratio (2:1) may be used to increase $PaO_2$ in severe hypoxemia |
| Plateau Pressure | < 30 cm $H_2O$ | • Non-invasive transpulmonary pressure<br>• Ideally kept low to ↓ risk of barotrauma |
| Peak Inspiratory Pressure (PIP) | < 45 cm $H_2O$ | • Keep low; less important than plateau pressure |

*(Continued)*

| Parameter | Suggested Initial Settings / Normal | Comments |
|-----------|-------------------------------------|----------|
| Positive End Expiratory pressure (PEEP) | 5 cm $H_2O$ (considered "physiologic") | • Improves oxygenation by preventing alveolar collapse and V/Q mismatch<br>• Titrate PEEP by 2.5 cm $H_2O$ increments until $FiO_2$ requirement ≤ 0.6 or plateau pressure > 35 cm $H_2O$ or ↓ compliance<br>• ↑ airway pressures and risk of barotrauma<br>• ↓ venous return and cardiac output |
| Compliance | 70-100 ml/cm $H_2O$ | • Δvolume/Δpressure = $V_T$ ÷(plateau pressure - PEEP)<br>• Decreased in CHF, pneumothorax, ARDS, effusions, pneumonia, chest wall disorders |
| Resistance | < 5-10 cm $H_2O$/L/sec | • Δpressure/flow rate = (PIP – plateau) ÷IFR<br>• ↑ in bronchoconstriction, mucous plugging |

## Acute hypoxemic respiratory failure
• **Common scenarios:** • ARDS • Pneumonia • CHF
  • Pulmonary fibrosis • Pulmonary contusion • Aspiration
• **Things to consider:**
  • Pulmonary overdistention ("**barotrauma**") promotes ventilator-associated lung injury, but can be prevented with lower tidal volumes (5-7 ml/kg) and plateau pressures (≤ 35 cm $H_2O$). Hypercapnia and respiratory acidosis ("permissive hypercapnia") may reduce barotrauma. pH as low as 7.2 is usually tolerated but increased sedation may be needed to suppress respiratory drive.
  • High respiratory rates (>20) needed to normalize $P_aCO_2$ may also ↑ auto-PEEP, ↑ physiologic dead space, and ↑ hypercarbia (*see page 71*)
• **PEEP** redistributes fluid from alveoli to interstitium, and recruits collapsed or flooded alveoli. In ARDS, PEEP 12-20 cmH$_2$O improves oxygenation. **Caveats:**
  • PEEP may reduce atrial filling, causing hypotension or tachycardia
  • In inhomogeneous lung disease (*e.g.* lobar pneumonia) PEEP may not improve oxygenation and may increase intrapulmonary shunt

- Interrupting the PEEP circuit even transiently (*e.g.*, manual bagging during transport) can cause deterioration in marginally oxygenated patients
- PEEP should be used to reduce $V_T \sim$ 6 mL/kg and plateau pressure <30 cmH$_2$O
- To reduce pulmonary edema, titrate PCWP to minimum that achieves an adequate cardiac output
- **Flow rate/wave-form:** Slower inspiratory flows (*e.g.* 40 L/min) and/or a decelerating flow pattern will ↑ inspiratory time and may improve oxygenation
- If **refractory hypoxemia** consider:
  - Trial of **prone position** for 20-40 min (if oxygenation is improved begin regular prone positioning 2-3 hr bid-tid). **Note** requires team effort to avoid dislodging ETT.
  - **Pressure control ventilation** (PCV) with inverse I:E ratio (1:1 or less) - will further increase inspiratory time and possibly oxygenation)
  - Inhaled nitric oxide, *see p 346.*
  - Recruitment maneuvers to open lung units: transient high ventilator pressures
  - Extracorporeal membrane oxygenation (ECMO)

## Severe airflow obstruction

- **Common clinical scenarios:** • Status asthmaticus or COPD • Thermal injury to upper airway • Central airway obstruction by mass/mucus plug •Tracheal stenosis

- **Things to consider:**
  - "Permissive" hypercapnia to pH as low as 7.2. This appears preferable to gas trapping, intrinsic PEEP and high airway pressures.
  - High PIPs may allow for lower plateau pressures
  - Intrinsic PEEP (**"auto-PEEP"**) reflects elevated alveolar pressure at end-expiration in severe airway obstruction. Measure at airway opening during an expiratory hold maneuver (*i.e.* while occluding the expiratory and inspiratory limbs of the ventilator). Intrinsic PEEP effectively raises the pressure needed to trigger ventilator,

increases work of breathing and muscle fatigue. Minimize intrinsic PEEP by:
- Lowering respiratory rate ($\leq$ 8/min) or lengthening expiratory time
- Increasing inspiratory flow rate (*e.g.* 80 L/min) to decrease inspiratory time and lengthen expiratory time (lowering respiratory rate is more effective).
- Avoiding extrinsic PEEP and sighs, since pressures are already excessive
- Diminished venous return is common on initiation of mechanical ventilation; hypotension responds to intravascular volume expansion or temporary disconnection from ventilator
- Early sedation & muscle relaxation decreases airway pressure, $O_2$ consumption and patient discomfort
- Refractory obstruction may respond to helium-oxygen (heliox) therapy. This strategy is controversial in small-airways obstruction (*e.g.* asthma)

## Restrictive lung disease
- **Indications:** • Progressive restrictive lung (*e.g.* pulmonary fibrosis) or chest wall (*e.g.* kyphoscoliosis) disease • Rarely, massive and tense fluid collection in the abdomen or recent abdominal surgery
- **Things to consider:**
  - Relieve restriction if possible (*e.g.* paracentesis, escharotomy)
  - Upright posture may improve restriction from intra-abdominal processes
  - Restriction increases risk of **(1)** reduced venous return impairing cardiac output and **(2)** increased physiologic dead space from high minute ventilation and PEEP, especially with concurrent hypovolemia

## Indications for sedation and muscle relaxation
- Patients at high-risk for ventilator-associated lung injury
  - Airway disease with increased airway pressure & intrinsic PEEP (*e.g.* status asthmaticus)
  - Hypoxemic respiratory failure and clinical instability

- Toxic $FiO_2$ (> 0.6) despite PEEP
- Hypoxemic respiratory failure with high intrinsic PEEP and increased work of breathing
- Bronchopleural fistula in patients with chest tubes
- Control of central neurogenic hyperventilation
- Modes that heighten discomfort: inverse ratio ventilation, permissive hypercapnia
- **Note:** prolonged neuromuscular blockade risks prolonged muscle weakness. Duration and dose should be minimized, ideally < 48 hr.
- Daily reduction of sedation leads to earlier extubation, reduced ICU stay

## Non-invasive ventilation[10]

- **Indications:** • Effective in hypoxemic respiratory failure due to CHF, COPD, complications of BMT, asthma; • Decreases ventilator-associated pneumonia; • May decrease need for endotracheal intubation, decrease mortality, and shorten length of stay
- **Contraindications:** • Uncooperative patient; • Impaired mental status; • Hemodynamic instability; • Inability to protect airway; • Upper airway obstruction; • Excessive secretions; • Facial deformity; • Absence of skilled respiratory therapist or appropriate monitoring • Risk of emesis
- **Administration:** • Usually delivered as bi-level positive airway pressure (BiPAP) via nasal mask/pillows or full face mask; • Critical care ventilator (rather than portable unit) allows higher and more precise $O_2$ delivery, higher inspiratory flow rate (improved patient comfort), and monitoring and alarms
- **Settings:** • Start with rate 10 bpm, rise time 0.4 sec, inspiratory pressure (IPAP) 8-10 $cmH_2O$ and expiratory pressure (EPAP=CPAP) 2-4 cm $H_2O$ • Titrate rate and IPAP to provide ventilation and EPAP to maintain $O_2$ sat and airway patency

[10] Hillberg RE, *et al.* Noninvasive ventilation. *N Engl J Med 1997; 337*: 1746-1752; Brochard L. Noninvasive ventilation for acute respiratory failure. *JAMA 2002; 288*: 932-935.

- **Complications:** • Local irritation from mask • Gastric distention (rare if peak pressure < 20 cm $H_2O$)
- **Alternative:** • High-flow oxygen via nasal cannula reduces mortality[11]

# Ventilator Emergencies

## High pressure

- If $O_2Sat \leq 80\%$ or hemodynamically unstable, **disconnect from ventilator and bag @ $FiO_2$ 100%**; check for causes as per below
- If stable oxygenation and hemodynamics, check ventilator peak and plateau pressures

**Peak (PIP):** max pressure registered with each volume cycled breath

**Plateau:** pressure at end-inspiration (may use 0.5 sec "hold" to measure)

| Increased resistance<br>Peak pressure elevated<br>(> 35 cm $H_2O$)<br>Plateau pressure normal<br>(≤ 35 cm $H_2O$) | Decreased compliance<br>Peak and Plateau pressures<br>elevated (> 35 cm $H_2O$) |
|---|---|
| • Endotracheal tube mucous or plugs<br>• Biting of endotracheal tube<br>• Tracheal obstruction<br>• Bronchospasm<br>**Interventions:**<br>• Check ventilator circuit<br>• Suction<br>• Bronchodilators<br>• Reposition tube<br>• Consider bronchoscopy | • Tube in main stem bronchus<br>• Asynchronous breathing<br>• Auto-PEEP<br>• Atelectasis, pneumonia, CHF<br>• Pneumothorax<br>• Abdominal compartment syndrome<br>**Interventions:**<br>• Stat CXR to find cause (decompress suspected pneumothorax if unstable)<br>• Decrease auto-PEEP by ↓ tidal volume:RR ratio or temporarily disconnect from ventilator circuit |

---

[11] Lemiale V, *et al.* Effect of Noninvasive Ventilation vs Oxygen Therapy on Mortality Among Immunocompromised Patients With Acute Respiratory Failure. *JAMA 2015; 314: 1711-1719;* Frat JP, *et al.* High-flow oxygen through nasal cannula in acute hypoxemic respiratory failure. *N Engl J Med 2015; 372: 2185-2196;* Stephan F, *et al.* High-Flow Nasal Oxygen vs Noninvasive Positive Airway Pressure in Hypoxemic Patients After Cardiothoracic Surgery. *JAMA 2015; 313: 2331-2339.*

**Low-pressure**
- If $O_2Sat \leq 80\%$ or hemodynamically unstable, **disconnect from ventilator and bag @ $FiO_2$ 100%**
- **Causes:**
  - Endotracheal tube slipped out of trachea → reintubate
  - Cuff leak → instill more air into cuff or reintubate
  - Tracheoesophageal fistula → attempt to reposition tube
  - Leak within mechanical ventilator circuit

# *Weaning from Mechanical Ventilation*[12]

**Daily Spontaneous Awakening & Breathing Trials**[13]
- Withdrawing sedative agents daily allows for spontaneous breathing trials and both reduces mechanical ventilation time and increases survival. Pain control can continue independently.

**Whom to consider for weaning: "wean screen"**
- Lung injury that is resolving or at least stable
- Gas exchange adequate with PEEP < 5-8 cm $H_2O$ and $FiO_2$ < 0.4-0.5
- Stable hemodynamics without vasopressors
- Able to initiate spontaneous breaths

**Spontaneous breathing trial, 30-120 min**
- Minimal ventilator assistance: T-piece or CPAP 1-5 cm $H_2O$ or PS 5-7 cm $H_2O$
- Rapid shallow breathing index (RSBI = respiratory rate {per min} ÷ tidal volume) < 105 during T-piece trial best predicts successful weaning [14]

---

[12] MacIntyre N. Discontinuing mechanical ventilatory support. *Chest* 2007; 132: 1049-1056; MacIntyre NR, et al. Evidence-based guidelines for weaning and discontinuing ventilatory support. *Chest* 2001; 120: 375S-395S.

[13] Girard TD, *et al.* Efficacy and safety of a paired sedation and ventilator weaning protocol for mechanically ventilated patients in intensive care. *Lancet* 2008; 371: 126-134.

- Adequate oxygenation: $PaO_2 \geq 60$ mmHg on $FiO_2$ $\leq 0.4$ ($PaO_2/FiO_2 = 150\text{-}300$) with PEEP $\leq 5$ cm $H_2O$
- Assess success based not on single parameter but integrated consideration of
  - Hemodynamic stability (without tachycardia, bradycardia, BP alteration)
  - Gas exchange (decrease in pulse-oximetry)
  - Patient comfort (diaphoresis or anxiety)

**After successful spontaneous breathing trial:**
- Assure ability to protect airway with good coughing strength and minimal need for suctioning (< q 2 hr)
- Alert and able to follow commands
- Anticipate difficulty of replacing airway if removed
- Consider possibility of obstructive upper airway inflammation
- Proceed with extubation
- Reintubation rate ~ 10-15% suggests appropriate balance of management considerations

**After unsuccessful spontaneous breathing trial**
- Consider etiology
  - Respiratory drive failure: drugs, CNS injury
  - Oxygenation failure: parenchymal disease, V/Q mismatch
  - Oxygen delivery failure: anemia, heart failure
  - Muscle failure: deconditioning, metabolic disease, nutrition
  - Systemic inflammation
- Ventilator support modes: SIMV, Pressure Control, Proportional assist, *etc.*
- Address failure mode
- Repeat "wean screen" q 24 hr.
- Consider tracheostomy if progress is inadequate

---

[14] Yang KL, *et al.* A prospective study of indexes predicting the outcome of trials of weaning from mechanical ventilation. *N Engl J Med* 1991; 324: 1445-1450.

# Targeted temperature management[15]

## aka therapeutic hypothermia

**Patient Selection**
- Return of spontaneous circulation, irrespective of "shockable" or "non-shockable" arrest
- Comatose (GCS < 8): Unable to follow verbal commands

**Induction**
- Pre-hospital cooling is NOT recommended
- Endotracheal intubation to allow neuromuscular blockade
- Goal core temperature 32-36°C
- Replace potassium to K > 3.8mEq/dL
- Vigilant search for seizures (especially continuous EEG) → anti-epileptic sedation
- Sedation and neuromuscular blockade for comfort, shivering, shock.
- Consider bispectral index surveillance of depth of awareness during paralysis. If sedation only, titrate "deep sedation"
- Cooling techniques:
  - Bolus fluid 30-40 mL/kg at 4°C; • Ice packs to neck, groin, axillae; • Rubber cooling blankets (avoid skin contact), dedicated surface cooling devices; • Intravascular (intracaval) cooling devices

**Maintenance**
- Individualize target temperature: higher T when risk of bleeding; lower T in cerebral edema or seizures
- Maintain at least 24 hr
- Inotropic support and/or intraaortic balloon pump more likely during hypothermia
- Correct hypothermia-induced polyuria
- Meticulous skin care against hypothermia wounds

---
[15] Callaway CW, *et al.* Post-Cardiac Arrest Care: 2015 AHA Guidelines Update. *Circulation 2015; 132: S465-482;* Donnino MW, et al. Temperature Management After Cardiac Arrest. *Circulation. 2015;132:2448-2456.*

- Consider higher likelihood of aspiration pneumonia
- Additional agents to suppress shivering: Magnesium sulfate to 3-4 mg/dL; Meperidine; Clonidine or dexmedetomidine

**Rewarming**

- Rewarm slowly 0.25-0.5°C/hr
- Volume repletion and monitoring/correction of potassium abnormalities
- Discontinue neuromuscular blockade but suppress shivering
- Suppress fever after cooling

# Endocrinology

## *Thyroid Function in Critical Illness*[1]

### Thyroid function tests

| TSH | Free T4* | Free T3* | Interpretation |
|---|---|---|---|
| Nml | Nml | - | Thyroid disease excluded |
| ↓ | Nml | ↓ or Nml | Non-thyroid illness (most common, esp. if TSH > 0.1 µU/mL) vs. subclinical hyperthyroidism (less common) |
| ↓ | ↑ | ↓,↑, or Nml | Non-thyroid illness vs. primary thyrotoxicosis. Nonthyroid illnes more likely if free T3 is Nml-low and asymptomatic. |
| ↓ | Nml | ↑ | T3 thyrotoxicosis |
| ↓ | ↓ | ↓ | Non-thyroid illness (most common) vs. central hypothyroidism (rare) |
| ↑ | Nml | ↓ or Nml | Recovery phase of non-thyroid illness (common) vs. subclinical hypothyroidism (more likely if pattern found early in critical illness) |
| ↑ | ↓ | ↓ to Nml | Primary hypothyroidism |
| ↑-Nml | ↑ | ↑ | Central hyperthyroidism (very rare) |

\* *Direct measurement or calculated index    Nml = normal*

### Non-thyroid illness ("sick euthyroid state")
- Most common cause of abnormal thyroid function in hospital inpatients (accounts for 80% of abnormal TSH levels)
- TSH usually low-normal, but may rise during recovery phase of illness
- Free and total T4 initially rise (decreased peripheral conversion and increased binding proteins) but become subnormal during severe or prolonged illness
- Total and free T3 characteristically fall due to decreased peripheral conversion
- No apparent benefit to supplementation with levothyroxine or liothyronine

---

[1] Haddady S, Farwell AP. Nonthyroidal Illness Syndrome in the Intensive Care Unit. In: Irwin RS, Rippe JM, eds. Irwin and Rippe's Intensive Care Medicine, 7/e. LWW; 2011.

**Etiology of abnormal TSH levels in hospitalized patients**[2]

| TSH level (µU/mL) | Thyroid Disease | Sick euthyroid | Glucocorticoid Rx |
|---|---|---|---|
| < 0.1 | 24 % | 41 % | 35 % |
| 0.1-0.34 | 0 % | 73 % | 27 % |
| 0.35-6.8 | – | – | – |
| 6.9-20 | 14 % | 72 % | 14 % |
| > 20 | 50 % | 45 % | 5 % |

## Non-thyroid causes of abnormal TSH
• Decreased: Acute or chronic illness; Glucocorticoids; Caloric restriction; Dopamine or adrenergic agonists; Opiates; Phenytoin
• Increased: Recovery phase of acute illness; Cimetidine; Dopamine antagonists; Neuroleptics; Metoclopramide

# *Myxedema Coma*[3]

## Etiology
• **Underlying thyroid disease:** • Autoimmune • Previous thyroid surgery or ablation (check for neck scars or history of [131]I administration) • Occasionally caused by 2° hypothyroidism (↓ TSH) or drugs (amiodarone, lithium)
• **Acute precipitants:** • Hypothermia (most cases in winter) • Stroke • CHF • Infection • Drugs: anesthetics, sedatives, narcotics • Trauma • GI bleed

## Manifestations:
• **Hypothermia:** Mortality increases as temperature falls
• **Neurologic:** • Lethargy → stupor → coma (↑ mortality if ↓ consciousness) • "Myxedema madness": depression, paranoia, hallucinations • Hyporeflexia
• **Respiratory:** • ↓ Hypoxic drive → hypoventilation → hypercapnia • Pleural effusions • Airway obstruction from macroglossia and myxedema infiltrate

[2] Spencer CA. Clinical utility and cost-effectiveness of sensitive thyrotropin assays in ambulatory and hospitalized patients. *Mayo Clin Proc* 1988; 63: 1214-1222.
[3] Klubo-Gwiezdzinska J, *et al.* Thyroid emergencies. *Med Clin North Am* 2012; 96: 385-403.

- **Cardiac:** • Bradycardia • Hypotension • Pericardial effusion ± tamponade • Systolic/diastolic dysfunction • ECG: block, ↓ voltage, QT ↑
- **Renal:** • Hyponatremia (impaired water excretion) • Intravascular volume contraction

## Management

- Replace **thyroid hormone**. Give IV initially (PO absorption ↓ from gut edema). Reduce dose if elderly or cardiac ischemia. Options: **(1) Levothyroxine (T4):** $T_{1/2}$ ~ 7 d, must be converted to T3 for activity. Load 300-500 mcg IV then 50-100 mcg qd. *See Levothyroxine on page 313.* **(2) Liothyronine (T3):** Active hormone, $T_{1/2}$ ~ 1 d. Controversial; high doses associated with increased mortality. Rationale: slow-onset of T4 monotherapy and inhibition of T4 → T3 conversion by concurrent non-thyroid illness. Load 10-20 mcg PO/IV, then 10 mcg q 4-6hr until clinical improvement[4]. Doses as low as 2.5 mcg appear to reverse metabolic abnormalities. *See Liothyronine on page 314.* **(3) Dual therapy:** Give T4 at slightly reduced dose (4 mcg/kg) plus T3 as above
- Concurrent **adrenal insufficiency** common (5-10%) → Initial stress dose IV glucocorticoids (draw cortisol level beforehand or use dexamethasone and perform ACTH stimulation test)
- Expedite mechanical ventilation for **respiratory failure** (progresses rapidly, with high risk for aspiration). Upper airway obstruction possible.
- If **hypotensive** give adequate volume prior to adding vasopressors (dopamine preferred over pure α-agonists). Consider pericardial tamponade or adrenal insufficiency in refractory hypotension.
- **Hypothermia:** Re-warm passively with blankets and warm room; active re-warming may cause distributive shock

---

[4] MacKerrow SD, *et al.* Myxedema-associated cardiogenic shock treated with intravenous triiodothyronine. *Ann Intern Med* 1992; 117: 1014-1015.

- **Hyponatremia:** Usually corrects with levothyroxine therapy. Avoid rapid correction and use of hypertonic saline unless Na < 120 mEq/L and/or symptoms.
- Search for precipitant; consider empiric antibiotics
- Adjust drug dosing for reduced drug metabolism

# *Thyroid Storm*[5]

### Etiology
- **Underlying thyrotoxicosis:** Usually Grave's disease
  - Acute thyroiditis; toxic multinodular goiter; Jod-Basedow (iodine-induced); factitious (thyroxine ingestion)
- **Acute precipitants:** Infection • Surgery or trauma • Iodine load (iodinated radiocontrast, kelp, amiodarone) • Childbirth • Thyroid manipulation or surgery • Psychiatric stress • Withdrawal of antithyroid drugs • Diabetic ketoacidosis • Pulmonary embolism • Stroke • Sympathomimetic drugs (pseudoephedrine) • Thyroiditis from [131]I-therapy with release of stored hormone

### Features: Mortality 20-30%
- **General:** Fever, tachycardia, diaphoresis (out of proportion to apparent infection)
- **Cardiopulmonary:** ↑ Metabolic demand, ↑ $O_2$ consumption, ↑ cardiac output • Hyperdynamic circulation → high-output CHF • Myocardial ischemia • Arrhythmias (usually SVT, esp. AF) • Systolic HTN with widened pulse pressure
- **Neuropsychiatric:** Delirium, stupor or coma, seizures • Myopathy > 50% • Ophthalmopathy (Grave's) • Agitation
- **GI:** • Vomiting, diarrhea, malabsorption • ↑ Gastrin → peptic ulcer disease • Abnormal LFTs
- **Rare:** aggravated myasth. gravis, thyrotoxic hypokalemic periodic paralysis (Asian men)
- **Labs:** ↑ glucose, ↑ WBC, ↓ Hct, ↓ platelets, ↓ $K^+$, ↑ $Ca^{++}$ (may be severe), ↑ LFTs

5  Klubo-Gwiezdzinska J, *et al.* Thyroid emergencies. *Med Clin North Am* 2012; 96: 385-403; Nayak B, *et al.* Thyrotoxicosis and thyroid storm. Endocrinol Metab Clin North Am 2006; 35: 663-686, vii.

## Treatment

**(1) Antithyroid**– effective for hyperfunctioning gland (*e.g.* Grave's) but not thyroiditis or exogenous thyroid hormone

- Inhibit new hormone synthesis with **propylthiouracil** (PTU; 200-250 mg PO/NG/enema q 4 hr) or **methimazole** (20 mg PO/NG q 4 hr). PTU preferred because it blocks peripheral T4 → T3 conversion.
- Inhibit hormone secretion with **iodine:** SSKI or Lugol's solution (8 gtts PO q 6 hr). **Caution:** Wait at least 2 hr after methimazole or PTU (iodine monotherapy can exacerbate thyrotoxicosis). **Iodine allergy:** Lithium carbonate 300 mg PO q 6 hr to keep lithium level ~ 1mEq/L

**(2) Block peripheral action and conversion of thyroid hormone**

- β-adrenergic blockade, *e.g.*, **propranolol** (0.5-1 mg IV/min to total of 2-10 mg, titrated to heart rate; then 20-80 mg PO q4-6 hr), propranolol also blocks T4 → T3 conversion
- Inhibit peripheral T4 → T3 conversion with glucocorticoids *e.g.*, dexamethasone (2 mg IV/PO q 6 hr) or hydrocortisone (100 mg IV q 8 hr). β-blockers & PTU also block T4 → T3.
- If intractable symptoms consider dialysis or plasmapheresis; or enteric binding of thyroid hormone with cholestyramine (4 g PO q 6hr)

**(3) Treat precipitating illness**, *e.g.* occult infection, CHF, diabetic ketoacidosis

**(4) General supportive care**

- Control hyperthermia with acetaminophen, cooling blankets
- Fluid resuscitation + dextrose for diaphoresis, vomiting, diarrhea, hypoglycemia
- Parenteral vitamin supplements (*e.g.* B-complex)
- Consider empiric glucocorticoids if adrenal insufficiency suspected

# Hyperglycemia[6]

| Features | | Diabetic ketoacidosis (DKA) | Hyperosmolar hyperglycemic state (HHS) |
|---|---|---|---|
| Type of diabetes | | 1 > 2 | 1 << 2 |
| Evolution | | Hours to days | Days to weeks |
| Dehydration | | Mild-moderate | Moderate to severe |
| Plasma glucose | | > 250; usually < 800 | > 600; can be > 1000 |
| Arterial pH | mild 7.25-7.3 | | > 7.3 |
| | moderate 7.00-7.24 | | (50% have mild |
| | severe < 7.0 | | anion gap) |
| Serum $HCO_3^-$ (mEq/L) | mild 15-18 | | |
| | moderate 10-15 | | > 15 |
| | severe < 10 | | |
| Ketones | | Positive | Trace |
| Serum osmolarity | | Variable (usually < 320 mOsm/kg) | > 320 mOsm/kg |
| Stupor or coma | | Variable based on severity | Common (25-50% of cases) |
| Mortality | | < 5% | 15% |

**Glycemic Control Background:** Hyperglycemia predicts bad outcomes. Exuberance about "tight" glycemic control[7] disproven in NICE-SUGAR:[8] excess ICU hypoglycemia and mortality.

**Blood glucose (BG) targets**
Threshold to initiate insulin: BG no higher than 180 mg/dL.
ICU Target: BG 140-180 mg/dL, probably closer to 140.
Non-ICU: Consider target BG 110-140 mg/dL.

**Estimate insulin daily, basal, prandial, correction doses[9]**
<u>Basal dose</u> = 50% of total daily dose as long-acting agent.

---

[6] Moghissi ES, *et al.* AACE and ADA consensus statement on inpatient glycemic control. *Diabetes Care* 2009; 32: 1119-1131; Kavanagh BP, *et al.* Glycemic control in the ICU. *N Engl J Med* 2010; 363: 2540-2546.

[7] Van den Berghe G, *et al.* Intensive insulin therapy in the medical ICU. *N Engl J Med* 2006; 354: 449-461.

[8] Finfer S, et al. Intensive versus conventional glucose control in critically ill patients. *N Engl J Med.* 2009;360:1283.

[9] Bode BW, *et al.* Intravenous insulin infusion therapy. *Endocr Pract* 2004; 10 Suppl 2: 71-80.

<u>Prandial dose</u> = 50% of daily dose divided among 3 meals, as short-acting insulin before meal.

<u>Correction factor</u> for individual insulin sensitivity = (1700 units ÷ total daily insulin dose).

<u>Correction dose</u>: [Actual BG – Target BG] * Correction Factor, before meal.

**ICU Intravenous Regimen, one example: Yale Protocol**[10]

Initial insulin bolus & infusion dose: [BG (mg/dL) ÷ 100] rounded up to 0.5 U administered as IV bolus + hourly infusion. Example BG 325mg/dL → 3.5 units IV bolus + 3.5 units/hour. Adjust hourly. Mix Insulin 1 unit / mL saline.

*See also* Joslin insulin infusion algorithm *page 306.*

**Inpatient who is not eating**

Insulin-treated DM: 80% of basal insulin or 0.2-0.3 unit/kg/d + Correction Dose every 6 hours of 1-4 unit for each BG 50 mg/dL above 150 mg/dL

Non-insulin-treated DM: Discontinue outpatient regimen + begin Correction Dose every 6 hours of 1-4 unit for each BG 50 mg/dL above 150 mg/dL

**Inpatient who is eating but poor control on outpatient regimen**

Basal insulin: increased from home regimen or 0.2-0.3 unit/kg/day

Prandial insulin: increased from home regimen or 0.05-1.0 unit/kg/meal +

Correction insulin: 1-4 unit for each BG 50 mg/dL above 150 mg/dL added to prandial

**Transition from IV to subcutaneous insulin**

Continue IV until able to tolerate food and 2 hr after first subcutaneous insulin

Calculate total daily dose (extrapolate from last 4-8 hr), reduce by 20% to be conservative, give half as basal (long-acting) dose and half divided among 3 meals. Use correction doses to target BG 140-180 mg/dL

---

[10] Goldberg PA, *et al.* Implementation of a safe and effective insulin infusion protocol in a MICU. *Diabetes Care* 2004; 27: 461-467.

## Hypoglycemia

Common risks: elderly, reduced oral intake, renal or liver disease, beta-blockers, interruption of parenteral nutrition, IV dextrose, dialysis, NPO

Nurse-driven hypoglycemia surveillance and treatment avoids more severe episodes.

Dose (mL) of 50% dextrose IV = (100-BG mg/dL) x 0.4

If altered sensorium and no IV access → IM glucagon 1 mg

### Pearls

Type I DM always requires basal insulin, even if NPO. Sliding-scale is not acceptable as a sole form of insulin therapy.

Target glucose < 110 mg/dL is probably unsafe in ICU.

Perform BG checks before every meal and bedtime, or every 6 hr if NPO.

Revisit insulin therapy with any change in caloric intake, procedure, transfer of service, glucocorticoids, vasopressors.

Check HbA1c at each hospital admission.

Add prandial insulin for patients with Type II DM, HbA1c > 8.5% and > 2 oral agents.

### Fasting patients for surgery or other procedures

Type II DM: Hold oral hypoglycemic agents. If on insulin, follow instructions on next line

Type I & Type II DM: reduce preceding bedtime glargine or detemir dose by 20%; give half of intermediate-acting (NPH) morning dose; suspend short-acting insulin except to correct BG > 180. Consider IV infusion 1-2 unit/hr with dextrose to achieve ICU target

### Diabetes Ketoacidosis or Hyperosmolar Hyperglycemic State[11]

(1) Identify the precipitant. (2) Volume resuscitation. (3) Check BG and electrolytes hourly. Insulin

<u>Standard approach</u>: 0.1 unit/kg bolus then 0.1 unit/kg/hr infusion to reduce BG 50-75mg/kg/hr

---

[11] Kitabchi AE, et al. Hyperglycemic crises in adult patients with diabetes. Diabetes Care 2009; 32: 1335-1343.

<u>Joslin DKA formula[12]</u>: • Start insulin infusion units/hr = (current BG – 60) x Multiplier. Starting multiplier = 0.02. • Adjust multiplier hourly based on BG measurements. • If BG=140-180 mg/dL or if $\Delta$BG > 50 mg/dL, no change. • If BG > 180 mg/dL, increase multiplier by 0.01. • If BG < 140 mg/dL, decrease multiplier by 0.01.

• When BG < 250mg/dL, add D10W. • If BG drops < 100 mg/dL, stop insulin, give D50 dose (100-BG mg/dL) x 0.4 mL, and resume insulin at ½ previous rate.

If unresponsive to insulin, seek other cause: sepsis, glucocorticoids, IV access, *etc.*

Add potassium once K<upper limit of normal, if renal function preserved

In DKA: When BG reaches 200 mg/dL (DKA) or 300 mg/dL (HHS), add D5W @100-200 mL/hr plus insulin 0.02-0.05 units/kg/hr until anion gap or acidosis are relieved

Transition to subcutaneous insulin after stabilization. Use estimated total daily dose 0.5-0.8 unit/kg/day. Be cautious about this highly variable estimate.

Conventional: NPH/Regular 0.4/0.2 total daily dose in AM + 0.2/0.2 total daily dose in PM

Alternative "basal bolus:" 0.5 total daily dose glargine daily or detemir once-twice daily + bolus lispro/aspart/glulisine 0.5 ÷ 3 total daily before each meal

[12] Ganda O. Joslin guideline for management of uncontrolled glucose in the hospitalized adult. *Boston; 2015.* www.joslin.org/joslin_clinical_guidelines.html.

# Adrenal Crisis[13]

### Setting
- Sudden extensive adrenal destruction (*e.g.* hemorrhage or infarction) **or**
- Major physiologic stress (*e.g.* surgery, infection, trauma) in unrecognized primary adrenal insufficiency **or**
- Inadequate "stress dose" corticosteroids in a patient with known or suspected adrenal insufficiency (*e.g.* chronic corticosteroid treatment, even at low doses)
- Septic shock causes relative (reversible) adrenal insufficiency

### Manifestations
- **Shock:** Both hypovolemic and distributive. Often out of proportion to severity of acute illness and refractory to fluids and pressors until adrenal hormone replacement.
- **GI:** Nausea and vomiting, anorexia; abdominal pain (may mimic acute abdomen)
- **Fever:** Accentuated by low cortisol but occult infection common
- **CNS:** Lethargy, confusion, coma
- **Physical/radiologic findings:** Hyperpigmentation of mucosae, creases, and sun-spared skin (1° insufficiency only) • Small cardiac silhouette on CXR • Calcified or enlarged adrenals on CT
- **Labs:** ↓ $Na^+$, ↑ $K^+$ (↓ aldo), ↑ BUN/Cr, ↓ glucose, ↑ $Ca^{++}$, eosinophilia
- **Secondary adrenal insufficiency differs:** • ACTH low-normal • No hyperpigmentation • Mineralocorticoid activity preserved (no hyperkalemia) • Hyponatremia from centrally increased ADH • Hypoglycemia common

---

[13] Cooper MS, *et al.* Corticosteroid insufficiency in acutely ill patients. N Engl J Med 2003; 348: 727-734; Puar TH, et al. Adrenal Crisis: Still a Deadly Event in the 21 Century. Am J Med 2015.

## Diagnosis

- **High dose ACTH (cosyntropin) stimulation:** Give 250 mcg IV. Cortisol ≥ 18-21 mcg/dL at baseline or within 60 minutes of injection accurately excludes chronic severe adrenal insufficiency. However, criteria may miss partial or recent onset insufficiency, especially in critically ill patients.
- **Relative adrenal insufficiency:** May contribute to hypotension in critical illness esp septic shock. Random cortisol < 15 mcg/dL is abnormal in critical illness, while random cortisol level > 34 mcg/dL is sufficient. If indeterminate, perform ACTH stimulation: incremental response < 9 mcg/dL is abnormal.
- **ACTH level:** Used to differentiate primary (ACTH >> normal) vs. secondary or tertiary disease (ACTH low-normal). Check random sample prior to empiric corticosteroids.

## Treatment

- Rapid volume resuscitation (30-50% of normal intravascular volume, typically 2-3 L NS) titrated to JVP or pulmonary edema. Replace K, glucose prn.
- Draw baseline cortisol and ACTH level
- Hydrocortisone 50-100 mg IV q 6-8 h. Taper ~ 50% per day after stabilized. Separate mineralocorticoid repletion not required acutely, but fludrocortisone should be added when daily hydrocortisone < 100 mg/day. Dexamethasone 4 mg IV restores vascular tone and will not interfere with ACTH testing but is less preferred.
- **Note:** Mineralocorticoids support intravascular volume; gluocorticoids support vascular tone.
- Perform ACTH stimulation test
- Identify and treat precipitating illness
- If primary adrenal insufficiency, will need chronic repletion with hydrocortisone (typically 15-20 mg q AM, 5-10 mg q PM) and fludrocortisone (0.1 mg qd, titrated to K$^+$).
- Routine glucocorticoids recommended in refractory septic shock, without ACTH stimulation testing

# Gastroenterology

## *Upper GI Hemorrhage*[1]

**Diagnosis**

- **Resuscitate during evaluation:** If orthostatic or hypotensive, active bleeding manifest as hematemesis, bright red blood per NG, hematochezia, hemoglobin ↓ 2 g/dL: need multiple large-bore IV access, volume infusion, intensive/ICU monitoring, expert consultation.
- **Key History:** NSAID or antiplatelet drugs; liver or variceal disease; weight loss; dysphagia; heartburn; prior AAA repair;
- **Stool color**[2]: 14% of UGI bleeds manifest as hematochezia (bright red blood per rectum or maroon stool) • Hematochezia predicts more transfusions, need for surgery and mortality (14 vs. 8%) compared with melena or brown stool
- **Nasogastric (NG) aspirate:** 90% sensitive in localizing bleeding to UGI tract (high (-) predictive value if non-bloody bile in NG aspirate) • No value to large volume lavage • Mortality: clear (6%) < coffee grounds (10%) < red blood (18%)
- **Etiology:** Peptic ulcer; gastric erosion; Mallory-Weiss tear; esophagitis; duodenitis; malignancy; varices and portal gastropathy; angiodysplasia; von Willebrand disease; Dieulafoy lesion; aorto-enteric fistula

---

[1] Barkun AN, *et al.* International consensus recommendations on the management of patients with nonvariceal upper gastrointestinal bleeding. *Ann Intern Med* 2010; 152: 101-113; Laine L, et al. Management of patients with ulcer bleeding. *Am J Gastroenterol* 2012; 107: 345-360; quiz 361.

[2] Wilcox CM, *et al.* A prospective characterization of upper gastrointestinal hemorrhage presenting with hematochezia. *Am J Gastroenterol* 1997; 92: 231-235.

**Prognosis in non-variceal upper GI hemorrhage:**
- **Pre-endoscopy (Blatchford score)[3]:** Low risk of re-bleeding & complications if **all** of following present:
  - BUN < 18 mg/dl; • SBP ≥ 110 mmHg; • HR < 100bpm; • Hgb > 13 g/dL (men), 12 g/dL (women). Possible outpatient management.
- **Post-endoscopy**

| Re-bleeding risk based on endoscopic findings[4] | | | |
|---|---|---|---|
| **Low Risk** | **Moderate Risk** | **High Risk** | **Highest Risk** |
| • PUD – no SRH<br>• M-W tear, non-bleeding;<br>• Erosive disease<br>• Normal | • PUD – black spot or clot;<br>• Erosive disease with SRH;<br>• Angiodysplasia | • PUD – non-bleeding visible vessel;<br>• PUD – SRH | • Active UGI bleeding;<br>• Varices<br>• Malignant lesion |

PUD= peptic ulcer disease; SRH= stigmata of recent hemorrhage;
M-W= Mallory-Weiss

**Rockall score[5]: Sum of all rows**

| Score | 0 | 1 | 2 | 3 |
|---|---|---|---|---|
| Age (yrs) | < 60 | 60-79 | ≥ 80 | — |
| Shock | HR < 100<br>SBP ≥ 100 | HR ≥ 100<br>SBP ≥ 100 | SBP < 100 | — |
| Co-morbidity | None | — | CAD, CHF, other major co-morbidity | Renal failure, liver failure, metastatic CA |
| Endoscopic Diagnosis | M-W lesion<br>No lesion/<br>no SRH | All other diagnoses | Malignant lesion of UGIT | — |
| Stigmata of recent hemorrhage | None or dark spot in ulcer base | — | Blood in UGIT, adherent clot, visible vessel | — |

SRH = stigmata of recent hemorrhage    UGIT = Upper GI Tract

3  Blatchford O, *et al*. A risk score to predict need for treatment for upper-gastrointestinal haemorrhage. *Lancet* 2000; 356: 1318-1321.
4  Hay JA, *et al*. Prospective evaluation of a clinical guideline recommending hospital length of stay in upper gastrointestinal tract hemorrhage. *JAMA* 1997; 278: 2151-2156.
5  Rockall TA, *et al*. Selection of patients for early discharge or outpatient care after acute upper gastrointestinal haemorrhage. *Lancet* 1996; 347: 1138-1140.

| Rockall score | % of Patients | Re-bleeding Rate | Mortality | Mortality in patients with re-bleeding |
|---------------|---------------|------------------|-----------|-----------------------------------------|
| 0-2  | 29 % | 4.3 % | 0.1 % | n/a  |
| 3-4  | 34 % | 13 %  | 3 %   | 12 % |
| 5    | 15 % | 17 %  | 8 %   | 21 % |
| 6    | 9 %  | 29 %  | 15 %  | 29 % |
| 7    | 8 %  | 40 %  | 20 %  | 35 % |
| ≥8   | 5 %  | 48 %  | 40 %  | 53 % |

## Treatment

- **Supportive:** Transfuse for Hb < 7 g/dL ("restrictive strategy"). Correct coagulopathy but do not delay endoscopy. Promotility agents not routinely indicated for endoscopy. 70-85% of patients stop bleeding without specific treatment.
- **Clopidogrel/prasugrel/ticagrelor & coronary stents:** Expert consultation before stopping, especially < 2-4 wk after bare-metal or < 3-12 mo after drug-eluting stent.
- **Acid suppression:** IV proton pump inhibitors control bleeding and reduce rebleeding. • H₂ blockers inadequate
- **Endoscopic therapy:** Indicated in most patients within 24 hr. For diagnosis & prognosis; biopsy if suspected tumor; mechanical and/or pharmacologic treatment;
- **Rebleeding:** Usually in first 3 days after endoscopic therapy. Second attempt at endoscopic therapy usually appropriate.
- **Surgery:** Required ~ 6%, and ¼ of rebleeding after initial endoscopic therapy. Catheter-based arterial embolotherapy: alternative to surgery, reduced success in coagulopathy, possibly superior in biliary or pancreatic source of bleeding.
- **Other medical therapy:** *H. pylori* testing and treatment. Bleeding interacts with testing; Negative *H. pylori* test should be repeated as outpatient.

• Somatostatin & octreotide not routinely indicated. Possible role in uncontrolled bleeding awaiting endoscopy or surgery, or in whom surgery is contraindicated • Restart cardiovascular-indicated ASA as soon as risk/benefit profile favorable. • ASA+PPI is preferred over clopidogrel alone to reduce rebleeding

## Variceal bleeding[6]

• **Prevent bleeding:**
  • Risk according to Child-Pugh Class (*see p 101*).
  • Identify varices by endoscopy; Endoscopic prophylactic variceal ligation favored at some centers.
  • Measure hepatic vein pressure gradient (HVPG, hepatic vein pressure – hepatic vein wedge pressure). HVPG>5mmHg elevated, > 10 predicts development of varices, > 20 predicts poor outcome esp < 24 hr of admission for bleeding. Reduction of HVPG to < 12 indicates a favorable therapeutic response.
  • Non-selective β-blockers (β1 reduce BP, β2 splanchnic vasoconstriction) such as propranolol, nadolol, or carvedilol for added α antagonism. Titrate to HR 50-60 bpm; Venodilators: nitrates > ACEI/ARB; Transjugular-intrahepatic portosystemic shunt (underline TIPS) may have prophylactic value in Child C or HVPG>20.
• **Arrest bleeding & related complications:** Minority stop spontaneously
  • Volume resuscitation with saline and PRBC
    • Platelet transfusion if < 50 K
  • Correct coagulopathy: vitamin K & FFP
    • Adequate airway prior to endoscopy
  • Octreotide 50 µg bolus then 50 µg/hr (*see page 331*) for 2-5 d • Endoscopic treatment of varices: cyanoacrylate obturation more effective than band ligation.
  • TIPS for refractory bleeding
  • Prophylaxis against bacterial peritonitis with fluoroquinolone or ceftriaxone

---

6 Garcia-Tsao G, *et al*. Management of varices and variceal hemorrhage in cirrhosis. *N Engl J Med* 2010; 362: 823-832.

- **Prevent recurrent variceal bleeding:**
  - Endoscopic variceal ligation + Nonselective β-blockers ± nitrates. Surveillance endoscopy periodically. Consider HVPG response. • TIPS for refractory bleeding

# Acute Lower GI Bleeding[7]

**Etiology:** Diverticulum; Angiodysplasia; Colitis (ischemic, infective, chronic inflammatory bowel disease, radiation); Neoplasia & postpolypectomy bleeding; NSAID colopathy; Hemorrhoids; Upper GI; Small bowel; Dieulafoy

**Resuscitate during evaluation**

Large-bore IV, volume and/or blood infusion as needed.

**Exclude upper GI bleeding as cause: NG tube lavage, melena, or endoscopy**

**Early or urgent colonoscopy:** After polyethylene glycol prep. Allows diagnosis & targeted therapy including coagulation, clips, local epinephrine.

**Alternative testing, or no source found after EGD and colonoscopy**

(1) Wireless capsule endoscopy (small bowel), contrast-enhanced CT

(2) Scintigraphy with $^{99}$Tc-sulfur colloid ($T_{1/2}$ 2-3 min, negative without active bleeding) or $^{99}$Tc-RBCs (detectable 12-24 hr later, detects 0.1mL/min bleeding). Can guide further examinations.

(3) Mesenteric angiography, requires ongoing bleeding (> 0.5 mL/min), best in diverticular bleeding, allows transcatheter embolotherapy

(4) Urgent surgical total or segmental colectomy, guided by above testing

---

[7] Pasha SF, *et al.* ASGE guideline: The role of endoscopy in the patient with lower GI bleeding. *Gastrointest Endosc 2014; 79: 875-885.*

# Acute Infectious Diarrhea[8]

**Evaluation**

If either <u>Colitis</u> (small-volume bloody stool, with/without mucus, urgency, tenesmus) OR <u>disabling or protracted</u> (≥ 48 hr) febrile diarrhea should prompt: • single stool specimen for SSYC or shiga-toxin-producing E. coli; • if febrile: blood culture; • if immunocompromised: stool inspection ("O&P"). Treat for specific identified pathogen.

If prior exposure to antibiotics, hospital, or nursing home: consider C. difficile *(see page 97)*

If persistent diarrhea ≥ 14 d, obtain single stool culture for bacteria and parasites; stool inspection for selected pathogens if immunocompromised

| Pathogen | Comments | Fever | Abd Pain | Bloody Stool | N/V | Fecal WBC |
|---|---|---|---|---|---|---|
| Toxins (staph, B. cereus, C. perfringens) | Incubation < 6 to 24 hr. | — | + | — | ++ | — |
| Salmonella, non-typhoidal | Community acquired, food-borne | ++ | ++ | + | + | ++ |
| Salmonella, typhoid | Community acquired in travelers. Often fever without diarrhea | ++ | + | — | + | — |
| Campylobacter | Community acquired, undercooked poultry | ++ | ++ | + | + | ++ |
| Shigella | Community acquired, person-to-person | ++ | ++ | + | ++ | ++ |
| Shiga toxin-producing E. Coli (e.g. O157:H7) | Food-borne outbreaks, under-cooked beef; bloody stool w/o fever | — | ++ | ++ | + | — |
| C. difficile | Nosocomial, post-antibiotics; marked leukocytosis in 50% | + | + | ± | — | ++ |

*++ Common  + Occurs  ± Variable  — Atypical or not characteristic*

*(continued)*

---

8 DuPont HL. Acute infectious diarrhea in immunocompetent adults. N Engl J Med 2014; 370: 1532-1540; Guerrant RL, et al. Practice guidelines for the management of infectious diarrhea. Clin Infect Dis 2001; 32: 331-351.

| Pathogen | Comments | Fever | Abd Pain | Bloody Stool | N/V | Fecal WBC |
|----------|----------|-------|----------|--------------|-----|-----------|
| Vibrio, non-epidemic | Seafood | ± | ± | ± | ± | ± |
| Vibrio cholera, epidemic | Epidemics in poor sanitary conditions. Stool mucus. | − | − | − | + | − |
| Yersinia | Community acquired, food-borne. Can resemble appendicitis. | ++ | ++ | + | + | + |
| E. histolytica | Tropical | + | + | ++ | ± | ± |
| Cryptospo-ridium | Waterborne outbreaks, travel, immune compromise; symptoms > 10 d | ± | ± | − | + | − |
| Cyclospora | Travel, food-borne; profound fatigue | ± | ± | − | + | − |
| Giardia | Water-borne, day care, IgA deficiency; symptoms >10 d | − | ++ | − | + | − |
| Norovirus | Winter outbreaks; nursing homes, cruise ships, schools, shellfish | ± | ++ | − | ++ | − |

++ *Common*  + *Occurs*  ± *Variable*  — *Atypical or not characteristic*

## Non-infectious differential diagnosis
• Medications • Tube feeding • Inflammatory bowel disease • Ischemic colitis • Factitious • Secretory: villous adenoma, gastrinoma, VIPoma

## Treatment
• The most important part of treating severe diarrhea is aggressive rehydration and appropriate electrolyte replacement

| WHO formula for oral rehydration solution (per L of water) | 3.5 g sodium chloride | 1.5 g potassium chloride |
|---|---|---|
| | 2.9 g trisodium citrate OR 2.5 g sodium bicarb | 20 g glucose OR 40 g sucrose |

• Anti-motility agents (loperamide, bismuth subsalicylate) OK to use in typical traveler's or watery diarrhea, but avoid if bloody or inflammatory diarrhea (may prolong fever, or predispose to toxic megacolon or hemolytic-uremic syndrome)
• Consider empiric fluoroquinolone if moderate-severe traveler's diarrhea or febrile community acquired diarrhea. Add erythromycin or azithromycin if suspected fluoroquinolone-resistant Campylobacter

infection (*e.g.* travel to southeast Asia), severely ill or immunocompromised. Avoid antibiotics if bloody stools without fever or other suspicion for shiga-toxin *E. coli* (may predispose to hemolytic-uremic syndrome)

# *Clostrodium Difficile Colitis*[9]

**Tests**
• Only test if diarrhea. • PCR superior to toxin EIA test. • Do not test to show cure.
• Seek routinely in inflammatory bowel disease admitted for flare, diarrheal illness peripartum or immunosuppressed

**Severe or complicated disease**
<u>Severe</u> = serum albumin < 3 g/dL plus either WBC > 15 k or abdominal tenderness
<u>Complicated</u>=Severe plus any of: ICU, hypotension, T ≥ 38.5°C, ileus or distention, altered sensorium, WBC > 35 k or < 2 k; Serum lactate > 2.2 mmol/L, any end organ failure (ventilator, dialysis, etc).

**Management**
• Empiric treatment if high clinical suspicion.
• Discontinue inciting antimicrobial if possible.
• Metronidazole if mild-moderate. • Oral vancomycin (125 mg qid x 10 d) if severe or metron. intolerant or treatment failure. • If colon inaccessible to oral (Hartmann pouch, ileostomy, colon diversion) use vancomycin by enema. • Avoid anti-peristaltic agents. • Consider avoiding PPIs

[9] Cohen SH, *et al.* Clinical practice guidelines for Clostridium difficile infection in adults. *Infect Control Hosp Epidemiol 2010; 31*: 431-455; Surawicz CM, *et al.* Guidelines for diagnosis, treatment, and prevention of Clostridium difficile infections. *Am J Gastroenterol 2013; 108*: 478-498; Leffler DA, et al. Clostridium difficile infection. *N Engl J Med 2015; 372*: 1539-1548.

- If <u>severe and complicated</u>: vancomycin 500 mg po q 6 h + metronidazole 500 mg IV q 8 h + rectal vancomycin (500mg in 500mL enema) q 6 h. • Obtain CT (for thickening, ascites, megacolon, ileus, or perforation)

**Early surgical consideration for subtotal colectomy recommended:**

- Hypotension requiring vasopressors; • Sepsis; • Altered sensorium; • WBC > 50 k; • Lactate > 5 mmol/L; • Complicated C diff and failiure to improve after 5 d therapy

**Recurrence (20% after first episode, 40-60% after second)**

- First recurrence: initial treatment regimen, guided by severity.
- Subsequent recurrences: vancomycin or fidaxomicin
- Caution: cumulative metronidazole neurotoxicity; do not use beyond 1st recurrence
- Consider <u>fecal microbiota transplant</u>[10] after 3 recurrences
- Prolonged taper: vancomycin 125 qid x 1 wk, bid x 1 wk, qd x 1 wk, q 2-3 d x 2-8 wk
- Fidaxomicin reduces recurrence (except common BI/NAP1/027 strain) at higher cost
- Role of tigecycline, rifaximin is unclear

**Other treatments**

- Colon-preserving surgery (diverting ileostomy and colonic lavage) is a promising colectomy alternative
- Probiotics are not recommended and may promote bloodstream infection
- IVIG is ineffective as monotherapy but may help in hypogammaglobulinemia
- Resins (cholestyramine, colestipol, etc) bind vancomycin and are likely ineffectiveare contraindicated
- Antitoxins and vaccines not currently available

---

[10] van Nood E, *et al.* Duodenal infusion of donor feces for recurrent Clostridium difficile. *N Engl J Med* 2013; 368: 407-415.

# Viral Hepatitis Serologies

| Scenario | ALT | HAV IgM | HAV IgG | HBs Ag | HBc IgM | HBc IgG | HBe Ag | HBeAb | HBsAb | HBV DNA | HCV Ab | HCV RNA |
|---|---|---|---|---|---|---|---|---|---|---|---|---|
| Acute HAV infection | ↑↑ | + | - | | | | | | | | | |
| Prior HAV infection or vaccination | Nml | - | + | | | | | | | | | |
| Acute HBV | ↑↑ | | | + | + | - | - | - | - | + | | |
| Acute HBV in "window period" | ↑↑ | | | - | + | - | - | - | - | +± | | |
| Chronic HBV, active replication | ↑ | | | + | - | + | + | - | - | + | | |
| Chronic HBV, "pre-core" mutant | ↑ | | | + | - | + | - | +± | - | + | | |
| Chronic HBV, minimally replicative (carrier) | Nml | | | + | - | + | - | + | - | - | | |
| Prior HBV infection | Nml | | | - | - | + | - | ± | + | - | | |
| Prior HBV vaccination | Nml | | | - | - | - | - | - | + | - | | |
| Acute HCV | ↑↑ | | | | | | | | | | - | + |
| Chronic HCV | Nml/↑ | | | | | | | | | | + | + |
| False positive HCV or prior infection with eradication | Nml | | | | | | | | | | + | - |

**Notes:** Ab = antibody  Ag = antigen  ALT = alanine aminotransferase  DNA = viral DNA
HAV = hepatitis A virus  HBe = hepatitis B "e"  HBs = hepatitis B surface  HBV = hepatitis B virus
HBc = hepatitis B core

# *Serum-Ascites Albumin Gradient*[11]

- Serum-ascites albumin gradient (SAAG) = serum albumin − ascitic fluid albumin
- SAAG ≥ 1.1 mg/dl predicts presence of **portal hypertension**
- 97% accuracy in classifying etiology (superior to "exudate-transudate" concept)

| SAAG ≥1.1 mg/dl (Portal hypertension present) | SAAG < 1.1 mg/dl (Portal hypertension absent) |
|---|---|
| • Cirrhosis (± co-existent infection or cancer); • Cardiac ascites (CHF, tricuspid regurgitation, constrictive pericarditis); • Massive liver metastases; • Portal vein thrombosis; • Budd-Chiari syndrome; • Fulminant hepatic failure; • Hepatocellular carcinoma; • Acute hepatitis (viral or alcoholic) superimposed on cirrhosis | • Peritoneal carcinomatosis • Peritonitis without cirrhosis (bacterial, TB) • Nephrotic syndrome • Pancreatic or biliary ascites • Malignant chylous ascites • Bowel infarction or obstruction • Hypothyroidism |

# *Spontaneous Bacterial Peritonitis*[12]

## Findings:

- Classic spontaneous bacterial peritonitis: ascitic fluid ≥ 250 PMN/mm$^3$ and single organism on Gram stain/culture, seen in 2/3 of infected ascites;
- Culture-negative neutrocytic ascites: ascites ≥ 250 PMNs, no organism on Gram stain/culture. Consider SBP, tuberculosis, peritoneal carcinomatosis, pancreatitis;
- Monomicrobial non-neutrocytic ascites: ascites ≤ 250 PMNs, single organism on Gram stain/culture. Treat as SBP if febrile or symptomatic, observe if asymptomatic.

---

[11] Runyon BA, *et al.* The serum-ascites albumin gradient is superior to the exudate-transudate concept in the differential diagnosis of ascites. *Ann Intern Med* 1992; 117: 215-220.

[12] EASL. Clinical practice guidelines on the management of ascites, spontaneous bacterial peritonitis, and hepatorenal syndrome in cirrhosis. *J Hepatol* 2010; 53: 397-417; Runyon BA, *et al.* Management of adult patients with ascites due to cirrhosis. *Hepatology* 2009; 49: 2087-2107.

- Secondary bacterial peritonitis: ascites ≥ 250 PMNs, polymicrobial Gram stain/culture, typically pneumoperitoneum, fluid has two of [protein > 1 g/dL, glucose < 50 mg/dL, LDH > serum upper limit]. Attributed to disrupted viscus, *i.e.* appendicitis, diverticulitis;
- Polymicrobial bacterascites: ascites ≤ 250 PMNs, polymicrobial gram stain/culture: Usually complication of puncture, can be observed if asymptomatic.
- Pathogens: *E. coli; Klebsiella spp; Enterobacter spp;* Enterobacteriacea; *S. pneumoniae;* Streptococci & enterococci; Polymicrobial; Anaerobes

## Evaluation

- Clinical signs may be subtle; • Consider SBP in all cirrhosis-related hospital admissions;
- Consider when a patient with cirrhosis develops hepatic encephalopathy, renal dysfunction, altered GI motility, nausea/vomiting, diarrhea;
- Treat empirically in GI hemorrhage.
- Except variceal hemorrhage, treatment without ascites culture is inappropriate.
- Blood culture bottle increases sensitivity of ascites culture.
- Alcoholic hepatitis (fever, peripheral leukocytosis): empiric antimicrobials can be discontinued after 48° if culture-negative
- Albumin infusion reduces mortality

# *Surgical Risk in Liver Disease*[13]

| Modified Child-Turcotte-Pugh[14] | 1 point | 2 points | 3 points |
|---|---|---|---|
| Encephalopathy# | None | Grade I-II | Grade III-IV |
| Ascites | Absent | Slight | Moderate |
| Bilirubin (mg/dL) - non-cholestatic | < 2 | 2-3 | >3 |
| cholestatic‡ | < 4 | 4-10 | > 10 |
| Albumin (g/dL) | > 3.5 | 2.8-3.5 | < 2.8 |

[13] Hanje AJ, *et al.* Preoperative evaluation of patients with liver disease. *Nat Clin Pract Gastroenterol Hepatol* 2007; 4: 266-276; O'Leary JG, *et al.* Surgery in the patient with liver disease. *Clin Liver Dis* 2009; 13: 211-231.

[14] Pugh RN, *et al.* Transection of the oesophagus for bleeding oesophageal varices. *Br J Surg* 1973; 60: 646-649.

| Modified Child-Turcotte-Pugh[14] | 1 point | 2 points | 3 points |
|---|---|---|---|
| INR | < 1.7 | 1.7-2.3 | > 2.3 |

[#] *Encephalopathy: (I) mild confusion or slowing; no asterixis (II) drowsy, asterixis present (III) marked confusion, somnolence; a sterixis present (IV) unresponsive or responsive only to painful stimuli; no asterixis;* [‡] *e.g. primary biliary cirrhosis*

## Implications of Child-Turcotte-Pugh Score[15]

| Class | CTP Score | Peri-op mortality | Description | Survival(%) | |
|---|---|---|---|---|---|
| | | | | 1 yr | 2 yr |
| A | 5-6 | 10% | Near-normal surgery response & regenerative ability. Risk ↑ if portal hypertension. | 100 | 85 |
| B | 7-9 | 31% | Moderate liver impairment. Tolerates non-cardiac surgery with pre-op preparation. Limited regeneration; sizable resections contraindicated. | 80 | 60 |
| C | ≥ 10 | 76% | Poor response to all operations regardless of preparation. Liver resection contraindicated regardless of size. | 45 | 35 |

## MELD[16] Score:

$MELD = 11.2 \times \ln[INR] + 9.57 \times 0 \ln[creatinine^{‡} \text{ mg/dL}] + 3.78 \times \ln[bilirubin \text{ mg/dL}] + 6.43$

[‡]Creatinine maximum = 4, applies for all renal replacement therapy

MELD score < 10, 10-14 and > 14 corresponds to Child-Turcotte-Pugh A,B,C

## MELD-Na Score[17] (Same range as MELD, better predicts mortality)

$MELD\text{-}Na = MELD - [Na \text{ mmol/L}] - [0.025 \times MELD \times (140\text{-}Na)] + 140$

[15] Garrison RN, *et al.* Clarification of risk factors for abdominal operations in patients with hepatic cirrhosis. *Ann Surg* 1984; 199: 648-655.

[16] Malinchoc M, *et al.* A model to predict poor survival in patients undergoing transjugular intrahepatic portosystemic shunts. *Hepatology* 2000; 31: 864-871.

[17] Kim WR, *et al.* Hyponatremia and mortality among patients on the liver-transplant waiting list. *N Engl J Med* 2008; 359: 1018-1026.

## Mortality after major surgery by MELD score[18]

7 d mortality best predicted by Am Society Anesthesia
class; subsequent mortality by MELD

| Score | 7d | 30d | 90d | 1yr | 5yr | 10yr |
|-------|-----|-----|-----|------|------|------|
| 0-7 | 2% | 6% | 10% | 20% | 51% | 73% |
| 8-11 | 3% | 10% | 18% | 29% | 59% | 78% |
| 12-15 | 8% | 25% | 32% | 45% | 70% | 87% |
| 16-20 | 15% | 44% | 56% | 71% | 94% | 94% |
| 21-25 | 23% | 54% | 67% | 85% | 92% | 100% |
| ≥26 | 30% | 90% | 90% | 100% | 100% | 100% |

## Contraindications to elective surgery

•Acute alcoholic or viral hepatitis; • Fulminant hepatic
failure; • Severe chronic hepatitis; • Child-Pugh class
C; • PT prolongation > 3 s despite vitamin K; • Platelet
count < 50 K; • Co-existing renal failure, cardiomyopathy or hypoxemia

## Optimizing medical therapy

•Adequate nutrition. Protein restriction has no prov-
en value, may be harmful.

• Correct coagulopathy: • PT may be less useful than
viscoelastography; • Correct PT (within 3s of normal)
with vitamin K, plasma, plasma concentrates;
• Maintain platelet count > 50 K by transfusion;
• Treat ↑ bleeding time with desmopressin (see page
274), possibly rFactor VII.

• Ascites & renal management: Risks perioperative
respiratory & wound complications. • Assure no
bacterial peritonitis by paracentesis if necessary;
• Restrict sodium; add K-sparing ± loop diuretic; avoid
unnecessary IV fluid • Large-volume paracentesis if
necessary pre- or intra-operatively, give albumin if
> 5L; • Role of TIPS controversial; • Avoid nephrotoxic
drugs (NSAIDs, aminoglycosides, radiocontrast);
• Correct hypokalemia and metabolic alkalosis • Keep
intraoperative central vein pressure low

• Encephalopathy: • Lactulose target 3-4 stool/d or
rifaximin 200-400 mg po q 8 h; • Avoid opiates,
benzodiazepines, constipation, infection, GI bleed

• Other: Alcohol abstinence; • Avoid acetaminophen

---

[18] Teh SH, et al. Risk factors for mortality after surgery in patients
with cirrhosis. Gastroenterology 2007; 132: 1261-1269.

# Hepatorenal syndrome[19]

**Diagnostic features: "functional" renal failure, and a diagnosis of exclusion**
- Cirrhosis with ascites; • Serum creatinine > 1.5 mg/dL; • No creatinine improvement despite ≥2d diuretic withdrawal and albumin (1 g/kg/d up to 100 g/d) volume expansion; • No shock; • No evident exposure to nephrotoxic drugs; • No evident parenchymal kidney disease (proteinuria > 500 mg/d; microhematuria > 50 rbc/hpf; abnormal ultrasound or biopsy) ; • No bacterial peritonitis

**Patterns:** • <u>"Type 1"</u> **Progressive oliguria with creatinine doubling ≤ 2 wks, usually triggered by event such as bacterial peritonitis. Ominous prognosis.**
- <u>"Type 2"</u> Slow/sustained azotemia, usually in refractory ascites. Less ominous.

**Treatment options for "Type 1" hepatorenal syndrome**
- <u>Diuretic withdrawal</u> and volume expansion with <u>albumin</u> and PRBC transfusion; • Stop nephrotoxic drugs. • Stop venodilators: nitrates, ACEI/ARB; • Search for and correct adrenal insufficiency
- Renal replacement therapy: standard indications (volume overload, intractable electrolyte or acid-base disorders).
- <u>Vasoconstrictors</u> to reverse splanchnic vasodilation. Dopamine is ineffective.
  - Midodrine 5-15 mg po tid plus octreotide 100-200 µg SQ tid to increase mean arterial pressure by 15 mmHg[20]. IV terlipressin used in Europe. **OR**

[19] Gines P, *et al.* Renal failure in cirrhosis. *N Engl J Med 2009; 361:* 1279-1290; Runyon BA, *et al.* Management of adult patients with ascites due to cirrhosis. *Hepatology 2009; 49:* 2087-2107; EASL. Clinical practice guidelines on the management of ascites, spontaneous bacterial peritonitis, and hepatorenal syndrome in cirrhosis. *J Hepatol 2010; 53:* 397-417; Nadim MK, *et al.* Management of the Critically Ill Patient with Cirrhosis: *A Multidisciplinary Perspective. J Hepatol 2015.*

[20] Esrailian E, *et al.* Octreotide/Midodrine therapy significantly improves renal function and 30-day survival in patients with type 1 hepatorenal syndrome. *Dig Dis Sci 2007; 52:* 742-748.

- Norepinephrine 0.1 µg/kg/min IV to ↑ MAP by 10 mmHg, titrate q 4 h to max 0.7 µg/kg/min; Albumin to maintain CVP > 10-15 mmHg. Treat until azotemia reversed or 2 wk.
- Liver transplantation; • Culture blood, urine, ascites even without evident infection

# *Acute Pancreatitis*[21]

## Diagnosis & Etiology
- **Amylase and lipase:** Value > 3x normal supports diagnosis; • Lipase more sensitive & specific; • Values or persistence do not predict severity, prognosis, or response;
- **Triglycerides:** Measure if not EtOH or gallstones; presume causal if > 1000mg/dL
- **ALT:** > 3x normal suggests gallstone pancreatitis; • Tumor: Seek if age > 40
- **Abdominal ultrasound:** Universally indicated: assess gallstones or bile duct dilatation
- **Contrast CT or MRI:** Assess local complications when failure to improve 48-72 hr

## Prognosis Difficult to define < 48hrs of onset
- Initial clinical findings associated with severe course
  - **Patient:** age > 55; obesity BMI > 30 kg/m$^2$; altered mental status; comorbid disease
  - **Systemic inflammatory response syndrome:** Two or more of • HR > 90 bpm; • T < 36° or 38°C; •WBC <4000 or > 12000/mm$^3$; •RR > 20/min or pCO$_2$ < 32 mmHg
  - **Labs:** BUN > 20 mg/dl or climbing; Hct > 44% or climbing; Creatinine elevated
  - **Radiology:** Pleural effusion; Pulm infiltrates; Multiple/extensive extrapancreatic collections
- **CT Severity Index**[22]: Sum of Size: Enlarged pancreas (1 point), pancreatic or peripancreatic inflammation

---

[21] Tenner S, *et al.* guideline: management of acute pancreatitis. *Am J Gastroenterol* 2013; 108: 1400-1415; 1416; Banks PA, *et al.* Classification of acute pancreatitis--2012. *Gut* 2013; 62: 102-111.

(2 pts), single peripancreatic fluid collection (3 pts), > 1 peripancreatic collections or air (4 pts); and Necrosis: < 30% (2 points), 30-50% (4 pts), > 50% (6 pts). Interpretation: Index > 7 predicts high morbidity/mortality

- Modified Marshall Score of organ failure

| Organ | 0 | 1 | 2 | 3 | 5 |
|---|---|---|---|---|---|
| $P_aO_2/FiO_2$ | > 400 | 301-400 | 201-300 | 101-200 | ≤ 101 |
| Creatinine | < 1.4 | 1.4-1.8 | 1.9-3.6 | 3.6-4.9 | > 4.9 |
| Systolic BP | > 90 | < 90 fluid responsive | < 90, not fluid responsive | < 90, pH < 7.3 | < 90, pH < 7.2 |

Nasal cannula: $FiO_2$ conversion: RA = 21%; 2L = 25%; 4L = 30%; 6-8L = 40%; 9-10L = 50%
Organ failure = score ≥ 2 in any system

## Treatment

- **Aggressive fluid** (250-500 mL/hr LR especially 1st 12-24 hr) aiming to reduce BUN
- **Supportive care:** ICU/stepdown; Fluids, pain control, nutrition support if NPO >1 week
- **Nutrition:** Enteral preferred over parenteral to avoid gut mucosal atrophy & bacterial flux. Oral, NG and nasojejunal are equivalent, continuous probably better than cyclic or bolus. Oral low-fat solids if pain resolved and no N/V.
- **Urgent ERCP papillotomy/stenting:** For cholangitis (within 24 hr), or jaundice + dilated common bile duct; otherwise MRI CP or endoscopic ultrasound preferred if not improving.
- **Prophylactic antibiotics and antifungals:** Not indicated.
- **Infected necrosis:** Suspect if deterioration or failure to improve after 7-10 d. Consider FNA for culture, or empiric antibiotics (agents known to penetrate pancreatic necrosis). Surgical debridement if unstable.

---

[22] Balthazar EJ, *et al.* Acute pancreatitis: value of CT in establishing prognosis. *Radiology* 1990; 174: 331-336.

- **Percutaneous aspiration:** Indicated to exclude superinfection in necrotizing pancreatitis with sepsis syndrome or if patient fails to improve clinically.
- **Surgical or Percutaneous intervention:** • Gallstones (cholecystectomy should be performed after resolution of episode; increased mortality if performed within first 48 hr) • Abscess or super-infected necrosis • Sterile necrosis with prolonged organ failure (*i.e.* 4-6 wk) • Symptomatic pseudocyst that fails conservative treatment and is not amenable to endoscopic or percutaneous drainage

# Nutrition: Enteral & Parenteral[23]

## Enteral Nutrition Prescription
- Enteral feeding preserves intestinal integrity, immune function ("trophic effect") and is more effective and safer than parenteral nutrition
- Begin enteral feeding ≤ 24-48 hr of admission, advance to goal next 48-72 hr
- Withhold enteral feeding during hemodynamic instability, catecholamines, etc

(1) Non-ICU: Estimate Basal Energy Expenditure (<u>Harris-Benedict</u> Equation)
- Male:
  BEE(kcal/d)= 66.5 + (13.8 x weight-kg) + (5.00 x height-cm) − (6.78 x age-years)
- Female:
  BEE(kcal/d)= 655. + (9.56 x weight-kg) + (1.85 x height-cm) − (4.68 x age-years)

(2) Determine <u>body weight</u> for dosing (*see* anthropometric equations *on p 4*):

[23] Kreymann KG, *et al.* ESPEN Guidelines on Enteral Nutrition. *Clin Nutr* 2006; 25: 210-223; McClave SA, *et al.* Guidelines for the provision and assessment of nutrition support therapy in the adult critically ill patient: SCCM and ASPEN. *JPEN J Parenter Enteral Nutr* 2009; 33: 277-316; O'Keefe SJ. A guide to enteral access procedures and enteral nutrition. *Nat Rev Gastroenterol Hepatol* 2009; 6: 207-215; Singer P, *et al.* ESPEN Guidelines on Parenteral Nutrition. *Clin Nutr* 2009; 28: 387-400; Casaer MP, *et al.* Nutrition in the acute phase of critical illness. *N Engl J Med* 2014; 370: 1227-1236.

- For BMI < 18.5, use actual weight to avoid over-feeding/refeeding syndrome
- For BMI 18.5-25 (normal) or 25-30 (overweight), use actual body weight (ABW)
- For BMI > 30, use IBW+ ¼ x (ABW-IWB), or use IBW x 1.1

**(3) Estimate <u>caloric</u> needs with stress correction**
- Simple: 20-25 kcal/kg/d
- <u>Permissive underfeeding in obese</u> (BMI > 30): 11-14 kcal/kg/d ABW or 22-25 kcal/kg IBW
- <u>Stress</u> addition: 25% (mild peritonitis, moderate trauma); 50% (severe infection, severe trauma, multisystem organ failure); 100% (burn >40%)
- Best: <u>indirect calorimetry</u> (measures $O_2$ consumption)
- Fluid: typically 30 ml/kg/d

**(4) Begin feedings**, typically start 20-30 mL/hr, increase every ~ 8hrs toward goal.
- Achieve > 50-65% of goal calories during 1st week; Failure to achieve 100% goal after 7-10 d may require supplemental parenteral nutrition.
- <u>Nitrogen balance</u> = Protein intake (grams) / 6.25 - (urine urea nitrogen + 4)
  Rationale: 6.25 reflects protein composition ≈ 16% nitrogen; 4 reflects obligatory nitrogen loss in skin and stool
  Goal of nitrogen balance = 0; Moderate stress 0-5; Severe stress > 5

**Formulations endorsed/described by society guidelines**
- Standard enteral formulations: ~ 1 kcal/mL, iso-osmolal (280-300 mOsm/kg).
- High caloric density formulations ~ 2 kcal/mL, high osmolality
- Hypertonic feeding may cause diarrhea and delayed gastric emptying
- "HN" = high nitrogen, only ~ 20% additional pro-tein "<u>Immune-modulating</u>" (*i.e.* supplemental argi-nine, glutamine, Ω3 fatty acids, anti-oxidant vita-

mins *etc.*) largely unsupported for high risk patients (mechanical ventilation, major elective surgery, trauma, burns, head & neck cancer). Avoid in severe sepsis whether surgical or medical. Other ICU patients should receive standard enteral formulations

- "<u>Anti-inflammatory</u>" lipids in ARDS & severe acute lung injury (*i.e.* Ω3 fatty acids, borage oil, anti-oxidant vitamins): largely unsupported
- "<u>Anti-oxidant</u>" vitamins & trace minerals including selenium for all EN via tube: largely disproven.
- "<u>Pro-biotic</u>" supplements may reduce infection in transplantation, major abdominal surgery, severe trauma. Avoid in pancreatitis. Caution in immunocompromised.
- <u>Fiber</u>: Insoluble fiber for all, soluble fiber for diarrhea. Avoid fiber in high risk for bowel ischemia or severe dysmotility.
- If <u>diarrhea</u>, consider formulations including soluble fiber or small peptides.

## Diarrhea during enteral tube feedings

- Hyperosmolar medications such as sorbitol, added to make liquid drugs palatable; • Antimicrobials; • *C. difficile* enterocolitis;
- Distinguish infective from osmotic diarrhea; Examine fecal volume and leukocytes, assay for *C. difficile*; Consider medications
- Do not automatically suspend enteral feeding, consider adding soluble fiber

**Measures to reduce aspiration risk**
- Elevate HOB 30-40°; • Continuous feeds may be preferred over bolus feeds; • Check gastric residual volumes q 4 h; • When residual volumes excessive (> 400-500 mL) reduce infusion to 20-25 mL/hr until residual volumes are acceptable; • Prokinetic agents when indicated (metoclopramide, erythromycin; caution about QT prolongation) or opiate antagonists: enteral naloxone 8 mg q 8 h[24], methylnaltrexone SQ (*see page 317*), alvimopan off-label. • Change to small bowel feeding if necessary. • Use chlorhexidine mouthwash bid; • Aspiration markers: Blue food coloring is toxic and contraindicated[25]; glucose oxidase test strips are insensitive

**Guide to Parenteral Nutrition (PN)**
- Nutrition may be withheld if preadmission nutrition status acceptable and enteral feeding not feasible for first 7 d. Otherwise parenteral nutrition reasonable upon admission and adequate resuscitation.
- For major upper GI surgery: If malnourished, 5-7 d preoperative PN continued into postop period is reasonable. PN should not be initiated in immediate post-op but rather delayed 5-7 d. PN should not be initiated if expected duration only 5-7 d.
- Consider initial mild "permissive underfeeding" to 80% energy requirements, which may reduce propensity to hyperglycemia, infection, prolonged ventilation
- Avoid soy-based lipids during first ICU week. Soy may contribute to infection and prolonged mechanical ventilation, but lipid may reduce hyperglycemia
- Consider intensity of glycemic control. Touted benefits of intensive glycemic control may indeed apply to patients receiving parenteral nutrition.

---

[24] Meissner W, *et al.* Enteral naloxone reduces gastric tube reflux and frequency of pneumonia in critical care patients during opioid analgesia. *Crit Care Med* 2003; 31: 776-780.
[25] Maloney JP, *et al.* Systemic absorption of food dye in patients with sepsis. *N Engl J Med* 2000; 343: 1047-1048.

- **Glutamine**: Consider in ICU, if not already provided in "immune modulating"
- Revisit <u>suitability for EN</u> often. Continue PN until ≥ 60% target energy via EN.
- Monitor triglycerides and liver enzymes during PN
- Consider increased risk of fungemia in PN

**Special populations**

<u>Pulmonary failure (ARDS)</u>

- Formulations to alter respiratory quotient (high lipid, low carbohydrate to reduce $CO_2$ production) are <u>not</u> indicated routinely; • Consider fluid-restricted, calorie-dense formulation; • Monitor phosphate

<u>Renal failure</u>

- Use standard enteral formulations and standard protein and calorie goals (no protein restriction); • Tailor electrolyte formulation as needed; • <u>Hemodialysis</u>: provide increased protein up to 2.5 mg/kg/d

<u>Hepatic failure</u>

- EN is preferred; • Protein restriction is undesirable; • Confine branched-chain amino acid formulations to refractory hepatic encephalopathy despite antimicrobials/lactulose; • Traditional nutrition assessment tests are limited in liver failure

<u>Acute pancreatitis</u>

- Enteral feeding usually improves outcome in pancreatitis
- Nasogastric tube & EN should be provided in severe acute pancreatitis, but nutrition support not necessary in mild-moderate pancreatitis unless unable to eat after 7 d; • Gastric or jejunal tube routes are acceptable;
- Measures to promote EN in pancreatitis: initiate EN early to prevent ileus; • Move feeding tube distally in GI tract; • Alter EN formula (change protein to small peptides; change lipid to medium-chain triglycerides or nearly fat-free elemental formulation; change from bolus to continuous feeding).

- If EN not feasible, PN should be initiated after 5$^{th}$ day of hospital admission

**Pearls**

- Bowel sounds indicate air introduced during eating, not GI motility. Absent bowel sounds or absent flatus do not preclude feeding.
- Enteral feeding should not necessarily be suspended for diarrhea, reflux, ileus
- Gastric residual volume up to 400-500mL is acceptable for enteral feeding; aspiration usually derives from pharyngeal contents
- Small bowel (duodenal, jejunal) feeding is indicated for persistently excessive gastric residual volume. Consider concurrent nasogastric decompression during small bowel feeding because of slowed gastric emptying.
- Jejunal feeding (*i.e.* to bypass pancreas) usually requires elemental/predigested feeding
- Traditional nutrition tests (prealbumin, anthropometry) not valid in ICU; instead use preadmission weight loss, nutrition, disease severity, GI function, comorbidity
- Account for calories in <u>propofol</u> (1.1 kcal/mL) and <u>clevidipine</u> (2.2 kcal/mL) infusion
- Consider risk of refeeding syndrome (marked hypophosphatemia and other electrolytes), and of thiamine deficiency, in severely malnourished.

# Hematology

## Anemia Differential Diagnosis

- **Kinetic classification:** • Blood loss; • Decreased RBC production (*e.g.* aplastic anemia); • Increased RBC destruction (*e.g.* megaloblastic anemia)
- **Morphologic classification:** • RBC size and shape;
  - • Reticulocyte response to anemia
- Reticulocyte count (normal 50 k/μL).
- Reticulocyte Production Index: RPI = % retics x (Hct ÷ 45) ÷ retic maturation time (d); [maturation time: Hct 45%: 1 d; 35%: 1.5 d; 25%: 2 d; 15%:2.5 d].
- Absolute reticulocyte count > 100 k/μL or RPI > 2 suggests active hemolysis and adequate marrow response.

| High reticulocyte count | Low reticulocyte count | | |
|---|---|---|---|
| | **MCV Low** | **MCV High** | **MCV intermediate** |
| Bleeding, Hemolysis | Fe-deficiency Other microcytic | Megaloblastic Other macrocytic | Chronic disease Underproduction |

## Hemolytic Anemia

**Immune Mediated: Direct Coombs Test Positive**
*Autoimmune hemolytic anemia*

- **Warm antibody autoimmune hemolytic anemia:** (usually IgG, rarely IgM): idiopathic (50-70%); lymphoproliferative disorder; SLE or other rheumatic; infection (HIV, EBV); congenital immunodeficiency; solid tumor (rare)
- **Cold antibody autoimmune hemolytic anemia**
- <u>Cold agglutinin</u> disease (usually IgM): • Acute: mycoplasma infection, EBV; • Chronic: idiopathic; primary lymphoproliferative

- <u>Paroxysmal cold hemoglobinuria</u> (polyclonal IgG: "Donath-Landsteiner"): • Acute: viral (rare in adults); • Chronic: idiopathic; CLL; $2°/3°$ syphilis

*Allo-immune hemolytic anemia*
- Hemolytic transfusion reaction; • Hemolytic anemia of the newborn: Rh; ABO;

**Drug-induced** immune hemolytic (autoantibody, hapten, immune complex)
- <u>Antibiotics</u>: Penicillins, cephalosporins, sulfa drugs, rifampin; • <u>Analgesics</u>: NSAIDs; Phenazopyridine • <u>Psychiatric</u> agents: Tricyclic antidepressants, phenothiazines; • <u>Cardiovascular</u> agents: $\alpha$-methyldopa, procainamide, thiazide diuretics; • <u>Endocrine</u> agents: Sulfonylureas; • <u>Methotrexate</u>, 5-FU

**Not Immune Mediated: Direct Coombs Test Negative**
- Trauma: • <u>Mechanical</u>: Paravalvular leak
- <u>Microangiopathic</u> hemolytic anemia: Thrombotic thrombocytopenia purpura (TTP); Hemolytic-Uremic Syndrome (HUS); Disseminated Intravascular Coagulation (DIC); Hemolysis Elevated Liver enzymes Low Platelets (HELLP, eclampsia-related); • Infection/Toxin: • <u>Infection</u>: malaria, babesiosis, bartonella, clostridia, sepsis; • Snake & spider <u>venom</u>; • Copper toxicity / Wilson's disease; • <u>Osmotic</u>: hypotonic infusions, freshwater drowning
- **Acquired membrane defects:** Paroxysmal nocturnal hemoglobinuria (PNH)
- **Congenital:** • <u>Hemoglobinopathy</u>: Sickle-cell disease; Thalassemia
- RBC membrane <u>fragility</u>: Hereditary spherocytosis or elliptocytosis
- RBC <u>metabolic defects</u>: G6PD deficiency; Pyruvate kinase deficiency

**Diagnosis: High reticulocyte count or index**
- **Smear:** Spherocytes (immune-mediated hemolysis or hereditary); reticulocytes (active marrow); schistocytes (microangiopathic hemolysis); RBCs with inclusions (*e.g.* malaria); "bite" cells (G6PD deficiency)

- **Haptoglobin:** Low level reflects intravascular hemolysis; elevated in inflammation (acute phase reactant); absent (ahaptoglobinemia) in 4-10% of African-Americans
- Serum or urine free hemoglobin, urine hemosiderin: High specificity
- **Coombs** (direct anti-globulin test): Confirms antibody-mediated process; pattern may suggest specific antigen
- **Cold agglutinins or paroxysmal cold hemoglobinuria-specific Ab:** If symptoms related to cold exposure

**Treatment of immune-mediated hemolytic anemia:** Glucocorticoids; Splenectomy; Immunosuppressives; If refractory[1], reports suggest trials of IVIG, danazol, mycophenolate, monoclonal antilymphocyte Ab.

### Glucose-6-phosphate-dehydrogenase (G6PD) deficiency[2]

- X-linked disorder (heterozygous females may have ≥ 50% affected RBCs)
- Minority have chronic hemolysis; majority suffer acute hemolysis triggered by infections (pneumonia, UTI, viral hepatitis, salmonella), metabolic stress (*e.g.* DKA), or drugs. Fava beans (favism) trigger attacks primarily in boys < 5 yr of Mediterranean descent.
- G6PD deficiency tests may be false-negative when most severely deficient RBCs have been lysed. Re-test 2-3 mo after acute episode.

---

[1] Hoffman PC. Immune hemolytic anemia. *Hematology Am Soc Hematol Educ Program 2009; 2009:* 80-86.

[2] Cappellini MD, *et al.* Glucose-6-phosphate dehydrogenase deficiency. *Lancet 2008;* 371: 64-74; Beutler E. Glucose-6-phosphate dehydrogenase deficiency. *N Engl J Med 1991;* 324: 169-174. www.G6PD.org

| Drugs *Unsafe* in G6PD Deficiency | Drugs Generally *Safe* in G6PD Deficiency |
|---|---|
| • acetanilide • dapsone • methylene blue • nalidixic acid• naphthalene (mothballs) • nitrofurantoin • phenylhydrazine • primaquine • pyridium • rasburicase • sulfamethoxazole • sulfacetamide • sulfanilamide • sulfapyridine | • acetaminophen • ascorbic acid • ASA • chloramphenicol • chloroquine • colchicine • diphenhydramine • isoniazid • L-DOPA • phenytoin • probenecid • procainamide • pyrimethamine • quinidine • quinine • streptomycin • sulfisoxazole • trimethoprim • vitamin K |

# *Iron-Deficiency Anemia*[3]

**Stages:** (1) Storage depletion (↓ marrow stores & ferritin); (2) Abnormal erythropoiesis (microcytosis & hypochromia); (3) Anemia & thrombocytosis. Hepcidin hormone regulates iron absorption and phagocytic recycling of senescent RBCs.

**Etiology**

- **Occult or manifest GI loss**[4]: 40% upper GI source (ulcers, esophagitis, AVM, cancer), 3 % small intestine, 22% colon (cancer, AVM, large polyps); 34% with no identifiable source, and 5% with lesions in both upper and lower GI tract. Only ~ 50% with identifiable source have heme positive stools.
- **Physiologic loss:** Menstruation, pregnancy, lactation, marathon running
- **Non-GI loss:** Genitourinary bleeding; intravascular hemolysis (paroxysmal nocturnal hemoglobinuria, cardiac valves); lung (hemosiderosis, bronchiectasis); severe trauma; surgical blood loss; repeated phlebotomy; elective blood donation
- **Increased utilization:** EPO administration
- **Decreased intake:** Primary malabsorption (*e.g.* celiac disease, lead poisoning); s/p gastrectomy (↓ transit time); s/p duodenal/jejunal resection/bypass; high

---

[3] Lopez A, *et al.* Iron deficiency anaemia. *Lancet 2015*; Camaschella C. Iron-deficiency anemia. *N Engl J Med 2015*; 372: 1832-1843; DeLoughery TG. Microcytic anemia. *N Engl J Med 2014*; 371: 1324-1331.

[4] Goddard AF, *et al.* Guidelines for the management of iron deficiency anaemia. *Gut 2011*; 60: 1309-1316.

gastric pH (achlorhydria, acid blockade; exacerbated by iron deficiency itself)

**Evaluation[4]:** Women (age > 50, menopausal, or strong family history colorectal cancer) and all men should undergo <u>GI investigation for malignancy</u>. Fecal occult blood testing has no value in this investigation. All should be screened for <u>celiac disease</u>. Note dual pathology > 10%. Only gastric CA or celiac should deter lower GI investigation.

**Assays of iron stores**
- **Direct:** Bone marrow biopsy; finding absence of stainable iron
- **Indirect:** Serum markers of iron stores

| Condition | Fe (µg/dl) | TIBC (µg/dl) | Fe/TIBC (transferrin saturation) | Ferritin (ng/ml) | Soluble transferrin receptor | Hepcidin (Future) |
|---|---|---|---|---|---|---|
| Normal | 60-150 | 250-450 | 20-50% | 40-200 | 10-30 nM/L | N.A. |
| Fe Deficiency | ↓ | ↑ | < 15 % spec 65% sens 80% | < 30 spec 98% * sens 92% | ↑ | ↓ |
| Fe-Overload | ↑ | ↓ | > 50% women > 60% men (90% sens) | > 300 women > 400 men (sens not specific) | | ↓ |
| Anemia of Chronic Disease | Nml/↓ | Nml/↓ | Typically ↓ | ↑ | Nml | ↑ |

*Fe = iron; TIBC = total iron binding capacity; * Specificity reduced in inflammation/infection*

**Iron supplementation**
- Generic oral 100-200 mg elemental iron/d divided in 3 doses x 4 wk ~ 2-3 g/dL Hb; • Fe-sulfate has 2x the elemental iron per weight as Fe-gluconate or fumarate; • Avoid enteric coated products, which impede duodenal absorption; • Separate in time from antiacids, tea & multivitamins; best qHS & between meals; • Reticulocytosis begins at 5-7 d, max 10 d; • Involve patient in dose-duration decisionmaking.

- Failure to respond: wrong diagnosis, non-adherence, ongoing bleeding, bone marrow suppression, malabsorption; consider intravenous iron (*see page 308*).

### Other causes of microcytic anemia

- Anemia of chronic disease: May be difficult to exclude co-existing Fe-deficiency (consider bone marrow bx with iron stain if serum markers non-diagnostic)
- Sideroblastic anemia: Confirmed by bone marrow biopsy with iron stain. Causes include lead poisoning.
- Thalassemia: Hb electrophoresis diagnostic in β-thal but usually normal in α-thal. Review of previous CBCs should show consistently low MCV (often < 70 fL). Free erythrocyte protoporphyrin (FEP) should be normal (elevated in Fe deficiency) and RBC count should be normal-high (low in Fe deficiency).

## *Macrocytic Anemia*

### Megaloblastic: impaired DNA synthesis, cell cycle arrest

- **Drugs** that impair DNA synthesis: • <u>Folate antagonists</u> (methotrexate, azathioprine, trimethoprim, pyrimethamine, ethanol) & anticonvulsants (phenytoin, valproic acid); • <u>Biguanides</u> (metformin, cholestyramine); • <u>Nucleoside antineoplastics</u> (5-FU, hydroxyurea, capecitabine, cladribine, alkylating agents); • <u>Nucleoside reverse transcriptase inhibitors</u> (zidovudine, lamivudine, stavudine); • <u>c-kit inhibitors</u>: sunitinib & imatinib
- **Vitamin B12** (cobalamin) deficiency: • <u>Inadequate diet</u> (vegan); • Deficiency of gastric <u>intrinsic factor</u>: gastrectomy, pernicious anemia, inherited; • <u>Malabsorption</u>: ileitis, bowel resection, tapeworms, bacterial overgrowth, lowered intestinal pH (Zollinger-Ellison), pancreatic insufficiency, drugs (colchicine, metformin, INH, PPIs, H2-blockers, cycloserine, aminosalicylic acid, sulfasalazine, sustained release KCl, cholestyramine), alcohol

- **Folate deficiency :** • <u>Increased requirements</u>: pregnancy, hemolysis, myeloproliferative syndromes, sickle cell; • <u>Malabsorption</u>: celiac, extensive small bowel disease/resection/fistulae, drugs (estrogens, tetracyclins, penicillins, erythromycin); • <u>Alcohol</u>
- **Myelodysplasia** (*e.g.* 5q⁻ syndrome); • **Red cell aplasia**

**Non-Megaloblastic:** • <u>Reticulocytosis</u> (*e.g.*hemolysis); • <u>Ethanol</u>, distinguished from B12/folate by serum levels; • Advanced <u>liver disease</u>; • <u>Hypothyroidism</u>; • <u>Spurious</u>: warm or cold agglutinins, hyperglycemia, leukocytosis

**Diagnosis**[5]

- **MCV:** May be normal; < 110 fL: non-specific; 115-130 fL: 50% have B12/folate deficiency; > 130 fL: most have B12/folate deficiency or HIV ART or hydroxyurea
- **Blood smear:** Evidence of megaloblastic "arrest" with hypersegmented neutrophils (98% sensitive for megaloblastic) and macro-ovalocytes. Target cells suggest liver disease.
- **Serum B12:** Low (100-250 pg/ml) suggests but does not prove deficiency. Automated tests often spuriously normal from intrinsic factor antibody.
- **Serum folate:** Poor correlation with tissues levels; RBC folate better test but may be spuriously low in B12 deficiency
- **Methylmalonic acid:** Elevated in 98% of B12 deficiency; normal in none; homocysteine elevated in both folate & B12 deficiency. Both respond rapidly to B12 replacement.
- **Intrinsic factor or anti-parietal cell antibody:** Highly specific but sensitivity only 50-70%; recent B12 injection or radioisotopes may cause false (+). Consider endoscopy

---

[5] Carmel R, *et al.* Update on cobalamin, folate, and homocysteine. *Hematology Am Soc Hematol Educ Program 2003: 62-81;* Carmel R, *et al.* Failures of cobalamin assays in pernicious anemia. *N Engl J Med 2012; 367: 385-386;* Stabler SP. Vitamin B12 deficiency. *N Engl J Med 2013; 368: 149-160.*

- **Marrow:** Discordance of nuclear/cytoplasmic maturation, evident in most mature cells. Hypercellular, erythroid population in marrow. Intramedullary hemolysis with ineffective erythropoiesis. Giant band forms and metamyelocytes.
- **Schilling test** (limited availability of radiopharmaceuticals): **(1)** Supraphysiologic B12 IM to saturate B12 binding sites **(2)** Oral administration of dual-radiolabeled B12 (IF-bound and unbound with different isotopes) **(3)** Urinary measurement of radiolabeled B12 excretion. ***Normal:*** Both isotopes excreted in urine. ***Pernicious anemia:*** Only IF-bound B12 excreted in urine. ***Malabsorption:*** Neither isotope excreted. Can repeat after tetracycline 250 mg qid x 10 d; if normalizes, suggests bacterial overgrowth.

# *Thrombocytopenia*[6]

### Differential diagnosis

- <u>Pseudothrombocytopenia</u>? Check for clumping (EDTA-dependent antibodies) by repeating platelet count in a citrated blood sample
- <u>Drug-induced</u> immune thrombocytopenia[7]: • Heparin (*see p 121*); • GPII$_b$/III$_a$ inhibitors (abciximab, eptifibatide, tirofiban); • P2Y12 platelet antagonists; •Acute ethanol toxicity; • Penicillin & beta-lactams; • Carbamazepine; • Linezolid; • Phenytoin; • Quinidine & quinine; • Rifampin; • Trimethoprim-sulfamethoxazole; • Valproic acid; • Vancomycin;
- <u>Hematopoietic nutrient deficiency</u> (*i.e.* acute folate deficiency )
- <u>Sepsis</u> especially with HIV or Disseminated Intravascular Coagulation (DIC);
- Major <u>hemorrhage</u> with <u>hemodilution</u>
- Mechanical <u>fragmentation</u> of platelets[7] • Mechanical circulatory support (ECMO, cardiopulmonary

---

[6] Hunt BJ. Bleeding and coagulopathies in critical care. *N Engl J Med* 2014; 370: 847-859.

[7] http://ouhsc.edu/platelets/ditp.html

bypass, intraaortic balloon pump); • Hemodialysis; • Nitinol intravascular occluder

- <u>Immune-mediated</u> thrombocytopenia. • <u>Primary</u>: • Immune thrombocytopenia purpura (ITP); • Antiphospholipid syndrome; • Post-transfusion purpura (antiplatelet alloAb)
- <u>Secondary</u> ITP: • Systemic lupus erythematosus; • Chronic lymphocytic leukemia; • HIV; • HCV
- <u>Microangiopathic hemolytic anemia</u> (associated with fragmented RBCs): • DIC; • Thrombotic thrombocytopenia purpura (TTP); • Hemolytic-uremic syndrome (HUS); • Pregnancy-hemolysis, elevated liver enzymes, low platelet (HELLP)
- <u>Other</u>: • Splenic sequestration; • Myelodysplastic syndrome; • Cancer;

**Platelet transfusion thresholds**
- Active bleeding: threshold 50 k/mm$^3$; High bleeding risk prophylaxis: 20 k/mm$^3$; Normal bleeding risk prophylaxis: 10 k/mm$^3$

# *Heparin-Induced Thrombocytopenia*[8]

### Setting & manifestations
- Highest risk in orthopedic surgery (3-5%), cardiac surgery (1-2%), then others.
- Typical early: Thrombocytopenia (50%) 5-10 d after heparin or reexposure, causing hypercoagulation or thrombosis from IgG-PF4 antibodies.
- Less common late: Abrupt onset on reexposure within 30-90 d, often anaphylactoid.
- Major surgery resets the

| Differential diagnosis |
|---|
| • Pseudothrombocytopenia (platelet clumping): examine smear, re-draw in citrate or heparin containing tube |
| • Sepsis • DIC/TTP • HELLP |
| • Immune: ITP, SLE, Post-transfusion |
| • Infections: HIV, EBV, hepatitis |
| • Drugs: chemotherapy, quinidine, NSAIDs, sulfa, GP IIb IIIa inhibitors |
| • Marrow suppression |
| • Ethanol • Splenomegaly |

[8] Greinacher A. Heparin-Induced Thrombocytopenia. *N Engl J Med* 2015; 373: 252-261; Linkins LA, *et al.* Treatment and prevention of heparin-induced thrombocytopenia, 9/e ACCP. *Chest* 2012; 141: e495S-530S.

clock despite recent heparin exposure. Distinguish from typical 40% ↓ Plt 1-2 days after cardiac surgery.
- 10-fold higher risk with unfractionated than LMWH
- Nadir Plt count is typically 40-80 k; lower suggest alternative diagnosis
- Monitor Plt count days 5,7,9 after heparin or surgery if considered high risk

**Diagnosis**
- 50% ↓ in platelets • Onset 5-10 d after heparin exposure, or within 8-10 hr if previous heparin exposure • Resolves after heparin stops • Exclusion of other causes • Confirmatory testing with *immunoassay* (*e.g.* anti-PF4, highly sensitive, nonspecific) AND *functional* assay (*e.g.* heparin-induced aggregation of washed platelets, specific but insensitive). • Negative result on complementary tests usually excludes diagnosis. • Overdiagnosis is probably more common than missed diagnosis

## 4T score[9] for risk of HIT

| 4Ts category | 2 points | 1 point | 0 points |
|---|---|---|---|
| Thrombocytopenia relative ↓ | Platelet count ↓ > 50% and nadir ≥ 20k/mm³ | Platelet count 30%-50% or nadir 10-19 k/mm³ | Platelet ↓ < 30% or nadir < 10 k/mm³ |
| Timing of onset | Platelet ↓ onset is clear d 5-10 or ↓ ≤ 1 d (prior heparin exposure within 30 days) | Platelet ↓ d 5-10 possible but missing platelet counts; onset > d 10; or ↓ ≤ 1 day (heparin 30-100 d ago) | Platelet ↓ ≤ 4 days without recent exposure |
| Thrombosis *etc.* | New thrombosis (confirmed); skin necrosis; acute systemic reaction after IV unfractionated heparin bolus | Thrombosis is progressive or recurrent; erythematous non-necrotizing skin lesions; suspected un-proven thrombosis | None |
| Other causes of platelet drop | None evident | Possible | Definite |

*(Continued)*

---

[9] Cuker A, *et al.* Predictive value of the 4Ts scoring system for heparin-induced thrombocytopenia: a systematic review and meta-analysis. *Blood* 2012; 120: 4160-4167.

| 4Ts category | 2 points | 1 point | 0 points |
|---|---|---|---|
| SUM=Probability of HIT | 6-8 = HIGH → further lab testing | 4-5 = INTERMEDIATE → negative rapid anti-PF4 antibody → HIT excluded[10] | 0-3 = LOW SCORE →No further evaluation |

## HIT Expert Probability (HEP) Sum Score[11] for risk of HIT, may outperform 4Ts

Magnitude of Fall

| < 30% | 30-50% | > 50% |
|---|---|---|
| -1 | +1 | +3 |

Timing of Fall with relation to heparin exposure, when typical onset HIT is expected

| < 4 d before | 4 d after | 5-10 d after | 11-14 d after | > 14 d after |
|---|---|---|---|---|
| -2 | +2 | +3 | +2 | -1 |

Timing of Fall with relation to heparin re-exposure, when rapid-onset HIT is expected (heparin in last 100d)

| < 48 h after | > 48 h after |
|---|---|
| 2 | -1 |

Nadir platelet count, x $10^{-9}$/L

| ≤ 20 | > 20 |
|---|---|
| -2 | +2 |

Thrombosis (choose 0 or 1)

| New venous or arterial thrombus ≥ 4 d (typical-onset) or immediately (rapid-onset) after heparin | Progression of VTE or ATE during heparin |
|---|---|
| +3 | +2 |

Skin necrosis at SQ heparin injection site or Acute systemic (anaphylactoid) reaction after IV heparin

+3 each

Bleeding, petechiae, or extensive bruising

-1

[10] Linkins LA, et al. Combination of 4Ts score and PF4/H-PaGIA for diagnosis and management of heparin-induced thrombocytopenia. Blood 2015.

[11] Cuker A, et al. The HIT Expert Probability (HEP) Score. J Thromb Haemost 2010; 8: 2642-2650.

Other causes of thrombocytopenia (include all that apply)

| Chronic ↓ Plt | New non-heparin known to cause ↓ Plt | Severe infection | Severe DIC fibrinogen < 100 & D-Dimer > 5 | Intraarterial device (IABP, VAD, ECMO) | Cardio-pulmonary bypass < 96 h | No other apparent cause |
|---|---|---|---|---|---|---|
| -1 | -2 | -2 | -2 | -2 | -1 | +3 |
| SUM= Probability of HIT | ≥2 = HIGH | | | <2 = LOW | | |

## Treatment

- Discontinue all heparin (including LMW heparin and line flushes) – platelet count should rise in 24-48 hr, with return to normal by 4-5 d.
- Among patients with HIT treated only by discontinuing heparin, symptomatic thrombosis rate is 25-50%, and fatal thrombosis rate is 5%.
- Avoid platelet transfusion – may induce thrombo-embolic complications.
- While awaiting confirmatory testing, treat with nonheparin anticoagulants (lepirudin, argatroban, bivalirudin; fewest data on fondaparinux) unless high risk of bleeding.
- In acute HIT, avoid warfarin without concomitant anticoagulants - may incite thrombosis; Delay warfarin until platelet count > 100 K.
- In patients with low platelet count considered unlikely to have HIT and not having an indication for anticoagulation, fondaparinux may be the safest agent.

# Transfusion of Blood Products[12]

**Whole blood:** Includes plasma, indicated for volume resuscitation in massive hemorrhage after > 5 u PRBC, volume 400-500 mL

**Packed red blood cells (PRBC):** Indicated in hemorrhage, symptomatic anemia. Limited benefit without ongoing hemorrhage or physiological evidence of inadequate oxygen delivery (tachycardia, hypotension, reduced urine output, *etc*). Hemoglobin "trigger" inadvisable: consider intravascular volume, evidence of shock or instability, extent & duration of anemia, physiology. "Restrictive" strategies of transfusion only for Hb <7 g/dL (in resuscitated critically ill trauma, mechanical ventilation, stable cardiac disease) are preferred, have equivalent or lower morbidity & mortality compared with permissive strategies, except ongoing myocardial ischemia. Sepsis: not indicated routinely. ARDS: transfusion should be avoided to ↓ acute lung injury. Caution: citrated-PRBC causes hypothermia, ↓ calcium, ↑ potassium, dilutional thrombocytopenia. Hyperkalemia reduced by using "fresh" PRBC or by washing before transfusion. Must be ABO-compatible. Risks: See transfusion reactions + transfusion-associated immunomodulation. Transfuse single units: each increases Hb ~ 1 g/dL. Volume 250-320 mL. Infuse over 1.5-4 hr.

**Types of PRBC products:** Leukoreduced: Expensive. Preferred to prevent alloimmunization in chronic repeat transfusion or future transplantation candidate, or after prior transfusion reaction, CMV-seronegative recipient. Washed: Requires an additional hour,

[12] Goodnough LT, *et al*. Concepts of blood transfusion in adults. *Lancet* 2013; 381: 1845-1854; Napolitano LM, *et al*. Clinical practice guideline: transfusion in adult trauma and critical care. *Crit Care Med* 2009; 37: 3124-3157; Kaufman RM, *et al*. Platelet transfusion. *Ann Intern Med* 2015; 162: 205-213; Roback JD, *et al*. Evidence-based practice guidelines for plasma transfusion. *Transfusion* 2010; 50: 1227-1239.

removes plasma and soluble antigens, leaked potassium. Used after prior transfusion reaction. <u>Irradiated</u>: prevents graft-versus-host disease in immunodeficiency or after transplantation or after donation from relatives. Reduces RBC viability.

**Platelets:** Indicated for bleeding, after cardio-pulmonary bypass (<100,000/µL), perioperatively (<50,000/µL, for CNS <100,000/µL), or spontaneously (<10,000/µL). Not suitable for HIT, TTP, DIC, ITP, uremia. <u>Other Risks</u>: GVHD. Infuse over 15-30 min. Increment should be 5,000/µL/unit, measured 10-60 min after transfusion. If smaller increment, request ABO-compatible platelets. Thereafter seek expert consultation.

**Fresh frozen plasma (FFP):** For bleeding (PT > 17s) or temporary reversal of warfarin, for example, before invasive procedures. Not indicated for volume replacement. Infuse over 30-60 min.

**Prothrombin Complex Concentrate (PCC):** Compared with FFP, more "balanced" ratio of VitK-dependent factors + Proteins C&S, lower volume, virus-inactivated.

**Cryoprecipitated antihemophilic factor:** Indicated for bleeding and low fibrinogen (< 100 mg/dL), von Willebrand disease, factor VIII replacement. Infuse over 15-30 min.

**Premedication:** No evidence of benefit of prophylactic acetaminophen+antihistamine.

# Transfusion Reactions[13]

**Acute Hemolytic:** 1-4 events/million units transfused preformed antibodies against major RBC antigens cause acute intravascular hemolysis; • *Symptoms*: fever, chills, back pain, N/V, hypotension, renal failure, DIC *Treatment*: Stop transfusion immediately; • Give diphenhydramine, acetaminophen ± hydro-

---

[13] Vamvakas EC, *et al.* Transfusion-related mortality. Blood 2009; 113: 3406-3417; Sihler KC, *et al.* Complications of massive transfusion. Chest 2010; 137: 209-220.

cortisone 50-100 mg IV; • Maintain urine output with alkalinized IVF; • Alert blood bank and send back product plus samples for Coombs, bilirubin, LDH, free Hb, DIC screen.

**Delayed Hemolytic:** 1/1000 units transfused; • 1-25 d post-transfusion • Sx similar to acute reaction but often less severe; • *Treatment:* Same as acute reaction if warranted by sx

**Non-hemolytic febrile:** Common (1-2 events/100 units transfused); • Platelets > PRBCs; • Onset ≤ 5 hr of transfusion; • Fever may be only 1-2 ° F > normal; • Other symptoms: chills, resp distress (usually self-limited); • Differential dx: hemolytic reaction, sepsis, contaminated blood product. *Treatment:* Stop transfusion & send back to blood bank; • Blood cultures; • Antipyretics ± meperidine 50-75 mg IV; • Consider leukocyte-reduced products if patient has had ≥ 2 febrile reactions

**Allergic:** Most common reaction (3-4 events/100 units transfused); • Immune response to plasma proteins; • *Symptoms:* pruritus, urticaria, bronchospasm, anaphylaxis (more likely if recipient is IgA-deficient) *Treatment:* Diphenhydramine if mild, standard treatment for anaphylaxis including epinephrine; • Unnecessary to stop transfusion if mild, but consider slowing infusion; • If severe or recurrent reactions use washed cells

**Transfusion-related acute lung injury (TRALI):** ARDS-like pulmonary leukoagglutination • 1-10 events/100,000 units transfused, with 3-5% mortality; • Acute $P_aO_2/FiO_2 ≤ 300$ + bilateral pulmonary infiltrates without volume overload within 72 hr; • *Treatment:* Supportive

**Post-transfusion purpura (PTP):** Rare, severe thrombocytopenia 5-10 d post-transfusion (usually RBC transfusion); • Due to anti-platelet alloantibodies

**Other:** • Volume Overload; • Infection (Viral, bacterial, tick-borne Babesia, endemic parasites: trypanosomiasis); • Transfusion-related immunomodulation (↑

nosocomial infection); • Acute hypothermia (massive transfusion); • Coagulopathy from massive transfusion & hypothermia; • Citrate-associated hypocalcemia; • Transfusion-associated systemic inflammation syndromes;

# Coagulation Tests[14]

### Phlebotomy conditions

• Discard catheter <u>dead-space</u> blood containing heparin; • If Hct > 0.55, tube citrate will over-dilute plasma & spuriously ↑ clotting time; • Clotting times are measured at room T, consider patient <u>temperature</u> & cold agglutins;

### Prothrombin time (PT):

• Sensitive to "<u>extrinsic pathway</u>:" Tissue factor, factor VII, and common pathway factors (II, V, X, fibrinogen); • Elevated in vitamin K antagonists (warfarin), liver disease, factor deficiency; • Normalized as <u>international normalized ratio</u>: INR=[(Patient PT) ÷ (Control PT)][ISI]

### Activated partial thromboplastin time (aPTT)

• "<u>Intrinsic pathway</u>:" HMWK, prekallikrein, factors XII, XI, IX, VIII, and common pathways (factors II, V, X, fibrinogen). aPTT sensitive to all clotting factors except factor VII; • Elevated in heparin (not LMWH) or bivalirudin or anti-factor $X_a$ therapy, antiphospholipid antibodies, factor deficiency.

### Thrombin Time (TT)

• Tests final step of coagulation, prolonged if low fibrinogen or thrombin inhibition; • Elevated by heparin, direct thrombin inhibitors (bivalirudin, hirudin, argatroban); fibrinogen disorders (deficiency/consumption, dysfibrinogen, elevated fibrinogen); presence of fibrin or fibrinogen degradation products; serum paraproteins such as myeloma or

---

[14] Zehnder JL. Clinical use of coagulation tests. In: Leung LLK, et al., editors. UpToDate. Waltham, MA.

amyloid; exposure to bovine thrombin; • NOT prolonged by direct $X_a$ inhibitors, fondaparinux, warfarin

## Reptilase Time (RT)

• Similar to thrombin time except <u>not sensitive to heparin</u>; • NOT prolonged by direct thrombin inhibitors. • Example: heparin or bivalirudin prolong TT not RT

## Ecarin Clotting Time (ECT)

• Monitors direct thrombin inhibitors such as dabigratran

## Anti-Factor-$X_a$ Activity[15] for therapeutic monitoring:

• <u>Unfractionated heparin</u>: 0.3-0.7 units anti-Xa ≈ 1.5 x PTT; • LMWH: therapeutic peak anti-$X_a$ measured 4 hr after dose: Twice-daily enoxaparin: 0.6-1.0 unit/mL; Once-daily enoxaparin: > 1.0 unit/mL; Tinzaparin: > 0.85 unit/mL; Dalteparin: > 1.05 Unit/mL.

## Whole blood activated clotting time (ACT) for therapeutic monitoring:

• Extends beyond range of aPTT, when heparin > 1.0 unit/mL, such as coronary or vascular intervention, heart surgery, dialysis; • Point-of-care tests *Hemochron* values exceed *Hemotec* for heparin; • ACT <u>sensitive</u> to unfractionated heparin, bivalirudin, argatroban, lepirudin; <u>insensitive</u> to enoxaparin, fondaparinux

## Fibrin D-dimer

• Indicates recent or active coagulation. Non-specific test combined with clinical suspicion (*i.e.* pulmonary thromboembolism) for decision-making

## Evaluation of coagulation

• PTT ↑ + PT normal: Intrinsic pathway defect. <u>Causes</u>: Heparin; Antiphospholipid antibody; Von Willebrand disease; factor deficiency

• PTT normal + PT ↑: Extrinsic pathway defect. <u>Causes</u>: Warfarin; Liver disease; Vitamin K deficiency (*e.g.*

---

[15] Garcia DA, *et al.* Parenteral anticoagulants: ACCP Guidelines. *Chest* 2012; 141: e24S-43S.

antimicrobials); acquired or congenital Factor VII deficiency.

• PTT + PT elevated: Probably final common pathway disorder. <u>Measure</u> thrombin time (TT) which if normal suggests factor II, V, X deficiency (liver disease, DIC, warfarin). See elevated TT above.

## Mixing study

Assumptions: (1) tests normal if ≥ 50% of factor is present; (2) Inhibitors are effective even diluted 50%; (3) Some inhibitors (*e.g.* FVIII) require delayed incubation.

• If 1:1 dilution <u>corrects defect</u>: factor deficiency is likely cause. • If 1:1 dilution <u>fails to correct</u> defect: inhibitors such as antiphospholipid antibody, heparin, acquired inhibitors (*e.g.* FVIII, IX, X) are likely cause.

## Antiphospholipid antibody

Assayed using • functional tests for lupus anticoagulant activity; • anticardiolipin antibody; • anti-β-glycoprotein-I antibody. • Dilute Russell's viper venom time sensitive to the latter, corresponds to clinically significant finding.

# Infectious Disease

## *New fever in the ICU*[1]

**Thresholds:** T > 38.3°C or T < 36.0°C
**Obtain 3-4 blood cultures within 24 hr**
- Povidone-iodine should dry 2 min; Alcohol-based preparations need dry 30 sec
- Wipe blood culture bottles with alcohol; Do not change phlebotomy needle to inoculate.

**Intravascular catheter infection suspected**
- Abrupt onset of sepsis without risk factor for nosocomial infection. Catheter inflammation or difficulty withdrawing blood. Certain pathogens: *Corynebacterium jeikeium*, *Bacillus* spp, atypical mycobacteria, *Candida*, or *Malassezia*
- Examine for peri-catheter purulence. Draw blood cultures from device and percutaneous site. Note high incidence of colonization of removed central venous catheters; routine culture is not advocated.
- All intravascular catheters should be removed or replaced in sepsis syndrome or embolic phenomena.

**Pulmonary infection suspected**
- Perform chest imaging (usually upright CXR); CT if immunocompromised·
- Inspection of expectorated, aspirated, or invasively-obtained specimen. Bronchoscopy useful for fungal, atypical bacteria (legionella spp, mycobacteria, nocardia), CMV. Process, culture, and examine specimens within 2 hr. Obtain before antibiotics.
- Consider thoracentesis if suspected parapneumonic, mycobacterial, fistulous
- Organisms almost always pathogens: *Legionella*, *Chlamydia*, *M. tuberculosis*, *Rhodococcus equi*, *Influenza virus*, *Respiratory syncytial virus*, *Parainfluenza virus*, *Strongyloides*, *Toxoplasma gondii*, *Pneumo-*

[1] O'Grady NP, *et al.* Guidelines for evaluation of new fever in critically ill adult patients. *Crit Care Med* 2008; 36: 1330-1349.

*cystis jiroveci, Histoplasma capsulatum, Coccidioides immitis, Blastomyces dermatitidis, Cryptococcus neoformans.*

- Organisms usually contaminants: enterococci, viridans streptococci, coagulase-negative staphylococci, Candida (sputum only, not bloodstream)
- Organisms that may be colonizers or pathogens (need good Gram stain or heavy growth): *Pseudomonas aeruginosa, Enterobacteriaceae, S. pneumoniae, Staph. aureus,* and *Haemophilus influenza*
- Immunocompromised (non-culture tests valuable for positive or negative diagnosis): CMV blood antigen if not infected with HIV, histoplasma, or cryptococcus; PCR for CMV, varicella-zoster virus, human herpes virus-6, and adenovirus; Galactomannan and β-D-glucan for aspergillosis and Candida

**Stool evaluation in ICU. (Diarrhea defined as > 2 container-conforming stools/d)** *(See pg 95)*

- Suspect *C. difficile* if fever/leukocytosis/diarrhea, antibiotics or chemotherapy within 60 d.
  - Immunoassays are rapid. Multiple specimens compensate for low sensitivity. PCR is more accurate. Pseudomembranes on procto-sigmoidoscopy are pathognomonic.
  - Empirical vancomycin if severely ill, but not if two negative tests using reliable assay.
- Alternatives: *Klebsiella oxytoca* antibiotic-associated colitis. • Norovirus; • Travel-related infection; • HIV-related diarrhea; • Tube-feed related; • Antimicrobial-associated
- Ova and parasites exam not usually useful if not admitted for diarrhea, or not HIV

**Urinary tract infection**

- Majority in ICU are related to urinary catheters and caused by multiresistant Gram(-) rods
- If indwelling urinary catheter, obtain specimen from sample port, not collection bag
- Examine & collect specimen within 1 hr of obtaining.

- Cultures from indwelling cathers > $10^3$ organisms/mL represent pyruria/candiduria but not necessarily etiology of fever
- Gram stains of centrifuged urine help select antimicrobial agent

## Sinusitis
- CT is useful if sinusitis is suspected to cause fever: nasogastric tubes, endotracheal tubes especially transnasal, maxillofacial trauma
- Puncture and aspiration of involved sinus is indicated if no response to empiric therapy

## Postoperative fever
- Early fever is usually non-infective; fever > 96 hr postoperatively is usually infective
- Atelectasis is a diagnosis of exclusion
- Wound infections 1-3 d post-op (group A streptococci, clostridia) evident on examination
- Abdominal surgery: new or persistent fever > 4 d suggest persistent or new pathology
- Consider deep or superficial vein thrombosis, pulmonary thromboembolism, suppurative phlebitis, malignant hyperthermia, drug-induced fever

## Surgical site infections
- Examine site daily. Open and drain incisions that appear infected.

## Central nervous system infection
- Lumbar puncture for fever and unexplained altered consciousness or focal neurological signs, unless contraindicated. Perform CT first if findings suggest intracranial process (*see page 139*) and consult neurosurgeon if there is a mass finding.
- Sample CSF prosthetic reservoirs and, if obstructed, lumbar space in fever evaluation
- Stupor or meningitis should trigger removal/culture of ventriculostomy

## CMV-related mononucleosis syndrome after blood transfusion

- Typically 1 mo after transfusion. High fevers, pancytopenia, atypical lymphocytosis in immuno-competent hosts. Immunocompromised hosts may suffer life-threatening disseminated infection with interstitial pneumonia, especially in primary infection.
- Uncommon after transfusion with leuko-reduced blood products

## Procalcitonin assay for early detection of bacterial infection

- Elevated within 2-3 hr, higher levels correspond to more severe clinical syndromes

## Non-infectious causes of fever in ICU

- Drug-fever
- Malignant hyperthermia: rigidity and fever, congenital, after halothanes, succinylcholine
- Neuroleptic malignant syndrome: muscle rigidity after neuroleptic antipsychotics
- Serotonin syndrome (*page 242*): resembles neuroleptic malignant syndrome, after SSRIs, noteworthy exacerbated by concomitant linezolid
- Drug withdrawal: • alcohol, • opiates, • benzodiazepines
- Other possibilities: • Acalculous cholecystitis; • Acute myocardial infarction; • Adrenal insufficiency; • Blood product transfusion; • Cytokine-related fever; • Dressler syndrome (pericardial injury syndrome); • Fat emboli; • Gout; • Immune reconstitution inflammatory syndrome; • Intracranial bleed; • Jarisch-Herxheimer reaction; • Pancreatitis; • Pulmonary infarction; • Pneumonitis without infection; • Stroke; • Thyroid storm; • Transplant rejection; • Tumor lysis syndrome; • Venous thrombosis

# Modified Duke Criteria for Endocarditis[2]

| Criteria for diagnosis of infective endocarditis (IE) | |
|---|---|
| **Definite** | • *Pathologic criteria:* <br> (1) Micro-organisms (demonstrated by culture or histology in a vegetation, embolized vegetation or intracardiac abscess) *or* <br> (2) Pathologic lesions (vegetation or intracardiac abscess confirmed by histology showing active endocarditis) *or* <br> • *Clinical criteria:* 2 major *or* 1 major plus 3 minor *or* 5 minor |
| **Possible** | • *Clinical criteria:* 1 major plus 1 minor *or* 3 minor |
| **Rejected** (negative predictive value ≥92%) | • Firm alternate diagnosis explaining evidence of IE *or* <br> • Resolution of endocarditis syndrome with antibiotic therapy for ≤ 4 days *or* <br> • No pathologic findings of IE at surgery or autopsy (after antibiotic therapy for ≤ 4 days) *or* <br> • Does not meet criteria for possible IE |

| Major Criteria | Minor Criteria |
|---|---|
| 1) Positive blood cultures for IE <br> • 2 separate blood cultures with organisms *typical* for IE* <br> • Persistently positive blood cultures with organism *consistent* with IE (2 drawn > 12 hr apart; or all of 3 or majority of ≥ 4 separate cultures, with 1st and last drawn ≥ 1 hr apart) <br> • Single positive blood culture for *Coxiella burnetii* or Ab titer > 1:800 <br> 2) Evidence of endocardial involvement: <br> • Echocardiogram (+) for IE**: Oscillating intracardiac mass# or abscess or new partial dehiscence of prosthetic valve <br> • New valvular regurgitation† | 1) Predisposing heart condition or IVDU <br> 2) Fever ≥ 38.0°C (100.4°F) <br> 3) Vascular phenomena: Major arterial emboli, septic pulmonary infarcts, mycotic aneurysm, intracranial hemorrhage, Janeway lesions, conjunctival hemorrhages <br> 4) Immunologic phenomena: Osler nodes, glomerulonephritis, Roth spots, rheumatoid factor <br> 5) Microbiologic evidence: (+) blood culture for organism that causes IE but not meeting major criteria *or* serologic evidence of active infection with organism consistent with IE, *e.g.* *Bartonella* spp. |

\* *Typical organisms include viridans streptococci, S. bovis, HACEK group, S. aureus; or community-acquired enterococci in the absence of a primary focus*

\*\* *Transesophageal echocardiogram (TEE) recommended in pts with prosthetic valves; those rated ≥ "possible IE" by clinical criteria; complicated IE (paravalvular abscess); transthoracic echocardiogram (TTE) first study in other patients*

\# *Mass on valve or supporting structures or in the path of regurgitant jets or on implanted material, in the absence of an alternative anatomic explanation*

† *Increase or change in preexisting murmur **not** sufficient*

---

[2] Li JS, *et al*. Proposed modifications to the Duke criteria for the diagnosis of infective endocarditis. *Clin Infect Dis* 2000; 30: 633-638.

# Surgery for Infective Endocarditis[3]

Mortality IE with heart failure 45% medically vs 21% surgical treatment

Mortality predictors in L-sided native valve IE:
• abnormal mental status; • ≥ moderate CHF; • non-Viridans infection; • non-surgical therapy

**Surgical strategy:** remove all infected tissue; repair > replacement but not usually possible

Early surgery during initial admission before completing antimicrobials

| Recommended | • all L-sided IE caused by *S.aureus*, fungal, or other highly resistant organisms.<br>• IE complicated by heart block, annular or aortic abscess, or destructive penetrating lesions<br>• persistent infection: persistent bacteremia or fever > 5-7 d after appropriate antimicrobials; abscess on TEE (CT scan helpful in posterior mitral abscess)<br>• prosthetic valve IE and relapsing infection after completion of appropriate antimicrobials |
|---|---|
| Probably helpful | • Recurrent emboli or persistent vegetation despite appropriate antimicrobial therapy. Note antimicrobials alone halve risk of embolization esp after 2 wk. |
| Possibly helpful | • Recurrent emboli or large (> 10 mm) or mobile vegetation (esp anterior mitral leaflet) despite appropriate antimicrobial therapy. Rationale: embolic events reduced, ultimately most survivors require surgery. |
| Attempt at non-surgical management | • Non-staphylococcal prosthetic valve endocarditis without complications or dysfunction<br>• Clinically improving and hemodynamically stable during antimicrobial therapy |

# Bacterial Endocarditis Prophylaxis[4]

**Prophylaxis recommended only for highest risk settings**
• Prosthetic cardiac valves
• Prior infective endocarditis

[3] Nishimura RA, *et al.* ACC/AHA 2008 guideline update on infective endocarditis. *Circulation* 2008; 118: 887-896.
[4] Nishimura RA, *et al.* 2014 AHA/ACC guideline for the management of patients with valvular heart disease. *J Am Coll Cardiol* 2014; 63: e57-185.

- Cardiac transplant recipients with valve regurgitation due to structurally abnormal valves
- Congenital heart disease (CHD):
  - Cyanotic CHD after repair, or repaired using palliative shunts or conduits
  - Completely repaired defects within 6 mo, using surgical or endoprosthesis, awaiting endothelialization
  - Residual defect at site of prosthetic repair or surgical/percutaneous implant
- Cardiac transplant valvulopathy

**Considerations**

- Prophylax only before dental procedures that manipulate gingivae or periapical teeth, or that perforate oral mucosae
- Bacteremia is common after chewing, toothbrushing, flossing. Benefit of prophylaxis is small, and the risk of adverse events outweighs benefit.
- Oral hygiene/ health probably more important to prevent IE than antibiotic prophylaxis

# Life-threatening Infective Rashes[5]

| Epidemiology | Manifestations | Diagnosis | Prognosis/Rx |
|---|---|---|---|
| **Rocky Mountain Spotted Fever (RMSF)** | | | |
| • *Rickettsia rickettsii*<br>• Tick-borne<br>• Occurs in almost all US states, but most cases in Southeast<br>• Most cases spring/summer | • Fever, myalgia, headache<br>• **Rash:** typically starts d 4 on wrists/ ankles, spreads to palms/soles then centrally. Initially pink-red macules that blanch; evolves to petechiae, purpura and gangrene of digits, nose and genitals<br>• 10%"spotless"<br>• Atypical rash in deeply pigmented pts | • Clinical diagnosis<br>• No early lab clues<br>• Triad of fever, rash & tick bite in only 60-70%<br>• Late serology confirmatory<br>• DFA of skin biopsy 70% sensitive, 100% specif<br>• ?PCR | • Mortality 5-25% (higher with delayed diagnosis)<br>• **Rx:** doxycycline (IV or PO); chloramphenicol in pregnancy or young child<br>• Broad-spectrum antimicrobials are ineffective. If there is clinical suspicion, promptly initiate directed therapy |
| **Meningococcal Sepsis** | | | |
| • *N. meningitidis*<br>• Transmission via respiratory droplets (close contact)<br>• Most cases winter/spring<br>• Patients usually < 20 y.o. | • Fever, headache, N/V, confusion, meningeal signs<br>• **Rash:** petechial, scattered on trunk/ extremities; evolves to palpable purpura ("gun-metal gray" with necrotic center). Petechiae clustered at pressure points.<br>• Purpura fulminans: cutaneous DIC with hemorrhagic bullae | • Gram stain/cx of blood, CSF, skin<br>• Gram stain of petechiae 70% sensitive<br>• Cx of skin bx may remain (+) after antibiotics given | • Mortality 10-20%<br>• **Rx:** PCN G IV<br>• Contacts: rifampin, ciprofloxacin or ceftriaxone |

*(Continued)*

---

[5]  Drage LA. Life-threatening rashes. *Mayo Clin Proc 1999*; 74: 68-72.

| Epidemiology | Manifestations | Diagnosis | Prognosis/Rx |
|---|---|---|---|
| **Staphylococcal Toxic Shock Syndrome (STSS)** | | | |
| • *Staph aureus* (toxin-producing)<br>• Most cases non-menstrual<br>• Associated with flu, childbirth, tracheitis, wound infection, nasal packing<br>• 40% recurrence | • Fever, malaise, myalgia, N/V, diarrhea<br>• Prominent confusion<br>• **Rash:** sunburn-like, diffuse macular erythroderm followed by desquamation of hands and feet in 5–14 d. Also causes conjunctival injection, oral-genital mucosal hyperemia, and "strawberry" tongue | • Isolation of *S. aureus* from blood unusual<br>• Diagnostic criteria:<br>1) fever or ↓ BP<br>2) typical rash<br>3) multi-organ involvement<br>4) exclusion of other causes | • Mortality 10–15% (5% in menstrual cases)<br>• **Rx:** anti-staph antibiotic, supportive care,<br>• Remove source<br>• Concurrent clindamycin may reduce toxin-release |
| Streptococcal Toxic Shock Syndrome<br><br>• Group A strep<br>• Soft tissue infections most common<br>• Most patients 20–50 y.o. and otherwise healthy | • Fever, hypotension, severe local pain<br>• **Rash:** highly variable; localized erythema, diffuse erythroderm or violaceous bullae<br>• Pain >> physical findings<br>• Can occur after blunt trauma or muscle strain | • Bacteremia in 60%, but open biopsy often necessary<br>• Diagnostic criteria: isolation of group A strep, ↓ BP and multi-organ involvement | • Mortality 30–70%<br>• **Rx:** PCN G plus aggressive surgical exploration and debridement<br>• Concurrent clindamycin may reduce toxin release<br>• Consider IVIG |

# *Bacterial Meningitis in Adults*

**Criteria for head CT prior to lumbar puncture, any of**[6]
• Immunocompromised (HIV, immunosuppressive tx, solid organ or hematopoietic stem cell transplant);
• CNS disease (mass lesion, stroke, focal CNS infection); • New onset seizure (< 1 wk); • Papilledema;
• Altered sensorium; • Focal neurological defect

---

[6] Tunkel AR, *et al.* Practice guidelines for the management of bacterial meningitis. *Clin Infect Dis* 2004; 39: 1267-1284. Hasbun R, *et al.* CT of the head before lumbar puncture in adults with suspected meningitis. *N Engl J Med* 2001; 345: 1727-1733.

## Data from 493 episodes in 445 adults at referral center 1962-1988[7]

| Finding | Community–Acquired | Nosocomial |
|---|---|---|
| Total cases | 296 episodes in 275 patients (60% of total) | 197 episodes in 175 patients (40% of total) |
| Recurrent cases | 38 episodes in 17 patients | 41 episodes in 19 patients |
| Predisposing factors | Otitis media (26%)<br>Sinusitis (12%)<br>Pneumonia (15%)<br>Immunocompromise (19%)<br>Diabetes (10%)<br>Alcoholism (18%)<br>CSF leak (8%) | Recent neurosurgery (68%)<br>Neurosurgical device (32%)<br>Immunocompromise (31%)<br>Recent head injury (13%)<br>CSF leak (13%) |
| Predisposing factors for recurrent meningitis | CSF leak (76%)<br>History of head trauma or neurosurgery (47%) | Neurosurgical procedure (100%)<br>CSF leak (47%) |
| Causative organism (in single episodes) | *Strep pneumonia* (38%)<br>*N. meningitidis* (14%)<br>Listeria (11%)<br>Streptococci (7%)<br>*Staph aureus* (5%)<br>*H. influenza* (4%)<br>Gram neg bacilli (4%)<br>Culture negative (13%) | Gram neg bacilli (38%)<br>Streptococci (9%)<br>*Staph aureus* (9%)<br>Coag neg staph (9%)<br>Mixed species (7%)<br>*Strep pneumonia* (5%)<br>*H. influenza* (4%)<br>Culture negative (11%) |
| Clinical findings (in community acquired cases) | Fever, nuchal rigidity and abnormal mental status  66%<br>Fever                                                                 95%<br>Nuchal rigidity                                               88%<br>Abnormal mental status                                  78%<br>Seizures                                                          23%<br>Focal neurologic findings                             28% ||
| **Cerebrospinal Fluid (CSF) Findings** |||
| Opening pressure (cm H$_2$O) | 0-13.9:  9%<br>14.0-29.9:  52%<br>> 30.0-39.9:  39% | 0-13.9:  23%<br>14.0-29.9:  52%<br>> 30.0:  26% |
| WBC per mm$^3$ | 0-99:  13%<br>100-4999:  59%<br>> 5000:  28% | 0-99:  19%<br>100-4999:  62%<br>> 5000:  20% |
| % PMNs | 0-19:  2%<br>20-79:  19%<br>> 80%:  79% | 0-19:  2%<br>20-79:  31%<br>> 80%:  66% |
| Protein (mg/dl) | 0-45:  4%<br>46-199:  40%<br>> 200:  56% | 0-45:  6%<br>46-199:  42%<br>> 200:  52% |
| Glucose < 40 mg/dl | 50% | 45% |
| Gram-stain, Cx (+) | 60%, 73% | 46%, 83% |

[7] Durand ML, *et al.* Acute bacterial meningitis in adults. *N Engl J Med* 1993; 328: 21-28.

- Overall fatality rate = 25% (19% meningitis-related)
- No significant change in mortality rate over time
- 98% of patients who died had at least one of: • age > 60yr • onset of seizures within 24 hr of admission • obtunded on admission

## Empirical treatment for community-acquired bacterial meningitis[8]

- **Adults < 50 yr:** Vancomycin + 3rd-generation cephalosporin (cefotaxime or ceftriaxone) against *S.pneumoniae* & *N.meningitides*. Add ampicillin if *Listeria monocytogenes* suspected.
- **Adults > 50 yr:** Vancomycin + ampicillin + 3rd-generation cephalosporin against above + *L.monocytogenes* + aerobic Gram-negative bacilli
- **Immunocompromised:** Vancomycin + ampicillin + either cefepime or meropenem, against above + *S.aureus*, Salmonella spp, *P.geruginosa*
- **Recurrent:** Vancomycin + 3rd-generation cephalosporin against *S.pneumoniae* & *N.meningitides* + *H.influenzae*.

**Dexamethasone** in suspected *S. pneumonia* or unknown etiology: 0.15 mg/kg q 6 h x 2-4 d until *S. pneumoniae* excluded. Initiate before or concomitant with first antimicrobial dose

# *Community Acquired Pneumonia*[9]

## Prognosis: CURB-65 Score[10]

Score 1 point each for • **C**onfusion; • blood **U**rea nitrogen > 20 mg/dL; • **R**espirations > 30/min; • **B**lood pressure < 90 systolic or ≤60 diastolic; • Age ≥ **65** years

| Score     | 0    | 1-2 | 3   | 4   | 5   |
|-----------|------|-----|-----|-----|-----|
| Mortality | 0.7% | 3%  | 17% | 42% | 57% |

---

[8] van de Beek D, *et al*. Advances in treatment of bacterial meningitis. *Lancet* 2012; 380: 1693-1702.

[9] Mandell LA, et al. IDSA/ATS consensus guidelines on the management of community-acquired pneumonia in adults. *Clin Infect Dis* 2007; 44 Suppl 2: S27-72.

[10] Lim WS, *et al*. Defining community acquired pneumonia severity on presentation to hospital. *Thorax* 2003; 58: 377-382.

## Prognosis: Pneumonia Severity Index/PORT Score[11]

| Characteristic | Score | Exam Findings | Score |
|---|---|---|---|
| Age | Age | Altered mental status | + 20 |
| Female Gender | - 10 | Resp rate ≥ 30 | + 20 |
| Nursing home resident | + 10 | SBP < 90 | + 20 |
| **Co-existing Illness** | | Temp < 35° or ≥ 40° C | + 15 |
| Malignancy | + 30 | Pulse ≥ 125 | + 10 |
| Liver disease | + 20 | **Laboratory/CXR findings** | |
| CHF | + 10 | Arterial pH < 7.35 | + 30 |
| Cerebrovascular disease | + 10 | BUN ≥ 30 mg/dl | + 20 |
| Renal disease | + 10 | $Na^+$ < 130 mmol/L | + 20 |
| **Exclusion criteria:** | | Glucose ≥ 250 mg/dl | +10 |
| • Age < 18  • HIV or AIDS | | Hct < 30 % | +10 |
| • 1° diagnosis other than | | $PaO_2$ < 60 mmHg | +10 |
|   pneumonia | | Pleural effusion | +10 |
| • Previous admission within | | | |
|   7 d | | | |

| PORT Score | Class | Mortality (%) | Admit Rate (%)[a] | ICU Admit (%) | Median Stay (days) | Recommended Site of Care |
|---|---|---|---|---|---|---|
| ≤ 50[b] | I | 0.1 | 5.1 | 4.3 | 5.0 | Outpatient |
| ≤ 70 | II | 0.6 | 8.2 | 4.3 | 6.0 | Outpatient |
| 71-90 | III | 0.9 | 16.7 | 5.9 | 7.0 | Inpatient (brief) |
| 91-130 | IV | 9.3 | 20.0 | 11.4 | 9.0 | Inpatient |
| > 130 | V | 27.0 | n/a | 17.3 | 11.0 | Inpatient |
| Total | | 5.2 | 7.4 | 9.2 | 7.0 | |

*a: Subsequent admission rate if initially treated as outpatient (no increased mortality)*
*b: Class I - age 50 or less and no co-existent illnesses or exam findings*

## More extensive diagnostic testing warranted[9]

- ICU admission, immunocompromised, cavitary infiltrates, failed outpatient therapy, leukopenia, alcoholism or liver disease, structural or obstructive lung disease, pleural effusion, recent travel
- Severe pneumonia: pretreatment blood cultures & good-quality expectorated or aspirated sputum Gram stain and culture, urinary antigen for legionella & pneumococcus
- Negative gram-stain & culture for staphylococcus & Gram negatives are compelling

---

[11] Fine MJ, et al. A prediction rule to identify low-risk patients with community-acquired pneumonia. N Engl J Med 1997; 336: 243-250.

## Likely etiology[9]

| Outpatient | Inpatient, non-ICU | ICU |
|---|---|---|
| Streptococcus pneumoniae; Mycoplasma pneumoniae; Haemophilus influenza; Chlamydia pneumoniae; Respiratory viruses* | S. pneumoniae; M. pneumoniae; C. pneumoniae; H. influenza; Legionella spp; Aspiration; Respiratory viruses* | S. pneumoniae; Staphylococcus aureus; Legionella spp; Gram-negative bacilli; H. influenza; |

*Respiratory viruses: Influenza A&B, adenovirus, respiratory syncytial virus, parainfluenza

**Treatment: administer first dose quickly *i.e.* in emergency department**

Outpatient

- Healthy: Macrolide or doxycycline
- Comorbidity (chronic heart, lung, liver, kidney disease, diabetes, alcoholism, cancer, asplenia, immunosuppressed or immunocompromised, recent antimicrobials in past 3 mo) or prevalent macrolide-resistant *S. pneumoniae*: (respiratory fluoroquinolone) or (β-lactam plus macrolide)

Inpatient, non-ICU: (respiratory fluoroquinolone) or (β-lactam plus macrolide)

ICU

- β-lactam (cefotaxime/ceftriaxone/ampicillin) plus (azithromycin or respiratory fluoroquinolone)
- β-lactam allergic: respiratory fluoroquinolone + aztreonam

If there is also a special consideration of

- *Pseudomonas*: (piperacillin/tazobactam, cefepime, imipenem, meropene) plus (cipro or levofloxacin) or (aminoglycoside and (azithromycin or fluoroquinolone)). If β-lactam allergic, substitute aztreonam for β-lactam.
- Community-acquired methicillin-resistant *Staph aureus*: add vancomycin or linezolid

**Special conditions or risk factors[9]**

Alcoholism: *S. pneumoniae*, oral anaerobes, *K. pneumoniae*, *Acinetobacter* spp, TB

Aspiration: Gram negative enteric organisms, oral anaerobes

COPD/tobacco: *H. influenza, Pseudomonas aeruginosa, Legionella* spp, *Moraxella catarrhalis, C. pneumoniae*

Lung abscess: Community-acquired MRSA, oral anaerobes, endemic fungi, TB, atypical mycobacteria

Bronchiectasis: *Pseudomonas aeruginosa, Burkholderia cepacia, S. aureus*

Obstructive lung tumor: Anaerobes, *S. pneumoniae, H. influenzae, S. aureus*

Bat or bird guano: *Histoplasma capsulatum*

Bird exposure: *Chlamydia psittaci*, Poultry: avian influenza

Rabbits: *Francisella tularensis*

Farm animals or parturient cats: *Coxiella burnetti* (Q fever)

HIV early: *S. pneumoniae, H. influenza*, TB

HIV late: early plus *Pneumocystis jirovecii, Cryptococcus, Histoplasma, Aspergillus*, atypical mycobacterium esp *kansasii, P aeruginosa, H. influenza*

Hotel or cruise ship last 2 wk: *Legionella* spp

Southwestern US travel or residence: *Coccidioides* spp, *Hantavirus*

SE or E Asia travel or residence: *Burkholderia pseudomallei*, avian influenza, SARS

Influenza active in community: Influenza, *S. pneumoniae*, Staph aureus, *H. influenza*

Cough > 2 wk with whoop or post-tussive emesis: *Bordetella pertussis*

Injection drug abuse: *S. aureus*, anaerobes, *M. tuberculosis, S. pneumoniae*

Bioterror: *Bacillus anthracis, Yersinia pestis, Francisella tularensis*

Narrow the antimicrobials based on cultures & sensitivity & response.

**Failure to respond to initial therapy**
• Common (6-15%) and high mortality (27-49%). Usually due to severity of initial illness. • Re-evaluate initial microbiological findings. • Consider special epidemiological or host risk factors. • Consider viral etiology. • Repeat blood cultures. • Utility of invasive

sputum sampling controversial; caution about colonization. • Urinary antigen tests for Legionella & pneumococcus. • Seek concomitant extrapulmonary infection source. • Chest CT to detect pneumonia complications or pulmonary thromboembolism. • Thoracentesis for effusion and empyema

**When to sample parapneumonic effusions[12] (*See pleural fluid analysis on p193*)**

• Loculated (not free-flowing); • Free-flowing but layers > 10 mm on lateral decubitus radiography; • Thickened parietal pleura on contrast-enhanced CT, suggesting empyema; • Accessible/evident by ultrasound

**Additional considerations**

- Consider influenza and pneumococcal vaccine upon discharge
- Consider follow-up chest x-ray to ensure resolution, with caveat that persistence of radiographic infiltrate (4-12 wk) is directly related to age, number of lobes involved and is slower in smokers
- Smoking cessation can eliminate an important risk for CAP

# *Pharyngeal swab technique*

*To swab the posterior pharynx properly (for example to test for bacteria), insert the sampling swab straight back, and not up the nostril.*

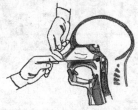

---

[12] Colice GL, *et al.* Medical and surgical treatment of parapneumonic effusions. *Chest 2000; 118: 1158-1171.*

# *Infections after Transplantation*

**Timing of common infections after allogeneic marrow transplant[13]**

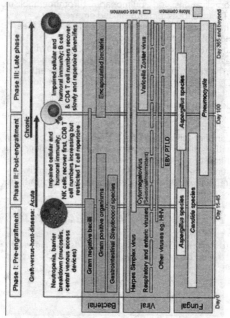

[13] Reproduced from Tomblyn M, *et al.* Guidelines for preventing infectious complications among hematopoietic cell transplantation recipients. *Biol Blood Marrow Transplant* 2009; 15: 1143-1238.

# Common infections after solid organ transplants[14]

| Timing after transplantation | Considerations |
|---|---|
| < 4 wk: nosocomial and technical | **Antimicrobial-resistant species:**<br>• MRSA; • VRE; • Non-albicans candida spp;• Aspiration pneumonia; • IV acces site infection;<br>• Wound infection;<br>• Anatomosis infection from ischemia or leak;<br>**Uncommon donor-derived:**<br>• HSV; • LCMV; • rabies; • West Nile<br>**From colonization of recipient:**<br>• Aspergillis; • Pseudomonas |
| 1-6 mo: activation of latent infections, relapsed, residual, & opportunistic infections | **Despite prophylaxis against PCP and antiviral (CMV, HBV):**<br>• BK polyomavirus nephropathy;<br>• C.difficile colitis; • HCV; • Adenovirus;<br>• Influenza; • Cryptococcus neoformans;<br>• Tuberculousis<br>Complications of anastomosis<br>In setting of no prophylaxis:<br>• Pneumocystis; • Herpesviridae (HVS, VZV, CMV, EBV); • HBV; • Listeria;<br>• Nocardia; • Toxoplasma;<br>• Strongyloides; • Lesihmania; • T. cruzi |
| > 6 mo: community-acquired | Community acquired pneumonia; Urinary tract infection; • Aspergillus; • atypical molds;<br>• mucormycosis; • Nocardia; • Rhodococcus;<br>**Late viral infections:**<br>• CMV (colitis or retinitis); • HBV or<br>• HCV (hepatitis); • SARS; • West Nile;<br>• JC polyomavirus (PML); • Lymphoma (posttransplant lymphoproliferative);<br>• Skin cancer |

[14] Fishman JA. From the classic concepts to modern practice. *Clin Microbiol Infect 2014; 20 Suppl 7: 4-9.*

# Fever & pulmonary infiltrates in solid-organ transplant patients

| Radiographic Abnormality | Acute Illness | Subacute or Chronic |
|---|---|---|
| Consolidation | • Bacteria (incl. legionella)<br>• Thromboembolism<br>• Hemorrhage<br>• Pulmonary edema | • Fungi, Nocardia, TB<br>• Tumor<br>• Viruses, PCP, radiation, drug reactions |
| Peribronchovascular abnormality | • Pulmonary edema<br>• Leukoagglutinin reaction<br>• Bacteria<br>• Viruses (influenza) | • Viruses, PCP<br>• Radiation<br>• Drug reactions<br>• Nocardia, tumor, fungi, TB |
| Nodular infiltrate (≥ 1 defects > 1 cm$^2$ with well-defined borders) | • Bacteria (incl. legionella)<br>• Pulmonary edema | • Fungi<br>• Nocardia, TB<br>• PCP<br>• PTLD |

# CNS infection in transplant recipients

| Pattern | Etiology |
|---|---|
| Acute meningitis | Bacterial esp. Listeria |
| Subacute/chronic meningitis | Cryptococcus (also TB, Listeria, Histoplasma, Nocardia, Strongyloides, Coccidioides, PTLD, HHV 6, VZV) |
| Focal brain infection | Aspergillus, listeria, toxoplasma, nocardia, PTLD |
| Progressive dementia | PML, HSV, CMV, EBV, demyelination due to drug reaction |

PTLD = EBV-associated post-transplant lymphoproliferative disease
PML = progressive multifocal leukoencephalopathy

# Neurology

## *Common Stroke Syndromes[1]*

### Ischemic Stroke Localization

| Syndrome | Arteries | Common Findings |
|---|---|---|
| Anterior Circulation | Internal carotid, middle cerebral, anterior cerebral | **Left:** Aphasia, right limb/face weakness<br>**Right:** Left visual neglect, denial of deficit, left limb/face weakness, poor visuospatial function |
| Posterior Circulation | Posterior cerebral | **Left:** Right hemianopsia, large lesions may lose ability to read but not write<br>**Right:** Left hemianopsia |
| Brainstem-cerebellum | Vertebral, basilar | Vertigo, cranial nerve findings especially extraocular movement palsies, quadriparesis, ataxia, nystagmus, crossed signs (ipsilateral cranial nerve palsies and contralateral limb weakness or sensory loss), coma |
| Lacunar motor stroke | Penetrating artery in pons or internal capsule | Pure hemiparesis |
| Lacunar sensory stroke | Penetrating artery in thalamus or posterior limb of internal capsule | Pure hemisensory symptoms |

### Common aneurysm sites

| Location (junction or bifurcation) | Signs of leak or rupture |
|---|---|
| Internal carotid-posterior communicating artery | • Ipsilateral 3rd nerve palsy |
| Anterior communicating artery | • Bilateral leg weakness, numbness and Babinski reflex |
| Middle cerebral bifurcation | • Contralateral face or hand weakness, aphasia (left) or visual neglect (right) |
| Basilar bifurcation | • Bilateral vertical gaze palsies, Babinski sign, coma |
| Vertebral-posterior inferior communicating artery junction | • Vertigo, lateral medullary syndrome |

---

[1] Caplan LR. Caplan's stroke : a clinical approach 4/e. *Philadelphia* Elsevier/Saunders; 2009.

## Common signs of hypertensive intracranial hemorrhage

| Location | Motor/sensory | Pupils | Eye Movements | Other |
|---|---|---|---|---|
| Putamen or internal capsule (40%) | Contralateral hemiparesis & sensory loss | Normal | Conjugate gaze paresis to opposite side ("eyes look toward lesion") | Aphasia (L), neglect (R) |
| Caudate (8%) | Transient contralateral hemiparesis | Ipsilateral Horner's* | Conjugate gaze paresis to opposite side * | Agitation, poor memory |
| Lobar (15%) | May include hemiparesis, aphasia | Normal | Conjugate gaze paresis to opposite sign | May include confusion, aphasia (L), hemianopsia, neglect (R) |
| Thalamus (20%) | Contralateral sensory >motor loss | Small, poorly reactive, 1- or 2-sided | Upgaze paralysis (eyes down &) in, ipsilateral conjugate gaze paresis * | Somnolence, aphasia (L), or neglect (R) |
| Pons # (8%) | Quadriparesis | Small, reactive | Absent horizontal gaze, ocular bobbing | Coma |
| Cerebellum (8%) | Ipsilateral ataxia, no paralysis | Ipsilateral pupil smaller * | Prominent nystagmus | Vomiting, postural instability |

*\* Variable finding    # Typical findings for large or bilateral lesions*

# Stroke mimics[2]

| Mimic | Features |
|---|---|
| Psychogenic | No objective CN findings, non-vascular distribution, inconsistent examination |
| Seizures | Prior or witnessed seizure, postictal period |
| Hypoglycemia | Prior hypoglycemic events, low serum Glc, ↓ consciousness |
| Migraine | Prior migraine, preceding aura, headache |
| Hypertensive encephalopathy | Headache, delirium, significant hypertension, cortical blindness, cerebral edema, seizure |
| Wernicke encephalopathy | Alcohol abuse, ataxia, ophthalmoplegia, confusion |
| CNS abscess | Drug abuse, endocarditis, endovascular device implant & fever |
| CNS tumor | Gradual symptom progression, other primary malignancy, seizure at onset |
| Drug toxicity | Lithium, phenytoin, carbamazepine |

[2] Jauch EC, *et al.* Guidelines for the early management of patients with acute ischemic stroke. *Stroke* 2013; 44: 870-947.

# Unusual Causes of Stroke[3]

| Condition | History or PE | Evaluation |
|---|---|---|
| Carotid or vertebral artery dissection | Neck injury or pain, Horner's syndrome ipsi- to dissection, contralateral to stroke | MRI (including T1 axial images of neck), MR angio, contrast angio |
| Aortic dissection | Chest or back pain | TEE, MRI, Chest CT |
| Paradoxical emboli | Co-existing DVT or PE, ASD or VSD findings | Echo with bubble contrast |
| Cardiac source emboli | A-fib, LV dysfunction, recent MI, rheumatic heart disease | Echo (preferably TEE) |
| Endocarditis (bacterial or marantic) | Fever, IVDU, end-stage cancer, heart murmur | Blood cultures, echo |
| Cholesterol emboli | Recent angiography, livedo, ischemic digital lesions | Retinal exam, eosino-philia/uria, ↓ complement |
| Venous sinus thrombosis | Postpartum, OCPs, hypercoagulability | MR venogram, angiography |
| CNS vasculitis | SLE, Behçet's, recent ophthalmic zoster | Angiography, brain or meningeal biopsy |
| Antiphospholipid antibody syndrome | Raynaud's, recurrent spontaneous abortion, prior thromboembolism | Anticardiolipin antibody, lupus anticoagulant |
| Thrombotic thrombo-cytopenic purpura | Thrombocytopenia, azotemia, purpura, fever | Blood smear, renal or skin biopsy |
| Drug-induced vasospasm | Drug abuse (cocaine, amphetamines) | Tox screen, angiography |

---

[3] Sigurdsson AP, *et al.* Stroke. In: Samuels MA, editor. Hospitalist Neurology. *Boston: Butterworth-Heinemann* 1999.

# NIH Stroke Scale[4]

| | |
|---|---|
| Level of consciousness (LOC) | 0: Alert; keenly responsive<br>1: Not alert, aroused by minor stimulation to obey or respond<br>2: Not alert, requires repeated stimulation, or is obtunded and requires strong stimulation to move (non-stereotyped)<br>3: Responds only with reflex motor or autonomic effects or totally unresponsive, flaccid, and areflexic. |
| LOC questions:<br>What is the month?<br>What is your age? | 0: Both correct<br>1: One correct<br>2: Neither correct |
| LOC commands:<br>Open & close your eyes. Grip & release best hand. | 0: Both performed correctly.<br>1: One performed correctly.<br>2: Neither performed correctly. |
| Best gaze | 0: Normal.<br>1: Partial gaze palsy; gaze is abnormal in one or both eyes, but forced deviation or total gaze paresis is not present.<br>2: Forced deviation, or total gaze paresis |
| Visual fields | 0: No visual loss<br>1: Partial hemianopia<br>2: Complete hemianopia<br>3: Bilateral hemianopia (blind including cortical) |
| Facial palsy | 0: Normal symmetrical movements<br>1: Minor paralysis (flattened N-L fold, smiling asymmetry)<br>2: Partial paralysis (total or near-total lower face paralysis)<br>3: Complete paralysis (absent facial movement in upper & lower face |
| Motor arm: Sitting: extend arms palms down, or Supine: extend arms 45°<br>Score each limb | 0: No drift for 10 sec<br>1: Drift; limb holds but < 10 sec<br>2: Some effort against gravity<br>3: No effort against gravity; limb falls<br>4: No movement |

*(Continued)*

---

[4] These are simplified elements of a formal assessment. Readers should first seek training detailed at http://www.ninds.nih.gov/doctors/NIH_Stroke_Scale.pdf

| | |
|---|---|
| Motor leg: 30° supine<br><br>Score each limb | 0: No drift 5 sec<br>1: Drift, limb holds < 5 sec<br>2: Some effort against gravity; limb falls < 5 sec<br>3: No effort against gravity; limb falls immediately<br>4: No movement |
| Limb ataxia: finger-nose or heel-shin if > weakness | 0: Absent<br>1: Present in 1 limb<br>2: Present in 2 limbs |
| Sensory | 0: Normal<br>1: Mild-moderate loss. Pinprick less sharp or loss of superficial pain, but aware<br>2: Severe: Not aware of being touched face, arm, leg |
| Best language | 0: No aphasia<br>1: Mild-moderate aphasia; loss of fluency or facility<br>2: Severe: all communication fragmentary<br>3: Mute, global aphasia |
| Dysarthria | 0: Normal<br>1: Mild-moderate: Slurs at least some words<br>2: Severe: Unintelligible speech >> dysphasia, or mute |
| Extinction and inattention ("Neglect") | 0: No abnormality<br>1: Visual, tactile, auditory, spatial, or personal inattention or extinction to bilateral simultaneous stimulation in 1 sensory modality<br>2: Profound hemi-inattention or extinction to >1 modality; does not recognize own hand or orients to only one side of space |

# Modified Rankin Score[5]

0 No symptoms at all
1 No significant disability despite symptoms; able to carry out all usual duties and activities
2 Slight disability; unable to carry out all previous activities, but able to look after own affairs without assistance
3 Moderate disability; requiring some help, but able to walk without assistance
4 Moderately severe disability; unable to walk without assistance and unable to attend to own bodily needs without assistance
5 Severe disability; bedridden, incontinent and requiring constant nursing care and attention
6 Dead

[5] Bonita R, *et al.* Recovery of motor function after stroke. *Stroke* 1988; 19: 1497-1500.

# Acute Ischemic Stroke[6]

## Background
- 80% of strokes are ischemic
- Consciousness impaired infrequently except posterior circulation strokes
- Unusual features (seizures at onset, impaired consciousness, gradual onset) should prompt search for stroke mimics *(see page 150)*
- Other diagnostic clues: contralateral ptosis/miosis: carotid dissection; fever & valve regurgitation murmur: endocarditis; headache & high ESR: giant cell arteritis

## Emergency evaluation and diagnosis
- Assess NIH Stroke Scale *(see page 152)* and activate emergency stroke service.
- Lab tests (should not delay tPA decisions): Glucose, emergency panel. Others: dabigatran → TT or ECT; intoxication → screen; subarachnoid hemorrhage and no CT blood → lumbar puncture; seizures → EEG).
- Immediate imaging for stroke: non-contrast CT (focal parenchymal hypodensity, Cortical swelling with sulcal effacement, loss of gray-white differentiation, hyperdense MCA sign) or MRI (diffusion-weighting). CT is adequate for lysis decision. Expert interpretation mandatory < 45 min of ED arrival.
- CT/MR angiography recommended if intra-arterial tPA or endovascular therapy contemplated, but should not delay IV tPA. Measures of infarct core & penumbra (*e.g.* ASPECTS score) may guide further therapy.
- Intravenous fibrinolysis recommended based on early imaging findings of ischemia irrespective of extent.

---

[6] Jauch EC, *et al.* Guidelines for the early management of patients with acute ischemic stroke. *Stroke 2013; 44: 870-947;* Powers WJ, *et al.* 2015 Update Guidelines for the Early Management of Patients With Acute Ischemic Stroke Regarding Endovascular Treatment. *Stroke 2015; 46: 3020-3035.*

- Frank hypodensity on non-contrast CT predicts hemorrhage from tPA; tPA should be withheld if > 1/3 MCA territory shows frank hypodensity.

## Management of arterial hypertension in acute ischemic stroke

- Otherwise eligible for tPA except BP > 185/110 mmHg: Labetalol 10-20mg IV over 1-2 min, may repeat once; Nicardipine 5 mg/h IV ↑ 2.5mg/h q 5-15 min until max 15 mg/h or target BP Consider other agents
  (hydralazine, enalaprilat, *etc.*) If BP is not maintained at or below 185/110 mmHg, do not administer tPA
- Maintain BP ≤ 185/110 mmHg during or after tPA or acute reperfusion. Check BP q 15 min x 8, taper. SBP > 180-230 or DBP > 105-120: labetalol 10 mg IV then 2-8 mg/min, OR nicardipine 5 mg/h ↑ 2.5 mg/h q 5-15 min until max 15 mg/h
- Consider nitroprusside if BP not controlled or DBP > 140 mmHg
- If no tPA, lower BP 15% during 1st 24 hr; No BP lowering if SBP > 220 or DBP > 120

## Criteria for tPA for acute ischemic stroke within 3 hrs of onset

<u>Inclusion criteria</u>

- Ischemic stroke causing measurable neurologic deficit; • Symptom onset (or last known normal) < 3 hr before fibrinolysis; • Age ≥ 18 yr

<u>Exclusion criteria</u>

- Head trauma or prior stroke < 3 mo; • Symptoms suggest subarachnoid hemorrhage; • Arterial puncture at noncompressible site < 7 d; • Previous intracranial hemorrhage; • Intracranial neoplasm, AVM, aneurysm; • Recent intracranial or intraspinal surgery; • SBP > 185 or DBP > 110 mmHg; • Active internal bleeding; • Bleeding diathesis: Platelet < 100 k/mm$^3$ (discontinue tPA infusion if already started when this is discovered); • Heparin < 48 hr causing aPTT > ULN; • Anticoagulant with INR > 1.7

or PT > 15 s; • Direct thrombin or Xa inhibitors with elevated sensitive tests (aPTT, INR, ECG, TT, Xa activity); • Glucose < 50 mg/dL; • CT evidence of multilobar infarction (hypodensity > 1/3 of a cerebral hemisphere)

<u>Relative exclusion criteria</u> (tPA may be tolerated despite 1 or more of these)
• Only minor or rapidly improving stroke symptoms (clearing spontaneously); • Pregnancy; • Seizure at onset with postictal residual neurological impairments; • Major surgery or serious trauma < 14 d;
• Recent GI or urinary tract hemorrhage < 21 d;
• Recent acute MI < 3 mo;

## Additional criteria for tPA 3-4.5 hr after onset
<u>Inclusion criteria</u>
• Ischemic stroke causing measurable neurologic deficit;
• Symptom onset (or last known normal) 3-4.5 hr before fibrinolysis

<u>Exclusion criteria</u>
• Age > 80 yr; • Severe stroke (NIHSS > 25); • Oral anticoagulant regardless of INR; • History both diabetes mellitus and prior ischemic stroke

## Eligibility for Endovascular interventions
<u>Incontrovertible:</u>
• Pre-stroke modified Rankin score 0-1 (no significant disability) *(see page 153)*
• tPA within 4.5 hr according to criteria above
• Causative occlusion of internal carotid or proximal (M1) middle cerebral artery
• Age ≥ 18 yr
• NIH Stroke Scale ≥ 6
• Alberta Stroke Program Early CT Score (ASPECTS) ≥ 6
• Groin puncture can begin ≤ 6 hr from symptom onset

Possible benefit (if initiated ≤ 6 hr from onset in selected patients):
- Anterior circulation occlusion with contraindications to tPA
- M2 or M3 middle cerebral, anterior cerebral, vertebral, basilar, or posterior cerebral artery causative occlusion
- ASPECTS < 6, Modified Rankin > 1, and causative ICA or M1 MCA occlusion

Other considerations
- Angioplasty/stenting cervical stenosis or complete occlusions has unproven value in acute ischemic stroke
- Data for intraarterial lysis for MCA occlusion is based on non-tPA agents.
- Endovascular stent-retrievers are preferred;
- Intraarterial tPA may be considered if systemic tPA is contraindicated but consequences are unknown.
- Not recommended to await tPA failure to proceed to endovascular intervention

Early and convalescent management
- Liberal airway support for decreased consciousness or bulbar dysfunction; • Maintain $SaO_2$ ≥ 94% but otherwise do not supplement $O_2$; • Treat fever > 38°C and cause; • Monitor seeking atrial fibrillation; • Arterial hypotension is poorly tolerated; • Use isotonic not hypotonic fluids to correct hypovolemia; • Target glycemia 140-180 mg/dL; • Treat hypoglycemia Glc < 60
- Urgent anticoagulation not recommended, irrespective of tPA; role of newer antithrombins unknown
- Aspirin 325 mg within 24-48 hr of stroke onset but not within 24 hr of tPA
- DVT prophylaxis if immobilized, including SQ antithrombins

- Non-cerebrovascular disease (such as atrial fibrillation) and moderate-severe strokes: urgent anticoagulation not recommended because of ↑ risk of intracranial bleeding
- Assess swallowing before starting to eat or drink; Defer PEG 2-3 wk
- Decompressive hemicraniectomy or evacuation of cerebellar space-occupying infarction are effective/lifesaving in preventing herniation & brainstem compression

**Urgent imaging after symptoms resolve**
- Cervical vessels should be imaged routinely after TIA (*e.g.* ultrasound); • MRI-DWI or contrast CT within 24 hr after TIA; • Intra-cranial MRA, CTA, or if indeterminate DSA in candidates for further intervention for intracranial disease;
- Usefulness of urgent carotid endarterectomy is not clear

# ABCD2 Stroke Risk after TIA[7]

|          | Age      | BP                        | Syndrome             | Duration   | DM      |
|----------|----------|---------------------------|----------------------|------------|---------|
| 0 points | < 60 yr  | < 140/90                  | Other                | < 10 min   | None    |
| 1 point  | ≥60 yr   | SBP ≥ 140 or DBP ≥ 90     | Speech disturbed only| 10-59 min  | Present |
| 2 points |          |                           | Unilateral weakness  | ≥ 60 min   |         |

### Risk of Stroke by ABCD2 score

| Score       | 1-3 (low) | 4-5 (moderate) | 6-7 (high) |
|-------------|-----------|----------------|------------|
| 2-day risk  | 1.0%      | 4.1%           | 8.1%       |
| 7-day risk  | 1.2%      | 5.9%           | 11.7%      |

[7] Johnston SC, *et al*. Validation and refinement of scores to predict very early stroke risk after transient ischaemic attack. *Lancet.* 2007; 369:283-92.

# Coma common reversible causes[8]

## Etiologies

| Structural brain disease | Usual treatment |
|---|---|
| Brain mass | Surgery, treat edema |
| Anoxic-hypoxic brain disease with return of spontaneous circulation after cardiac arrest | Targeted temperature management |
| Raised intracranial pressure | Trendelenburg, mannitol, hypertonic saline, hyperventilation and corticosteroids |
| Subdural or epidural hematoma | Consider evacuation |
| Intracerebral hemorrhage | Correct coagulation and consider evacuation |
| Acute ischemic stroke | Fibrinolytic therapy |
| Hydrocephalus | Ventriculostomy and drainage |
| Cerebral or cerebellar edema from stroke | Decompressive craniectomy |
| Cerebral venous sinus thrombosis | IV heparin and possible endovascular intervention |
| Sepsis | Antimicrobial & surgical treatment; resuscitation and support |
| Pituitary apoplexy | Possible surgery, hormone replacement |
| CNS infection | Antimicrobials, drain abscess, consider steroids for meningitis |
| Non-convulsive or minimally convulsive status epilepticus | Anti-epileptic drugs guided by EEG |
| Diffuse encephalopathy | |
| Hypoglycemia | 50% dextrose |
| Hyperglycemia, diabetic or alcoholic ketoacidosis | IV saline, insulin |
| Hyponatremia | Hypertonic saline |
| Hypercalcemia | IV saline, furosemide, other drugs |
| Hyperammonemia | Treat underlying condition |
| Renal failure | Dialysis |
| Hepatic encephalopathy | Lactulose |
| Thyroid storm | Anti-thyroid medications and β-blockers |
| **Structural brain disease** | **Usual treatment** |
| Myxedema coma | Hormone replacement |
| Adrenal crisis | Hormone replacement and IV fluids |
| Wernicke's encephalopathy | IV thiamine |
| Toxins | |
| Sedative hypnotics (EtOH, barbiturates, benzos) | Supportive care |
| Opioids (heroin, oxycodone, hydrocodone) | Naloxone |

---

[8] Edlow JA, *et al.* Diagnosis of reversible causes of coma. *Lancet* 2014; 384: 2064-2076.

| Structural brain disease | Usual treatment |
|---|---|
| Dissociatives (ketamine, phencyclidine) | Supportive care |
| MDMA | Treat hyponatremia if present |
| Inhalants (Alkyl nitrites, nitrous oxide, hydrocarbons) | Treat methemoglobinemia if present (alkyl nitrites) |
| Toxic alcohols (methanol, ethylene glycol) | Fomepizole, bicarbonate |
| Cyanide, hydrogen sulfide | Hydroxocobalamin for cyanide |
| Carbon monoxide | Hyperbaric oxygen |
| Methemoglobinemia (alkyl nitrites, nitrous oxide, hydrocarbons) | Oxygen and methylene blue |
| Antipsychotics, antidepressants | Bicarbonate (wide QRS interval on ECG) |
| Antiepileptic drugs (phenytoin, valproate, carbamazepine) | Supportive care |
| Clonidine | Naloxone |
| β-adrenergic blockers | Glucagon, high dose insulin/glucose, IV lipid emulsion |
| Cholinergic agents (organophosphates, carbamates) | Atropine, pralidoxime |
| Fumigants (methyl bromide) | Supportive care |
| Hypoglycemics (sulfonylureas, insulin, unripe ackee fruit, meglitinides) | Dextrose, octreotide (sulfonylureas) |
| Herbicides (glufosinate, not glyphosate) | Supportive care |
| Isoniazid | Pyridoxine |
| Salicylates (ASA, oil of wintergreen) | Bicarbonate |
| Neuroleptic malignant syndrome | Benzodiazepines |
| Serotonin syndrome | Benzodiazepines, cyproheptadine |
| Snake envenomation | Antivenins |

## Clues

### History

• <u>Sudden</u> onset: Stroke, seizure, drug overdose; • <u>Gradual</u> onset: Tumor or inflammatory CNS disease; • Preceding <u>thunderclap</u> headache: Subarachnoid hemorrhage, intracranial hemorrhage, cerebral venous sinus thrombosis, pituitary apoplexy, cerebellar stroke; • <u>Seizure</u> at onset: Convulsive or non-convulsive status epilepticus, carbon monoxide, cyanide, hypoglycemics, organophosphates, bu-

propion, γhydroxybutyrate, baclofen, tricyclic antidepressant, carbamazepine, propoxyphene; • History of
<u>cancer</u>: Brain metastases; • <u>Bleeding</u> diathesis: In-
tracerebral hemorrhage, subdural hematoma; • <u>Hy-
percoagulable</u>: Cerebral venous sinus thrombosis;

**Vital signs**

• <u>Fever</u>: Sepsis, focal infection (including CNS),
phencyclidine or ketamine, neuroleptic malignant
syndrome, serotonin syndrome, massive pontine
hemorrhage, subarachnoid hemorrhage, heat stroke,
hypothalamic injury, salicylates, organophosphates,
MDMA; • <u>Hypothermia</u>: Hypoglycemia, alcohol,
sedative/hypnotics, sepsis, myxedema, adrenal crisis,
pituitary apoplexy; • <u>Tachycardia</u>: Antidepressants,
antipsychotic or ketamine, hyper-adrenergic from
acute brain injury; • <u>Bradycardia</u>: β-adrenergic
blockers, clonidine, organophosphates, sedative-
hypnotics, γ-hydroxybutyrate, opioids, intracerebral
pressure (including hydrocephalus); • <u>Hypertension</u>:
Hypertensive encephalopathy, posterior reversible
encephalopathy syndrome, eclampsia, phencyclidine,
ketamine, MDMA, clonidine (early), general acute
CNS disease. HTN+bradycardia may reflect raised
intracranial pressure; • <u>Hypotension</u>: Sepsis, tricyclic
antidepressants, sedative-hypnotic, cyanide,
phenothiazines, and clonidine; • <u>Tachypnea</u>: Early
sepsis, metabolic acidosis, diencephalic damage,
salicylates; • <u>Slow respirations</u>: Sedative-hypnotic or
opioids, organophosphates, terminal event with
medullary involvement;

**Breath**

• Dirty <u>restroom</u>: Uremia; • <u>Fruity</u>: Ketoacidosis;
• Musty or <u>fishy</u>: Hepatic encephalopathy; •<u>Garlic</u>:
Organophosphates;

**General exam**

• <u>Cachexia</u>: Brain metastases; • Tongue laceration: Seizure; • <u>Goiter</u>: Myxedema coma; • <u>Meningismus</u>: Meningitis or subarachnoid hemorrhage; • <u>Ascites</u>, jaundice, caput medusa : Hepatic failure; • <u>Peripheral edema</u>: Renal and hepatic failure, myxedema; • <u>Increased secretions</u>: Organophosphates, ketamine; • <u>Decreased bowel sounds</u>: Opioids; • <u>Increased bowel sounds</u>: Organophosphates;

**Skin**

• <u>Bullae</u>: Coma-bullae non-specific, classically associated with barbiturates; • <u>Puffy</u> cool skin: Myxedema; • <u>Pigmentation</u> of mucosae & creases: $1°$ Adrenal crisis; • <u>Dry</u> skin: Anticholinergic agents such as tricyclic antidepressants and antipsychotics; • <u>Purpura or petechiae</u>: TTP, vasculitis, DIC, mengococcus, rickettsia; • <u>Sweating</u>: Organophosphates, hypoglycemia, thyroid storm, sympathetic hyperactivity, neuroleptic malignant syndrome, serotonin syndrome; • Needle <u>track marks</u>: Opioid overdose; • <u>Jaundice</u>, caput medusa, palmar erythema, spider angiomata: Hepatic encephalopathy;

**Neurological** (seek lateralizing or focal defect or brainstem dysfunction)

• <u>Miosis</u>: Opioid, organophosphates, clonidine; • <u>Mydriasis</u>: Tricyclic antidepressant or MDMA; • Horizontal <u>nystagmus</u>: Ethanol, anti-epileptic drugs, dissociative agents; • Vertical <u>nystagmus</u>: Brainstem lesions, dissociative agents;

**Laboratory findings**

• <u>Hypoglycemia</u>: Insulin, sulfonylureas, β blockers, meglitinides, unripe ackee fruit; • <u>Hyperglycemia</u>: Diabetic ketoacidosis, non-ketotic hyperosmolar coma; • <u>Hyponatremia</u>: MDMA, carbamazepine; • <u>Hypernatremia</u>: Dehydration; • Raised <u>ammonia</u>: Liver failure, valproic acid;

**Blood gases**
- Metabolic acidosis: GOLDMARK; • Respiratory acidosis: CNS depressant (opioid, benzodiazepine, barbiturate), hypercarbic respiratory failure; • Respiratory alkalosis: Central hyperventilation, salicylates; • Methemoglobinemia: Alkyl nitrates; • Anion gap metabolic acidosis: Cyanide, hydrogen sulfide, toxic alcohols, salicylates, all causes of lactic acidosis; • Osmolar gap: Methanol and ethylene glycol;

**ECG**
- Prolonged QTc: Tricyclic antidepressant or antipsychotics, acute structural brain injury; • Prolonged QRS: Tricyclic antidepressants, phenothiazines, carbamazepine, propoxyphene, acute structural brain injury; • Osborne waves: Hypothermia; • Deep T wave inversion: Subarachnoid hemorrhage, acute structural brain injury;

# Status Epilepticus[9]

**Definition:** Continuous generalized convulsive seizure lasting > 5 min, or two seizures without intercurrent recovery to baseline consciousness.

**Precipitants:**
- **Acute structural injury**: Trauma, tumor, stroke, hemorrhage, anoxia
- **Remote structural injury**: Head trauma, prior stroke or neurosurgery, AVM
- **CNS infection**: Encephalitis, meningitis

---

[9] Meierkord H, *et al.* EFNS guideline on the management of status epilepticus in adults. *Eur J Neurol 2010; 17: 348-355;* Riviello JJ, Jr., *et al.* Treatment of status epilepticus. *Neurocrit Care 2013; 18: 193-200;* Brophy GM, *et al.* Guidelines for the evaluation and management of status epilepticus. *Neurocrit Care 2012; 17: 3-23;* Lowenstein DH, *et al.* Status epilepticus. *N Engl J Med 1998; 338: 970-976.*

- **Toxic:** Penicillins, imipenem, fluoroquinolones, metronidazole, isoniazid, cyclic antidepressants, lithium, antipsychotics, lidocaine, bupivacaine, flumazenil, clozapine, meperidine, theophylline, cyclosporine, cocaine
- **Drug withdrawal:** Ethanol, opiates, barbiturates, benzodiazepines (flumazenil)
- **Metabolic:** Hypo- or hyperglycemia; electrolytes (↓ Na, ↓ Ca, ↓ Mg); hyperosmolar state; hypoxia; uremia; hepatic encephalopathy
- **New-onset or inadequately controlled chronic epilepsy:** change in anti-convulsant drug levels (drug interactions, non-adherence, altered absorption); intercurrent infection or metabolic abnormality; ethanol excess or withdrawal

**Complications: High mortality**
- Neuronal death after ≥ 30 min of continuous seizure
- Related also to rhabdomyolysis, aspiration, metabolic/lactic acidosis, respiratory failure, neurogenic pulmonary edema, myocardial injury

**Choice of initial drug therapy**
- Roughly equal efficacy lorazepam vs. phenobarbital vs. phenytoin vs. diazepam followed by phenytoin, in RCT[10]
- Benzodiazepines first line: rapid, accessible, diverse routes (mucosal, IM, IV); limited by sedation/respiratory depression
- Lorazepam and diazepam have similar onset (3 vs. 2 min) but diazepam has shorter $T_{1/2}$ by redistributing out of CNS;
- Benzodiazepines and phenytoin incompatible through same IV
- Fosphenytoin (water-soluble phenytoin prodrug) may be given more rapidly than phenytoin, although time to onset of clinical effect is similar

---

[10] Treiman DM, *et al.* A comparison of four treatments for generalized convulsive status epilepticus. VA Status Epilepticus Cooperative. *N Engl J Med* 1998; 339: 792-798.

## Suggested management algorithm

| Time | Intervention |
|---|---|
| 0-5 min | • Assess ABCs; cardiac monitor • Give $O_2$, intubate if necessary<br>• Obtain history and examine<br>• Start IV and draw chemistries (including Mg/Ca), CBC, renal/liver function, tox screen and anticonvulsant drug levels<br>• Check fingerstick glucose; give thiamine 100 mg IV prior to dextrose<br>• Teat hyperthermia promptly with antipyretics or cooling blankets<br>• **Lorazepam** 0.1 mg/kg IV at 2 mg/min; Diazepam if no IV<br>• Call for EEG monitoring |
| 5-25 min | *If seizures continue:*<br>• **Phenytoin** 20 mg/kg IV at 50 mg/min **or** **fosphenytoin** 20 mg/kg PE* IV at 150 mg/min<br>• Monitor EKG and vital signs |
| 25-30 min | *If seizures continue:*<br>• **Phenytoin** additional 5-10 mg/kg IV at 50 mg/min **or** **fosphenytoin** additional 5-10 mg/kg PE* IV at 150 mg/min |
| 30-50 min | *If seizures continue:*<br>• **Phenobarbital**‡ 20 mg/kg IV at 50-75 mg/min **or**<br>• Consider proceeding directly to anesthesia with **midazolam** or **propofol** or pentobarbital if **(1)** patient already in ICU or **(2)** severe systemic disturbance (*e.g.* hyperthermia) or **(3)** seizures continue > 60-90 min |
| 50-60 min | *If seizures continue:*<br>• **Phenobarbital**‡ additional 5-10 mg/kg IV at 50-75 mg/min |
| > 60 min | *If seizures continue, begin anesthesia in ICU with:*<br>• **Midazolam** 0.2 mg/kg IV followed by 75-100 mcg/kg/hr **or** **propofol** 5 mg/kg IV followed by 30-100 mcg/kg/min<br>• Adjust dosing to EEG response • Additional agents¥<br>• Therapeutic levels will likely require intubation and pressor support<br>• Therapeutic hypothermia proposed for neuroprotection |

\* *Fosphenytoin dispensed in phenytoin equivalents (PE)*
‡ *Barbiturates may require vasopressor support*
¥ *Additional (off-label) agents (off-label) for refractory status epilepticus may include IV pentobarbital, valproate, levetiracetam, magnesium, ketamine, inhalational anesthetics*

# Alcohol Withdrawal Syndromes[11]

**Normal ethanol clearance** $\cong$ 20 mg/dl/hour; more rapid in chronic alcoholics. Symptoms may occur with ethanol level.

| Syndrome | Timing * | % pts# | Symptoms |
|---|---|---|---|
| Minor or early withdrawal | Onset 8 hr Peak 24-36 hr | ≥ 80% | • Irritability/agitation but no delirium<br>• Sleep disturbance, hypervigilance<br>• ↑ HR, ↑ BP, ↑ T°, tremor |
| Hallucinosis | Onset 8 hr Peak 24-72 hr | 25% | • Visual > auditory hallucinations<br>• Sensorium typically intact<br>• Does **not** predict DTs |
| Withdrawal seizures | Onset 8-24 hr Peak 24 hr | 25% | • Generalized tonic-clonic seizures (partial seizures suggest alternative diagnosis)<br>• Status epilepticus uncommon<br>• More common with prior seizures |
| Delirium tremens (DTs) | Onset 48 hr, up to 2 wk | 5% | • Chronic alcoholics only, rare if age < 30<br>• Often precipitated/ masked by other illness<br>• Delirium and clouded consciousness<br>• Hyperadrenergic state (↑ HR, ↑ BP, ↑ T°, tremor, sweating)<br>• Mortality 1- 5% (historically 20%)<br>• Also arrhythmia, sepsis, aspiration, volume depletion, electrolyte disturbances |

\* Timing since last drink of alcohol
# % of pts with chronic alcoholism admitted to hospital not given prophylactic treatment

## Differential diagnosis

• **Drug withdrawal:** barbiturate, benzos, amphetamine, narcotics • **Metabolic:** hypoglycemia, ketoacidosis, thyroid storm, hepatic encephalopathy • **Infection:** sepsis, meningitis • **Toxic:** methanol, ethylene glycol • **Psychiatric**

---

[11] Schuckit MA. Recognition and management of withdrawal delirium (delirium tremens). *N Engl J Med* 2014; 371: 2109-2113; Mayo-Smith MF, *et al.* Management of alcohol withdrawal delirium. *Arch Intern Med* 2004; 164: 1405-1412; Turner RC, *et al.* Alcohol withdrawal syndromes. *J Gen Intern Med* 1989; 4: 432-444.

## Depressant drug therapy

<u>First-line:</u> <u>Benzodiazepines</u> reduce symptoms, seizures, DTs. Use prophylactically and to treat symptoms. Examples:

| Drug | Dose for severe sx | Fixed dose regimen * |
|------|-------------------|---------------------|
| Chlordiazepoxide | 50-100 mg PO q 1 hr | 50 mg q 6 hr x 4, then 25 mg q 6 hr x 8 |
| Diazepam | 10-20 mg PO/IV q 1 hr | 10 mg q 6 hr x 4, then 5 mg q 6 hr x 8 |
| Lorazepam | 2-4 mg PO/IV/IM q 1hr | 2 mg q 6 hr x4, then 1 mg q 6 hr x 8 |
| Oxazepam | 30-60 mg PO q 1 hr | 30 mg q 6 hr x 4, then 15 mg q 6 hr x 8 |

*Taper short-acting agents 30-50%/d after 48 hr; longer acting agents "self-taper"

<u>Second line:</u> Propofol (intubated) or dexmedetomidine.

## Additional management

- Liberal access to ICU; • Administer thiamine & folate prior to glucose;
- Treat <u>hyperadrenergic symptoms</u> with β-blockers or labetalol titrated to HR
- Treat uncontrolled <u>agitation or hallucination</u> with antipsychotics, *e.g.* haloperidol
- All <u>alcoholics</u> should also receive thiamine (100 mg IV qd x 3 d) plus folate
- Hypoglycemia, ↓ Mg and ↓ $PO_4$ common, especially if malnourished

## Other alcohol-related syndromes

- Wernicke's encephalopathy: Triad of ataxia, confusion and ophthalmoplegia & nystagmus. Caused by thiamine deficiency. Risk of irreversible deficits if not treated promptly. Dextrose may exacerbate symptoms if given prior to thiamine.
- Korsakoff's psychosis: chronic dementia with severe memory impairment and confabulation out of proportion to other cognitive deficits. Sensorium usually intact. Also caused by thiamine deficiency; may occur with/without Wernicke's.
- Cerebellar degeneration/ataxia; • Central pontine myelinolysis; • Polyneuropathy

- **Alcohol ketoacidosis:** Binge + starvation, Anion-gap (β-hydroxybutyrate) acidosis, medical precipitant common, profound volume depletion, treat with dextrose, thiamine, volume

# Cerebrospinal Fluid Data[12]

## Total protein in CSF from 4200 patients

| CSF protein range (mg/dL) | < 45 | 45-75 | 75-100 | 100-500 | >500 | Average (mg/dL) |
|---|---|---|---|---|---|---|
| Diagnosis | Percent of patients with each disease | | | | | |
| Purulent meningitis | 2 | 4 | 8 | 64 | 22 | 418 |
| Aseptic meningitis | 46 | 25 | 9 | 21 | - | 77 |
| Brain abscess | 27 | 45 | 9 | 18 | - | 69 |
| TB meningitis | 1 | 12 | 15 | 68 | 5 | 200 |
| Neurosyphilis | 46 | 29 | 11 | 13 | - | 68 |
| Acute ethanol | 92 | 6 | 2 | - | - | 32 |
| Uremia | 58 | 25 | 15 | 2 | - | 57 |
| Myxedema | 24 | 55 | 6 | 16 | - | 71 |
| Epilepsy (idiopathic) | 90 | 10 | - | - | - | 31 |
| Brain tumor | 31 | 25 | 12 | 31 | 1 | 115 |
| Cord tumor | 14 | 11 | 8 | 39 | 28 | 425 |
| Cerebral trauma | 54 | 18 | 9 | 15 | 4 | 100 |
| Multiple sclerosis | 68 | 24 | 6 | 3 | - | 43 |
| Polyneuritis | 51 | 16 | 8 | 21 | 5 | 74 |
| Poliomyelitis | 47 | 28 | 10 | 15 | - | 70 |
| Cerebral thrombosis | 66 | 26 | 4 | 3 | - | 46 |
| Cerebral hemorrhage | 14 | 17 | 13 | 38 | 18 | 270 |

## Hypoglycorrhachia syndromes (CSF/serum glucose < 0.5)

- **Infectious:** • acute bacterial meningitis • TB meningitis • fungal meningitis • amebic/helminthic meningitis (*Naegleria, Cysticerca, Trichinella*) • acute syphilitic meningitis and generalized paresis • specific viruses: lymphocytic choriomeningitis, mumps, herpes simplex/zoster meningitis (uncommon)
- **Rheumatologic:** • meningeal sarcoid • rheumatoid meningitis • SLE myelopathy
- **Hypoglycemia**

---

[12] Adapted from Merritt HH, *et al*. The cerebrospinal fluid. *Philadelphia: Saunders*; 1938.

- **Other:** • leptomeningeal carcinomatosis • subarachnoid hemorrhage • chemical meningitis after intrathecal infusion, myelogram, spinal anesthesia, etc.

## Lumbar fluid changes in 99 patients with brain abscess

| Pressure (cm H$_2$O) | | | Protein (mg/dL) | | |
|---|---|---|---|---|---|
| | < 20 | 38% | | < 50 | 29% |
| | 20-30 | 35% | | 50-100 | 38% |
| | > 30 | 26% | | > 100 | 33% |

| WBCs (per mm$^3$) | | | Glucose (mg/dL) | | |
|---|---|---|---|---|---|
| | < 5 | 29% | | > 40 | 79% |
| | 5-100 | 38% | | < 40 | 21% |
| | > 100 | 33% | One WBC / 500-1000 RBC is normal in CSF | | |

## Admission CSF findings in 35 patients with TB meningitis[13]

| Finding | | Total | Died | Finding | | Total | Died |
|---|---|---|---|---|---|---|---|
| WBCs (per mm$^3$) | < 50 | 3 | 1 | Glucose (mg/dL) | 0-20 | 14 | 5 |
| | 51-200 | 12 | 2 | | 21-40 | 12 | 4 |
| | 201-1,000 | 19 | 7 | | 41-60 | 7 | 1 |
| | > 1,000 | 1 | 1 | | > 60 | 2 | 1 |
| PMNs (%) | 0 | 5 | 2 | Protein (mg/dL) | 0-50 | 5 | 3 |
| | 1-25 | 20 | 5 | | 21-100 | 7 | 1 |
| | 26-50 | 5 | 1 | | 101-200 | 13 | 4 |
| | 51-75 | 4 | 3 | | > 200 | 10 | 3 |
| | > 75 | 1 | 0 | | | | |
| AFB Smear | + | 7 | 1 | TB culture | + | 26 | 8 |
| | - | 25 | 10 | | - | 8 | 3 |
| | Unknown | 3 | 0 | | Unknown | 1 | 0 |

# *Muscle Innervation*[14]

| Muscle | Nerve | Root * |
|---|---|---|
| Trapezius | Spinal accessory | C3-4 |
| Deltoid | Axillary | C5-6 |
| Brachioradialis | Radial | C5-6 |
| Ext carpi radialis longus | Radial | C6-7 |

*(continued)*

[13] Adapted with permission from Hinman AR. Tuberculous meningitis at Cleveland Metropolitan General Hospital 1959 to 1963. *Am Rev Respir Dis* 1967; 95: 670-673.

[14] Adapted from Brain. Aids to the examination of the peripheral nervous system. *London: W.B.Saunders; 2000.* Brazis PW, *et al.* Localization in clinical neurology. *Boston, Mass.: Little, Brown; 1996.*

| Muscle | Nerve | Root * |
|---|---|---|
| Triceps | Radial | C6,7,8 |
| Extensor digitorum | Posterior interosseous | C7-8 |
| Biceps brachii | Musculocutaneous | C5-6 |
| Flexor carpi radialis | Median | C6-7 |
| Abductor pollicis brevis | Median | C8,T1 |
| Opponens pollicis | Median | C8,T1 |
| Flexor digit profundus 1&2 | Anterior interosseous | C7-8,T1 |
| Flexor digit profundus 3&4 | Ulnar | C7-8,T1 |
| Flexor carpi ulnaris | Ulnar | C7-8,T1 |
| Interossei | Ulnar | C8,T1 |
| Abductor digiti minimi | Ulnar | C8,T1 |
| Iliopsoas | Femoral | L2,3,4 |
| Quadriceps femoris | Femoral | L2,3,4 |
| Adductors | Obturator | L2,3,4 |
| Gluteus med/minimus | Superior gluteal | L4,5,S1 |
| Gluteus maximus | Inferior gluteal | L5, S1,2 |
| Hamstrings | Sciatic | L5, S1,2 |
| Gastrocnemius/soleus | Tibial | S1,2 |
| Flexor digitorum | Tibial | L5,S1 |
| Interossei | Med/lateral plantar | L5, S1,2 |
| Tibialis anterior | Deep peroneal | L4,5 |
| Extensor digitorum | Deep peroneal | L4,5 |

\* Bold denotes predominant root

# Spinal & Peripheral Nerves[15]

## Spinal root and selected peripheral nerve lesions

| Root | Disc | Muscles | Weakness | Reflex loss |
|---|---|---|---|---|
| C4 | C3-4 | Trapezius, scalene | Shoulder shrugging | None |
| C5 | C4-5 | Deltoid, biceps, brachioradialis | Shoulder abduction, external rotation of arm, elbow flexion | Biceps, brachio-radialis |
| C6 | C5-6 | Brachioradialis, biceps, pronator teres, extensor carpi radialis | Elbow flexion, arm pronation, finger and wrist extension | Biceps, brachio-radialis |
| | | Radial nerve injuries produce similar findings except brachioradialis function is normal | | |

(continued)

[15] Adapted from *Aids to the examination of the peripheral nervous system. London: W.B.Saunders; 2000.* Brazis PW, *et al.* Localization in clinical neurology. *Boston, Mass.: Little, Brown; 1996.*

| Root | Disc | Muscles | Weakness | Reflex loss |
|------|------|---------|----------|-------------|
| C7 | C6-7 | Triceps, pronator teres, extensor digitorum | Elbow extension, finger and wrist extension | Triceps |
| C8 | C7-T1 | Flexor digitorum, flexor/abductor pollicis, interossei | Long flexors of fingers, intrinsics of hand (finger abduction, palmar abduction of thumb) | Finger flexor |
| | | Ulnar nerve injuries similar but also weaken thumb adductor | | |
| T10 | T9-10 | | Beevor's sign (sit-up → umbilicus pulled up-wards) | |
| L2 | L1-2 | Iliopsoas | Hip flexion | Cremaster |
| L3 | L2-3 | Iliopsoas, adductors | Hip flexion, thigh ad-duction | Knee jerk |
| L4 | L3-4 | Quadriceps, sartorius, tibialis anterior | Knee extension, ankle dorsiflexion and inversion | Knee jerk |
| | | Femoral nerve injury limited to knee extension; associated hip flexion and adduction weakness localizes to plexus | | |
| L5 | L4-5 | Glutei, hamstrings, tibialis, extensor hallux/digiti, peronei | Thigh adduction and internal rotation, knee flexion, plantar and dorsiflexion of ankle and toes | None |
| | | Deep peroneal nerve weakness limited to ankle/toe extensors; posterior tibial nerve lesions weaken foot inversion | | |
| S1 | L5-S1 | Gluteus maximus, hamstrings, soleus, gastrocnemius, extensor digitorum, flexor digitorum | Hip extension, knee flexion, plantar flexion of ankle and toes | Ankle jerk |
| S2 | S1-2 | Interossei | Cupping and fanning of toes | |

## Anterior aspect: Peripheral segments on left Spinal segments on right [16]

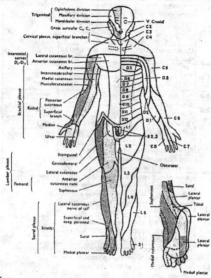

Key
C: cervical
D: dorsal (thoracic)
L: lumbar
S: sacral

[16] Figures reproduced from *Brain's Diseases of the Nervous System*, 10th ed. Walton J (ed.). p 47, by permission of Oxford University Press.

## Posterior aspect: Spinal segments on left, Peripheral on right

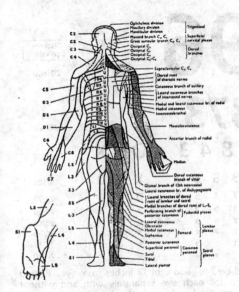

# *Visual Acuity Screen*[17]

| | Distance Equivalent |
|---|---|
| **96** | 20/800 |
| **873** | 20/400 |
| **2 8 4 3    O X X** | 20/200 |
| **6 3 8 5 2    X O O** | 20/100 |
| **8 7 4 5 9    O X O** | 20/70 |
| **6 3 9 2 5    X O X** | 20/50 |
| **4 2 8 3 6 5  O X O** | 20/40 |
| 3 7 4 2 5 8  X X O | 20/30 |
| 9 3 7 8 2 6  X O O | 20/25 |
| 4 2 8 7 3 9  o o x | 20/20 |

Hold card in good light 14 inches from eye. Record vision for each eye separately with and without glasses. Presbyopic patients should read through bifocal segment. Check myopes with glasses only.

**Pupil Diameter (mm)**

. •₂ ❸ ➍ ➎ ➏ ❼ ❽ ❾

[17] Adapted with permission from J.G. Rosenbaum MD, Pocket Vision Screen, Beachwood, Ohio.

# Folstein Mini-Mental State[18]

| Area | Points | Task |
|------|--------|------|
| Orientation | 5 | Year, Season, Date, Day, Month |
| | 5 | State, County, Town, Hospital, Floor |
| Registration | 3 | Patient recites three consecutive objects named (*e.g.* ball, flag, tree) |
| Attention, Calculation | 5 | Serial 7's (5 responses: 93-86-79-72-65); alternatively spell "WORLD" backwards |
| Recall | 3 | Three objects registered above, 5 minutes later |
| | 2 | Name a pencil and watch |
| | 1 | Repeat "No ifs, ands, or buts." |
| Language | 3 | 3-stage command: "Take a paper in your right hand, fold it in half, and put it on the floor." |
| | 1 | Read and obey, "Close your eyes." |
| | 1 | Write a sentence |
| | 1 | Copy design below |
| Level of consciousness | 0 | Assess along continuum: Alert-Drowsy-Stuporous-Comatose |

Close Your Eyes

***Interpretation:*** Score 0-23 (or score of 23-29 with altered mental status) suggests cognitive dysfunction. No identifiable pathology in 1/3.

---

[18] Folstein MF, *et al.* "Mini-mental state". A practical method for grading the cognitive state of patients for the clinician. *J Psychiatr Res* 1975; 12: 189-198.

# Glasgow Coma Scale[19]

| Best Motor Response | Obeys | 6 |
|---|---|---|
| | Localizes | 5 |
| | Withdraws | 4 |
| | Abnormal flexion | 3 |
| | Extends | 2 |
| | Nil | 1 |
| Verbal Response | Oriented | 5 |
| | Confused conversation | 4 |
| | Inappropriate words | 3 |
| | Incomprehensible sounds | 2 |
| | Nil | 1 |
| Eye Opening | Spontaneous | 4 |
| | To speech | 3 |
| | To pain | 2 |
| | Nil | 1 |

| Score | Mortality in Head Injury |
|---|---|
| 3-5 | > 60% |
| 6-8 | 12% |
| 9-12 | 2% |

[19] Teasdale G, et al. Assessment of coma and impaired consciousness. A practical scale. Lancet 1974; 2: 81-84; Jennett B, et al. Predicting outcome in individual patients after severe head injury. Lancet 1976; 1: 1031-1034.

# Neurologic Prognosis After Cardiac Arrest[20]

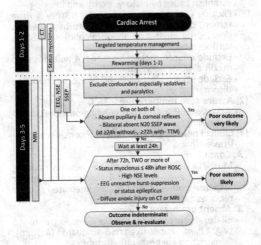

NSE=Neuron specific enolase blood chemistry
SSEP=Somatosensory evoked potential after median nerve stimulation

[20] Sandroni C, *et al.* Prognostication in comatose survivors of cardiac arrest. *Resuscitation* 2014; 85: 1779-1789; Circulation. 2015 Nov 3; 132(18 Suppl 2):S465-82. Callaway CW, *et al.* Part 8: Post-Cardiac Arrest Care. *Circulation.* 2015; 132:S465-482.

# Brain Death Exam[21]

**(1) Establish an irreversible and proximate cause of coma:**
- Establish cause by history, exam, and imaging
- Exclude CNS depressant drugs by history & drug screen, clearance 5 half-lives, note hypothermia slows drug clearance. Blood alcohol < 0.08% is sufficient.
- Exclude neuromuscular blockade: 4 twitches with maximal ulnar nerve stimulation
- Exclude severe electrolyte, acid-base, or endocrine disorder.

**(2) Assure core temperature > 36°C**
- Achieve SBP ≥ 100 mmHg using vasopressors if necessary

**(3) Clinical neurologic assessment if considered irreversible**

**A. Coma.**
- Must lack responsiveness to noxious stimuli, including eye opening & movement, motor response other than spinally-mediated (latter requires expertise)

**B. Absent brainstem reflexes.**
- Bilateral absence of pupillary response to to bright light. Pupils fixed mid- or dilated (4-9mm). Constriction suggests intoxication.
- Ocular movement absent with head-turning (only if c-spine is stable), no eye deviation with 50mL ice $H_2O$ each ear 5 min apart (head of bed 30°, observe 1 min)

**B. Absent brainstem reflexes**
- Absent corneal reflex (cotton swab, squirts of water)
- Absent facial muscle movement to noxious stimuli (*e.g.* supraorbital ridge & TMJ)

---

[21] Wijdicks EF, *et al.* Evidence-based guideline update: determining brain death in adults. *Neurology 2010; 74: 1911-19180;* Booth CM, *et al.* Assessing outcome for comatose survivors of cardiac arrest. *JAMA 2004; 291: 870-879.*

- Absent gag (pharyngeal blade) and tracheal reflexes (suctioning to carina).

**C. Apnea**
- Achieve systolic blood pressure ≥100 mmHg with vasopressors
- Preoxygenate > 10 min with 100% $O_2$ to PaO2 > 200 mmHg
- Reduce ventilator frequency to 10/min
- Set positive end-expiratory pressure (PEEP) to 5 cm and assure no desaturation
- Assure eucapnea with arterial blood gas, as long as pulse-oximetry > 95% oxyHb
- Disconnect from ventilator, supplying 100% $O_2$ > 6 L/min at level of carina
- Examine for respiratory movements (abdominal or chest) for 8-10 min
- Abort if SBP < 90 mmHg • Abort if pulse-oximetry < 85% oxyHb for > 30 sec. Repeat with T-piece/CPAP 10 cm H2O, and 100% $O_2$ 12 L/min
- If no respiratory drive, repeat ABG after 8 min
- Apnea test suggest brain death if no respiratory movements, $PaCO_2$ ≥ 60 mmHg or increases ≥ 60 mmHg over baseline.
- Inconclusive tests may be repeated with longer observation (10-15 min), adequate preoxygenation

**(4) Ancillary tests are optional**
- EEG, angiography, HMPAO SPECT brain blood flow, transcranial Doppler ultrasound, MRI all can support inconclusive clinical testing

**Pitfalls in diagnosis of brain death (consider confirmatory testing)**
Severe facial trauma • Pre-existing pupillary abnormalities • Toxic levels of drugs affecting neuromuscular or ocular function (sedatives, aminoglycosides, tricyclics, anticholinergics, anticonvulsants, chemotherapeutic agents, neuromuscular blockers) • Chronic $CO_2$ retention (COPD, sleep apnea, morbid obesity)

**Observations compatible with brain death**
(*i.e.* diagnosis still valid)
• Respiratory-like movements (shoulder elevation, back arching) *without* tidal volumes • Sweating, blushing, tachycardia • Normal BP without pressors • Spinal reflexes (*e.g.* Babinski) or spontaneous limb movements

**Consider Organ Donation!** http://www.unos.org

# Pulmonary

## *Chest Anatomy - Radiographs*[1]

**Posteroanterior Chest View**

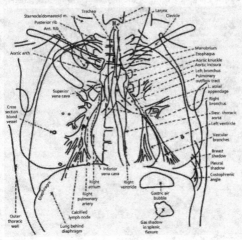

1 Meschan I. *Roentgen Signs in Diagnostic Imaging*, 2nd ed.
Boston: Saunders; 1987. Reproduced with permission.

## Lateral Chest View

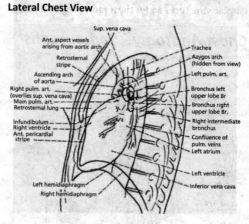

## Cardiac structures on PA chest radiograph

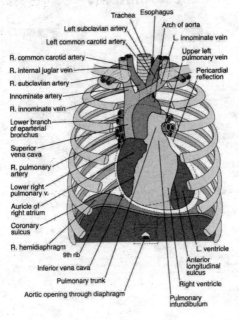

# Chest Anatomy - CT[2]

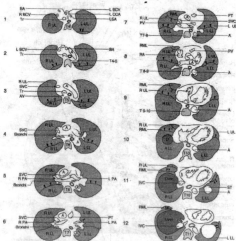

A=Aorta; AV=Azygos vein; BA=brachiocephalic artery; BCV=brachiocephalic vein; CCA=common carotid artery;
D=Diaphragm; IVC=Inferior vena cava; L=left; LA=L atrium; LL=Lower Lobe; PA=Pulmonary artery; PT=Pulmonary trunk;
R=right; RML=R middle lobe; ST=Stomach; SVC= Superior vena cava; Tr=Trachea; UL=Upper Lobe

[2]Meschan I. *Roentgen Signs in Diagnostic Imaging*, 2nd ed. Boston:
Saunders; 1987.  Reproduced with permission.

# Bronchoscopic Anatomy[3]

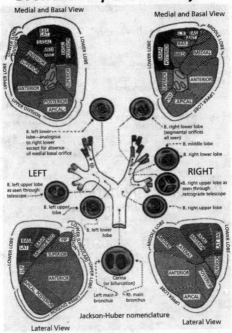

Jackson-Huber nomenclature

[3] Am J Surg. 1955 Feb;89(2):319-23. Segmental bronchi and the bronchopulmonary segments. JACKSON CL. Adapted with permission by Elsevier. See also HG Colt, "Bronchoscopy step by step" at www.bronchoscopy.org

# Fleishner Score: Incidental Pulmonary Nodules[4]

Applies to newly- and incidentally-detected nodule on CT age > 35 yr

Size=average of length + width

| Nodule size | Low-risk patient (No or minimal smoking or other risk factors) | High-risk patient (Smoking or other risk factors) |
|---|---|---|
| ≤ 4-6 mm | No-follow-up: risk < baseline CT of asymptomatic smoker | FU 12 mo, if no change → no follow-up unless ground-glass or partly solid |
| > 4-6 mm | FU 12 mo, if no change → no follow-up unless ground-glass or partly solid | Initial FU CT 6-12 mo then 18-24 mo. If no change → no follow-up unless ground-glass or partly solid |
| > 6-8 mm | Initial FU 6-12 mo and then 18-24 mo if no change | Initial FU CT 3-6 mo then 9-12 and 24 mo if no change |
| > 8 mm | FU CT 3, 6, 24 mo; Dynamic contrast CT, PET, biopsy | |

# Pulmonary Function Testing[5]

## Lung volumes in a healthy individual

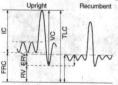

**Abbreviations**

**ERV** = expiratory reserve vol.
**FEF$_{25-75\%}$** = forced expiratory flow from 25-75% VC
**FEV$_1$** = forced expiratory volume in 1 second
**FRC** = functional residual capacity
**FVC** = forced vital capacity
**IC** = inspiratory capacity
**RV** = residual volume
**TLC** = total lung capacity
**VC** = vital capacity

---

[4]  MacMahon H, et al. Guidelines for management of small pulmonary nodules detected on CT scans. Radiology 2005; 237: 395-400.

[5]  Figures courtesy of John L. Johnson, MD. Pellegrino R, et al. Interpretative strategies for lung function tests. Eur Respir J 2005; 26: 948-968.

## Spirometry Patterns

- **Normal:** FVC, $FEV_1$, PEFR and $FEF_{25-75\%} > 80\%$ predicted; $FEV_1/FVC > 95\%$ predicted • Can be seen with intermittent disease (*e.g.* asthma), pulmonary emboli and pulmonary vascular disease

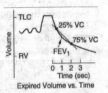

- **Obstructive:** Obstruction to airflow prolongs expiration • $FEV_1/FVC < 95\%$ predicted and increased airway resistance • Differential diagnosis: asthma, COPD, bronchiectasis, cystic fibrosis, bronchiolitis, proximal airway obstruction

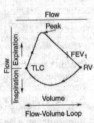

Flow-Volume Loop

- **Restrictive:** Reduced volumes without changes in airway resistance • Decreased VC and TLC, $FEV_1$ and FVC decreased proportionately ($FEV_1/FVC$ ratio $> 95\%$ pred)

- Must confirm lung volumes by helium dilution or plethysmography (reduced FVC on spirometry not specific for restrictive disease, although normal FVC predicts normal TLC) • Differential diagnosis: interstitial disease, CHF, pleural disease, pneumonia, neuromuscular disease, chest wall abnormalities, obesity, lung resection

- **Bronchodilator response:** Positive if FVC or $FEV_1$ increase 12% *and* $\geq 200$ mL

- **Poor effort:** Most reliably diagnosed by technician performing test rather than spirometric values. Forced expiratory time (FET) < 6 sec suggests inadequate expiration.

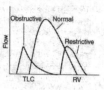

## Grading of PFT abnormalities

| Obstruc-tion | % Predicted FEV₁ |
|---|---|
| Mild | 70 - 100% |
| Moderate | 60 - 69% |
| Mod-severe | 50 - 59% |
| Severe | 35 - 49% |
| Very Severe | < 35% |

| Restriction | % Predicted TLC# | % Predicted FVC |
|---|---|---|
| Mild | 70% - LLN* | 70% - LLN* |
| Moderate | 50 - 69% | 60 - 69% |
| Mod-severe | | 50 - 59% |
| Severe | < 50% | 35 - 49% |
| Very Severe | | < 35% |

\# TLC superior to FVC in assessing restrictive disease
\* LLN = lower limits of normal

## Diffusion capacity (DL_CO)

- Evaluates • Pulmonary vascular disease; • pulmonary hemorrhage; • change in collagen-vascular or drug-related pulmonary disease. Adjust for hemoglobin & alveolar ventilation (VA). Imprecise.
- **Reduced:** emphysema, interstitial lung disease, pulmonary embolism, pulmonary vascular disease, lung resection, severe CHF
- **Increased:** pulmonary hemorrhage, mild CHF
- **Normal:** asthma, chronic bronchitis, chest wall and pleural abnormalities, neuromuscular disease

## Mechanical upper airway obstruction

- Diagnosed by contour of flow-volume loop and re-producibility (see below). If suspected, alert technician to emphasize performance of inspiratory limb of loop.
- **Variable extrathoracic:** • Uni-/Bilateral vocal cord paralysis • Rheumatoid arthritis • Post-intubation vocal cord adhesions • Obstructive sleep apnea • Burns

- **Variable intrathoracic:** Non-circumferential tracheal tumors making walls "floppy" • Relapsing polychondritis; • Tracheomalacia after surgery; • Mainstem bronchus tumors
- **Fixed upper airway obstruction:** Benign stricture after prolonged intubation • Tracheal tumor; • Goiter; • Small endotracheal or tracheostomy tube; • Bilateral stenosis of mainstem bronchi (rare)

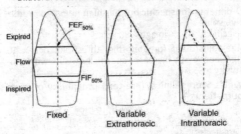

## Predicted Peak Expiratory Flow (L/min)[6]

| Age | Women (height in inches) | | | | | Men (height in inches) | | | | |
|-----|-----|-----|-----|-----|-----|-----|-----|-----|-----|-----|
| (yrs) | 55 | 60 | 65 | 70 | 75 | 60 | 65 | 70 | 75 | 80 |
| 20 | 390 | 423 | 460 | 496 | 529 | 554 | 602 | 649 | 693 | 740 |
| 25 | 385 | 418 | 454 | 490 | 523 | 543 | 590 | 636 | 679 | 725 |
| 30 | 380 | 413 | 448 | 483 | 516 | 532 | 577 | 622 | 664 | 710 |
| 35 | 375 | 408 | 442 | 476 | 509 | 521 | 565 | 609 | 651 | 695 |
| 40 | 370 | 402 | 436 | 470 | 502 | 509 | 552 | 596 | 636 | 680 |
| 45 | 365 | 397 | 430 | 464 | 495 | 498 | 540 | 583 | 622 | 665 |
| 50 | 360 | 391 | 424 | 457 | 488 | 486 | 527 | 569 | 607 | 649 |
| 55 | 355 | 386 | 418 | 451 | 482 | 475 | 515 | 556 | 593 | 634 |
| 60 | 350 | 380 | 412 | 445 | 475 | 463 | 502 | 542 | 578 | 618 |
| 65 | 345 | 375 | 406 | 439 | 468 | 452 | 490 | 529 | 564 | 603 |
| 70 | 340 | 369 | 400 | 432 | 461 | 440 | 477 | 515 | 550 | 587 |

6 Leiner GC, *et al.* Expiratory Peak Flow Rate. Standard Values for Normal Subjects. Am Rev Respir *Dis* 1963; 88: 644-651.

## *Pulmonary thromboembolism (PE)*[7]

### Symptoms are nonspecific[8]

One study of PE vs no-PE when suspected in an emergency department: no difference in incidence of dyspnea, pleuritic chest pain, cough, substernal chest pain, fever, hemoptysis, syncope, unilateral leg pain, and unilateral leg swelling.

### D-dimer is nonspecific but has high negative predictive value[9]

Specificity ~ 10% in age > 80 yr.

Age-adjustment for abnormal threshold: age x 10 µg/L above 50y increases specificity > 35% with sensitivity > 95%

### Well's Score: clinical (pre-test) probability of PE in outpatients[10]

| Criterion | Points | Criterion | Points |
|---|---|---|---|
| Suspected DVT | 3 | Previous DVT or PE | 1.5 |
| Alternative diagnosis less likely than PE | 3 | Hemoptysis | 1 |
| Heart rate > 100 bpm | 1.5 | Malignancy | 1 |
| Immobilization or surgery in past 4 wk | 1.5 | | |

[7] Konstantinides SV, *et al.* 2014 ESC guidelines on the diagnosis and management of acute pulmonary embolism. *Eur Heart J* 2014; 35: 3033-3069, 3069a-3069k; Konstantinides S, *et al.* Management of venous thrombo-embolism. *Eur Heart J* 2014; 35: 2855-2863.

[8] Pollack CV, *et al.* Clinical characteristics, management, and outcomes of patients diagnosed with acute pulmonary embolism in the emergency department. *J Am Coll Cardiol* 2011; 57: 700-706.

[9] Schouten HJ, *et al.* Diagnostic accuracy of conventional or age adjusted D-dimer cut-off values in older patients with suspected venous thromboembolism. *BMJ* 2013; 346: f2492.

[10] Wells PS, *et al.* Derivation of a simple clinical model to categorize patients probability of pulmonary embolism. *Thromb Haemost* 2000; 83: 416-420.

| Category | Total Points | % of patients | Probability of PE |
|---|---|---|---|
| Low probability | 0-2 | 40 % | 3.6 % |
| Moderate probability | 3-6 | 53 % | 20.5 % |
| High probability of PE | > 6 | 7 % | 66.7 % |

## Revised Geneva Score[11]: clinical (pre-test) probability of PE

| Criterion | Points |
|---|---|
| Previous DVT or PE | 3 |
| HR 75-98/min | 3 |
| HR ≥95/min | 5 |
| Surgery or fraction < 1month | 2 |
| Hemoptysis | 2 |
| Active cancer | 2 |
| Unilateral leg pain | 3 |
| Pain on leg vein palpation & unilateral edema | 4 |
| Age≥65y | 1 |

| Category | Score | PE Incidence |
|---|---|---|
| Low | 0-3 | ~ 10% |
| Intermediate | 4-10 | ~ 30% |
| High | ≥ 11 | ~ 65% |

## Diagnostic Algorithm

<u>Shock or hypotension</u>: seek immediate diagnosis

- Option: Bedside echocardiography evidence of acute pulmonary hypertension & RV dysfunction;
- Option: CT angiography (CTA)
- Option: Compression ultrasound + high clinical suspicion

These are sufficient to confirm or exclude diagnosis and proceed to therapy

<u>Hemodynamically stable</u>:

- High probability of PE: CTA
- Low-intermediate probability of PE: D-Dimer, and if positive, CTA

---

[11] Le Gal G, *et al.* Prediction of pulmonary embolism in the emergency department: the revised Geneva score. Ann Intern Med 2006; 144: 165-171.

**Prognostication**

- Simplified PE severity index (PESI)[12]: Any of
  (• Age > 80; • Chronic heart failure or COPD; • HR ≥
  110/min; • BP < 100; $SaO_2$ < 90%) confers 30-day
  mortality of 10.9% vs 1%. In these patients, echo RV
  dysfunction and troponin evidence of acute RV
  overload favor aggressive observation and management.

**Treatment**[13]

<u>Hemodynamically unstable ("massive PE"):</u>

- Immediate anticoagulation
- Fibrinolysis if bleeding risk is acceptable
- Surgical embolectomy if bleeding risk unacceptable
  or failed fibrinolysis
- Catheter-based (mechanical, ultrasound-mediated
  fibrinolysis, catheter-fibrinolysis) is an acceptable
  alternative to surgery above
- Hemodynamic support: Norepinephrine, epinephrine, dobutamine, and volume may each have
  a role. Percutaneous RV mechanical circulatory
  support devices are commercially available.
- Respiratory support: PEEP can exacerbate LV
  underfilling

<u>Intermediate-risk ("submassive PE"):</u>

- Definition: hemodynamically stable + simplified
  PESI ≥ 1 + (abnormal troponin/proBNP ± echo RV
  dysfunction)
- Inpatient anticoagulation and monitoring for
  hemodynamic deterioration
- Concomitant RV dysfunction & elevated tro-
  ponin/proBNP suggest instability, and may justify
  reperfusion, although this remains controversial.
- Hemodynamic deterioration should trigger prompt
  reperfusion as for "massive PE"

[12] Jimenez D, *et al*. Simplification of the pulmonary embolism severity index for prognostication in patients with acute symptomatic
pulmonary embolism. *Arch Intern Med 2010; 170: 1383-1389.*
[13] Kearon C, et al. Antithrombotic Therapy for VTE Disease: CHEST
Guideline. *Arch Chest 2016; 149: 315-352.*

## Anticoagulation in low- or intermediate-risk patients

- If <u>cancer-associated thrombosis</u>: LMWH recommended over warfarin or NOACS
- If <u>not cancer-associated</u>: dabigatran, rivaroxaban, apixaban, or edoxaban preferred over warfarin.
  - If dabigatran or edoxaban, first initiate parenteral LMWH or UFH
  - If rivaroxaban or apixaban, do NOT use parenteral LMWH or UFH
  - If warfarin (target INR 2.5, range 2.0-3.0), first overlap LMWH or UFH.
- Note avoid rivaroxaban, apixaban, dabigatran, edoxaban in CLCr < 30mL/min
- <u>Malignancy</u> or pregnancy: unfractionated heparin
<u>Duration</u> of anticoagulation: • Provoked/reversible cause: 3 mo; • Unprovoked: ≥ 3 mo especially if low bleeding risk; • Second unprovoked: indefinite; • Malignancy: 3-6 mo or indefinite or until cure
- Venous insufficiency is a common morbid late complication
- Surveillance is warranted for chronic thromboembolic pulmonary hypertension, an uncommon serious treatable late complication.

# Pleural Fluid Analysis[14]

### Light's Criteria

| | |
|---|---|
| • Any of following **excludes** transudates (98% sensitive, 83% specific for exudative effusion): <br> (1) Pleural/serum LDH > 0.6 <br> (2) Pleural LDH > 2/3 upper limit for serum LDH <br> (3) Pleural/serum Protein > 0.5 | **Always transudative** <br> • CHF <br> • Cirrhosis with ascites <br> • Hypoalbuminemia <br> • Nephrotic syndrome <br> **Sometimes transudative** <br> • PE (35%) <br> • Malignancy (10%) <br> • Sarcoidosis <br> **Sometimes exudative** <br> • Diuretic-treated CHF |

[14] Light RW. Pleural effusion. *N Engl J Med* 2002; 346: 1971-1977; Wilcox ME, *et al.* Does this patient have an exudative pleural effusion? *JAMA* 2014; 311: 2422-2431.

- Serum albumin - pleural albumin < 1.2 g/dL: more specific for exudate (92%) but should not be used as only criteria

**Appearance**
- Bloody: fluid hematocrit < 1% is non-significant; hematocrit 1-20 suggests cancer, PE, trauma; fluid hematocrit > 50% of serum hematocrit suggests hemothorax
- Turbid despite centrifugation suggests chylothorax or pseudochylothorax
- Putrid: suggests empyema • Viscid: mesothelioma
- "Anchovy paste" or "chocolate sauce": amebiasis

**Additional useful tests for exudative effusions**

*Leukocytes*
- Total WBC count rarely helpful
- Neutrophil predominance: pneumonia, PE, pancreatitis, abdominal abscess
- Lymphocyte predominance: tumor, TB, resolving acute process
- Eosinophilia (> 10%): blood or air in pleural space • asbestos • drug reaction • paragonimiasis • uncommon in TB and malignancy

*Cytology (cell block and smears)*
- 70% yield for metastatic adenocarcinoma, lower for other cancers
- Mesothelial cells nonspecific, but > 2-3% makes tuberculosis unlikely
- Send flow cytometry if lymphoma suspected

*Glucose:*
- Glucose < 60 mg/dL: complicated parapneumonic effusion (< 40 mg/dL → chest tube) • neoplasm • TB • hemothorax • Churg-Strauss syndrome • rheumatoid arthritis or SLE • paragonimiasis

*Amylase:*
- Elevated in: esophageal perforation • pancreatic disease • malignancy

### Triglycerides
- Elevated in chylous effusions: > 110 mg/dl is 100% specific, < 50 mg/dl excludes

### LDH:
### Nonspecific indicator of inflammation pH
- < 7.0: complicated parapneumonic effusion (empyema)
- < 7.20: empyema, systemic acidosis, esophageal rupture, rheumatoid arthritis, TB, neoplasm, hemothorax, paragonimiasis

**Tests for tuberculous pleuritis:** • Interferon $\gamma$ > 140 pg/mL; • PCR; • Pleural biopsy with AFB stain and culture; • Adenosine deaminase > 40 unit/L (neither sensitive nor specific)

**Avoid reexpansion pulmonary edema:** keep pleural pressure > -20cm $H_2O$

**Useful tests for effusion of unknown cause**

• PE evaluation; • Serial LDH measurement (reassuring if decreasing); • Thoracoscopy

# Pulmonary Hypertension[15]

## WHO Classification

| |
|---|
| **Group 1:** Pulmonary arterial hypertension (PAH) Idiopathic PAH (classic); Heritable (familial, specific genetic defects); Drug -and toxin- induced; Associated with HIV; with Portal hypertension (aka porto-pulmonary HTN); with Congenital heart disease; with Schistosomiasis; 1': Pulmonary veno-occlusive disease or pulmonary capillary hemangiomatosis; 1'': Persistent pulmonary hypertension of the newborn |
| **Group 2:** PH due to left heart disease L heart failure: with reduced LV ejection fraction; with preserved LV ejection fraction; Valvular heart disease; Acquired or congenital LV inflow or outflow (valve) disease or cardiomyopathy |

[15] Galie N, et al. 2015 ESC/ERS Guidelines for the diagnosis and treatment of pulmonary hypertension. Eur Respir J 2015; 46: 903-975; Simonneau G, et al. Updated clinical classification of pulmonary hypertension. J Am Coll Cardiol 2013; 62: D34-41.

| **Group 3:** PH due to lung disease |
| --- |
| COPD; Interstitial lung disease (ILD); Other mixed restrictive & obstructive; Sleep apnea disorders; Alveolar hypoventilation; High altitude; Developmental lung disease |

| **Group 4:** Chronic thromboembolic pulmonary hypertension (CTEPH) |
| --- |

| **Group 5:** Other |
| --- |
| Hematologic disorders: chronic hemolytic (eg sickle-cell) anemia; myeloproliferative disease; splenectomy |
| Systemic: Sarcoidosis, LAMS, histiocytosis |
| Metabolic: Glycogen storage; Gaucher; Thyroid disease |
| Other: Tumor obstruction; Fibrosing mediastinitis; Chronic renal failure; Segmental PH |

**Hemodynamic Confirmation Required (echo alone not sufficient):** mPAP > 25 mmHg at rest + PAWP or LVEDP ≤ 15 mmHg + PVR > 3 Wood Units

Controversies: • Use of pulmonary vascular resistance (PVR) combining PA pressure with cardiac output (high PVR at high versus low CO are different); • Correction for BSA (PVR index vs PVR, analogous to cardiac index vs CO, higher BSA → higher PVRI); • Correction for systemic blood pressure (high PA pressure with high versus low SBP are different)

**Treatment:** Seek expert guidance[16]
**General:** Avoid pregnancy; Supervised exercise training; Immunization; Oral anticoagulation for most Group 1 & Group 4; Oxygen; Digoxin?; Diuretics
**Vasoreactivity test:** If vasoreactive during cath, initiate long-acting calcium channel blocker; otherwise monotherapy 4-6 wk with advanced agent
**Strategy:** Functional Class IV or rapid-progression: prostanoid. Class II-III: oral agent (if not calcium blocker then consider ambrisentan+tadalafil[17]). Refractory: combination therapy.

---

[16] Galie N, et al. Updated treatment algorithm of pulmonary arterial hypertension. J Am Coll Cardiol 2013; 62: D60-72; Taichman DB, et al. Pharmacologic therapy for pulmonary hypertension in adults. Chest 2014; 146: 449-475.

[17] Galie N, et al. Initial Use of Ambrisentan plus Tadalafil in Pulmonary Arterial Hypertension. N Engl J Med 2015; 373: 834-844.

**Advanced agents:**

*(See Pulmonary Vasodilators on page 348.)*

- Prostanoids: First-line for functional class IV or rapid progression. Epoprostenol/prostacyclin IV; Treprostinil (IV, SQ, inhaled); Iloprost (inhaled). Limitations: Short half-life, pain, variability, R → L IV embolization in Eisenmenger
- Endothelin receptor antagonists: Oral nonselective bosentan; oral selective ET1A: ambrisentan, macicentan. Limitations: Teratogenic; Hepatotoxicity; Edema
- PDE5 inhibitors: Sildenafil, tadalafil
- Guanylate cyclase stimulant: Riociguat: effective groups 1 & 4; Contraindicated pregnancy

# Preoperative Pulmonary Evaluation[18]

## ACCP Risk for perioperative pulmonary complications

| | |
|---|---|
| • COPD<br>• Age > 65<br>• Congestive heart failure<br>• ASA Class ≥ II<br>• Tobacco smoking<br>• Poor nutrition, albumin < 3.5 g/dL<br>• Obstructive sleep apnea<br>• Symptomatic pulmonary hypertension, or 6 min walk < 330 m | • Thoracic, abdominal, neuro, head & neck, vascular, AAA repair<br>• Surgery > 3 hr<br>• Emergency surgery<br>• General anesthesia<br>• Long-acting neuromuscular blockers<br>• Interstitial lung disease |

[18] Qaseem A, *et al.* Risk assessment for and strategies to reduce perioperative pulmonary complications for patients undergoing noncardiothoracic surgery: ACP guideline. *Ann Intern Med* 2006; 144: 575-580. Smetana GW, *et al.* Preoperative pulmonary risk stratification for noncardiothoracic surgery. *Ann Intern Med* 2006; 144: 581-595.

## American Society of Anesthesia (ASA) Classification

| ASA Class | Definition | Pulm. complication risk |
|---|---|---|
| I | Normal healthy patient | 1.2% |
| II | Mild systemic disease | 5.4% |
| III | Systemic disease that is not incapacitating | 11.4% |
| IV | Incapacitating systemic disease, constant threat to life | 10.9% |

## Respiratory Failure Index[19]: Another predictor of post-op respiratory failure

| Factor | Score | Factor | Score |
|---|---|---|---|
| Type of surgery | | Albumin < 3 g/dL | 9 |
| AAA | 27 | BUN > 30 mg/dL | 8 |
| Thoracic | 21 | History of COPD | 6 |
| Neuro, upper abdomen, peripheral vascular | 14 | Functional status: partially or fully dependent | 7 |
| Neck | 11 | Age > 70 | 6 |
| Emergency surgery | 11 | Age 60-69 | 4 |

| Class | Points | Post-op respiratory failure |
|---|---|---|
| 1 | ≤ 10 | 0.5 % |
| 2 | 11-19 | 1.8 % |
| 3 | 20-27 | 4.2 % |
| 4 | 28-40 | 10.1 % |
| 5 | > 40 | 26.6 % |

## Interventions to reduce perioperative risk
- Reduce or treat incisional pain.
- Postoperative lung expansion maneuvers: <u>deep breathing</u> exercises, incentive <u>spirometry</u>, and/or continuous positive airway pressure (CPAP)

---

[19] Arozullah AM, *et al.* Multifactorial risk index for predicting postoperative respiratory failure in men after major noncardiac surgery. *Ann Surg* 2000; 232: 242-253.

- Selective use of <u>postoperative nasogastric tube drainage</u> to avoid pneumonia and atelectasis in (1) postoperative nausea/vomiting, (2) unable to tolerate oral intake, (3) symptomatic abdominal distention
- Preoperative <u>spirometry</u> and <u>radiography</u> should be applied only in at-risk patients
- Routine PA catheterization and total parenteral nutrition are not indicated
- Preoperative smoking cessation, supportive data are marginal
- Inhaled ipratropium if clinically apparent COPD; β-agonists if wheezing
- Oral or inhaled steroids if COPD or asthma and pulmonary function not optimal (does not increase rate of infections or other postoperative complications, but potential adrenal suppression if ≥ 20 mg/d prednisone for ≥ 3 wk)
- Defer elective surgery for acute exacerbations of pulmonary disease
- In high risk patients consider laparoscopic or shorter (< 3 hr) procedures, and spinal/epidural or regional rather than general anesthesia
- Avoid long-acting neuromuscular blockers (*e.g.* pancuronium)

**Lung cancer resection surgery[20]**

- Age is not a contraindication; • ABG hypercapnia ($pCO_2$ > 45 mm) & hypoxemia are insufficiently predictive
- Preoperative cardiac assessment if planned pneumonectomy, established or suspected cardiac or coronary disease, or functional capacity < 4 mets.

---

[20] Brunelli A, *et al.* Physiologic evaluation of the patient with lung cancer being considered for resectional surgery: Diagnosis and management of lung cancer, 3rd ed. Chest 2013; 143: e166S–190S.

- Perform <u>spirometry</u>. • Perform nuclear <u>perfusion</u> (Q) scan if pneumonectomy planned. • Calculated <u>predicted postop</u> (ppo) $FEV_1$ & $ppoDL_{CO}$ as product of baseline x ppo intact perfusion.
- <u>Low risk</u> (predicted mortality < 1%):
  - $ppoFEV_1$ and $ppoDL_{CO}$ > 60%, or
  - $ppoFEV_1$ and $ppoDL_{CO}$ between 30-60%, and climbs 3 flights stairs (22m) or
  - cardiopulmonary exercise test (CPEX) $VO_2max$ > 20 mL/kg/min
- <u>Moderate risk</u>
  Not low risk, or high-risk findings on preoperative cardiac assessment, or
  $ppoFEV_1$ and $ppoDL_{CO}$ < 30%, and CPEX $VO_2max$ 10-20 mL/kg/min
- <u>High risk</u> (mortality > 10%, high morbidity and predicted loss of function)
  Moderate risk + CPEX $VO_2max$ < 10 mL/kg/min
  High risk implies surgical goals be tempered, or nonsurgical options considered

# Renal

*See Acid-Base Rules of Thumb, Acid-Base Map, & Other Renal Equations on pp 1-2.*

## Gaps and Deltas

### Useful equations

Anion gap = $[Na^+] - [HCO_3^-] - [Cl^-]$ = Unmeasured anions – unmeasured cations

Albumin-derived anion gap = $[2 \times albumin] + [0.5 \times PO_4]$

Reflects non-volatile acids (*e.g.* lactate)

Calculated osmolarity = $2 \times Na^+ + \dfrac{Glucose}{18} + \dfrac{BUN}{2.8} + \dfrac{Ethanol}{4.6}$

Osmolar gap = Measured osmolality – calculated osmolarity

$\Delta$gap ("gap gap") = $\dfrac{\Delta \text{Anion gap (measured-average normal)}}{\Delta HCO_3 \text{ (average normal-measured)}} \approx \dfrac{(AG-12)}{(24-HCO_3)}$

### Causes of an elevated anion gap (> 7-11 mEq/L)

| Acidosis present ("MUDPILES") | Acidosis present ("GOLDMARK")[1] |
|---|---|
| • Methanol<br>• Uremia<br>• Diabetic ketoacidosis (also alcoholic and starvation ketoacidosis)<br>• Paraldehyde<br>• Iron or isoniazid<br>• Lactic acidosis (including metformin)<br>• Ethylene glycol<br>• Salicylates<br>• Other: CO, CN⁻, H₂S, sulfur, theophylline, toluene (glue-sniffing) | • Glycols (ethylene & methylene)<br>• Oxoproline chronic acetaminophen metabolite in malnourished women<br>• L-lactate<br>• D-lactate<br>• Aspirin<br>• Renal failure<br>• Ketoacidosis whether diabetic, alcoholic, or starvation |

*Acidosis absent:* • Dehydration; • Alkalosis; • Sodium salts of unmeasured anions (citrate, lactate or acetate); • Certain antibiotics (sodium penicillin, carbenicillin); • Decrease in unmeasured cations (severe combined hypomagnesemia, hypocalcemia and hypokalemia)

---

[1] Mehta AN, *et al.* GOLD MARK. *Lancet* 2008; 372: 892.

201

## Causes of a decreased anion gap (< 3 mEq/L)

| Increase in unmeasured cations | Decrease in unmeasured anions |
|---|---|
| • Hypercalcemia; • Hypermagnesemia; • Hyperkalemia; • Lithium intoxication; • Monoclonal IgG gammopathy; • Bromide or • Iodide intoxication | • Hypoalbuminemia; • Dilution |

## Causes of an elevated osmolar gap (> 10 mOsm/l)

| With anion gap metabolic acidosis | No metabolic acidosis |
|---|---|
| • Ethylene glycol; • Methanol; • Formaldehyde; • Uremia without dialysis (atypical); • Paraldehyde; • Alcoholic or diabetic ketoacidosis; • Lactic Acidosis; • Propylene glycol | • Isopropyl alcohol; • Diethyl ether; • Mannitol; • Severe hyperlipidemia or hyperproteinemia; • Sorbitol, glycerin or fructose; • Radiocontrast |

## Causes of a "gap gap" or "delta-delta" gap

| Δ Anion gap/Δ HCO₃ < 1 | Δ Anion gap/Δ HCO₃ > 1.5 |
|---|---|
| • Non-anion gap acidosis or chronic respiratory alkalosis superimposed on anion gap acidosis, e.g. diarrhea and ESRD, salicylate intoxication • DKA with urinary ketone losses • Some cases of chronic renal failure | • Metabolic alkalosis superimposed on anion gap acidosis, e.g. vomiting and diabetic ketoacidosis • Lacidosis (typical Δ/Δ = 1.6) |

## Pearls

- Absent anion gap does not exclude typical causes of anion gap acidosis, i.e. DKA[2]. Correction for albumin increases diagnostic sensitivity.
- No cause found for elevated anion gap in 1/3 of patients
- Large anion gaps (e.g. > 30 mEq/L) are usually DKA, lactic acidosis, alcohols. Higher anion gaps correlate with increased severity of illness.
- "Normal" anion gap is lab-dependent. The traditional value of 12 ± 4 mEq/L is high compared with results from newer instruments (normal range

---

[2] Kamel KS, et al. Acid-base problems in diabetic ketoacidosis. N Engl J Med 2015; 372: 546-554.

$7 \pm 4$ mEq/L). Time trends (comparison with individual patient baseline) may be useful.

- High AG and normal lactate in alcoholism suggests AKA, not detected using urinary ketone tests for acetoacetate

# Metabolic Acidosis[3]

| Mechanism | Anion Gap? | Etiology |
|-----------|------------|----------|
| Increased acid production | Usually | • See anion gap acidoses (page 201) |
| Loss of $HCO_3$ | No | • Dilutional from IV fluids<br>• GI loss: diarrhea, ileal loop or tube/fistula drainage<br>• Renal loss: carbonic anhydrase inhibitors, Type II RTA (proximal) |
| Decreased renal acid excretion | No | • Type I RTA (distal)<br>• Type IV RTA (hypoaldosteronism)<br>• Chronic renal failure (some cases) |
| Exogenous acid | No | • Hyperalimentation<br>• Lysine or arginine therapy<br>• Toluene ingestion (hippuric acidosis)<br>• Ammonium chloride or hydrochloride ingestion |

## Non-anion gap metabolic acidosis
AKA "hypochloremic." Use below surrogate measures of urinary ammonium to determine intrinsic versus extrinsic renal causes

|  | Urinary anion gap | Urinary osmolal gap |
|--|-------------------|---------------------|
| Calculation | Urinary AG = $U_{Na} + U_K - U_{Cl} - U_{HCO3}$ | Urinary OG = Measured osmolality $-2 \times [U_{Na} + U_K]$ + urine urea nitrogen (mg/dL)/2.8 + urine glucose (mg/dL)/18 |
| Unreliable in | • Urine pH > 6.5' • other urine anions (ketoacids, ASA, D-lactate, high-dose PCN); • urinary Na < 20 mmol/L. | Heavy nondissociated acid load, e.g. ketoacidosis |
| Intrinsic renal disease | Urinary AG > 0 | Urinary osmolal gap < 40 mmol/L |
| Normal or GI $HCO_3$ loss | Urinary AG < 0 | Urinary osmolal gap > 40 mmol/L |

[3] Berend K, et al. Physiological approach to assessment of acid-base disturbances. N Engl J Med 2014; 371: 1434-1445.

## Bicarbonate therapy
*(See Bicarbonate on page 268.)*

- Should be limited to following scenarios:
  - Bicarbonate loss (*e.g.* diarrhea, Type I RTA) with moderate acidosis
  - Severe acidosis (*e.g.* pH < 7.15 or $HCO_3$ < 8 mEq/L) with hemodynamic consequences. Bicarbonate generally temporizes only until underlying cause is treated. Effectiveness in organic acidoses (*e.g.* diabetic ketoacidosis) unclear. Do not use in hypercarbic respiratory acidosis.
  - Salicylate or tricyclic antidepressant toxicity (even if not acidemic)
- Bicarbonate should be administered as near-isotonic infusion (rather than bolus) to achieve pH > 7.20 or $HCO_3$ > 8-10 mEq/L *(See bicarbonate page 268)*.
- Calculated $HCO_3$ deficit (mEq)
    = [$HCO_3$ deficit/liter] x $V_D$ of $HCO_3$
    = [(target− actual $HCO_3$)] x [ (0.4 + 2.6/$HCO_3$) x lean body wt]

  **Note:** Calculation is approximate; assess actual pH change 30 min after infusion

- Consequences of $NaHCO_3$ administration include hypernatremia, volume overload, "overshoot" alkalosis, paradoxical worsening of intracellular acidosis.

# *Lactic Acidosis*[4]

### Diagnosis: lactate > 2 mEq/L.
- Suspect in $\Delta$Anion gap/$\Delta HCO_3$ > 1; Exclude other causes of AG acidosis (page 201)

### Type A: Tissue hypoxia
- Etiology: • Shock Sepsis • Anemia/hemorrhage • CO poisoning • $PaO_2$ < 30mmHg • Anemia Hb < 5g/dL
- Acidosis itself worsens cardiac, renal and hepatic dysfunction, which may in turn increase lactate production or reduce clearance

---

4  Kraut JA, *et al*. Lactic acidosis. *N Engl J Med* 2014; 371: 2309-2319.

## Type B: No tissue hypoxia

- Liver disease: Fulminant or acute-on-chronic liver failure (*e.g.* sepsis, GI bleeding). Correcting hypoglycemia may improve acidosis. Portends very poor prognosis.
- Diabetic or alcoholic ketoacidosis: Etiology unclear; may relate to hypoglycemia or thiamine deficiency in alcoholics
- Seizures: Usually transient unless underlying Type A mechanism
- Renal failure
- Cancer (Warburg effect): Usually acute leukemia or lymphoma
- Drugs: • propofol (high dose) • propylene glycol diluent (IV diazepam, lorazepam, esmolol, nitroglycerin, phenytoin; yields D- and L-lactate) • metformin (treat with dialysis) • nitroprusside (cyanide toxicity) • β-adrenergic agonists • Lactated Ringer's solution • nucleoside reverse transcriptase inhibitors (*e.g.* didanosine and stavudine) • vasopressors • fructose and sorbitol (used as insulin-sparing sugars in TPN) • isoniazid • paraldehyde • salicylates
- Toxins: • ethanol • methanol • cyanide • cocaine (restraints, seizures)
- Short gut syndrome: D-lactate absorbed but not metabolized
- Hereditary enzyme deficiencies (gluconeogenesis, pyruvate oxidation, mitochondrial myopathies)

## Management

- Treat underlying condition; Target central venous oximetry > 70% (unproven)
- Consider NaHCO3 to keep pH > 7.15-7.20 *(see bicarbonate therapy, above).*

**Note:** increased pH may cause increased lactate production.

# Renal Tubular Acidosis[5]

Consider in unexplained acidosis with normal anion gap

|  | Distal (Type 1) | Proximal (Type 2) | Hyporeninemic hypoaldosteronism (Type 4) |
|---|---|---|---|
| Defect | Inadequate distal acidification | Inadequate proximal $HCO_3$ reabsorption | Aldosterone deficiency or resistance |
| Etiology | • Autoimmune dis. (esp. Sjögren's) • Hypercalciuria • Cirrhosis • Obstruction • Sickle cell disease • 1° hyperPTH • Amphotericin B, lithium | • Myeloma • Heavy metals • Drugs: carbonic anhydrase inhibitors, ifosfamide, nucleoside-analog reverse transcriptase inhibitors; topiramate; • Cystinosis • Idiopathic | • Diabetic nephropathy • Chronic interstitial nephritis • Drugs: ACE inhibitors, NSAID, heparin, K+-sparing diuretics, cyclosporine |
| Urine pH | > 5.3 (exclude urease-splitting pathogen and extreme hypovolemia) | > 5.3 if above re-absorptive threshold; otherwise < 5.3 | Usually < 5.3 |
| Untreated plasma [$HCO_3$] | May be < 10 mEq/L | > 12 mEq/L | > 15 mEq/L |
| Fractional [$HCO_3$] excretion when plasma [$HCO_3$] > 20 mEq/L | < 3% | > 15-20% | < 3% |
| Plasma [$K^+$] | Usually low-normal; ↑in Na-reabsorption defect (sickle-cell, obstruction) | Normal or ↓ | ↑ |
| Urine anion gap (< 0 in GI loss) | Positive | Variable | Positive |

*(Continued)*

[5] Gluck SL. Acid-base. *Lancet* 1998; 352: 474-479; Rodriguez Soriano J. Renal tubular acidosis. *J Am Soc Nephrol* 2002; 13: 2160-2170.

|  | Distal (Type 1) | Proximal (Type 2) | Hyporeninemic hypoaldosteronism (Type 4) |
|---|---|---|---|
| Diagnosis | Response to $NaHCO_3$[a] or $NH_4Cl$[b] | Response to $NaHCO_3$[a] | ↓ Plasma aldosterone & renin activity; TTKG < 5[c] suggestive in ↑ K |
| Amount $NaHCO_3$ to normalize plasma [$HCO_3$] | 1-3 mEq/kg/d | 10-15 mEq/kg/d | 1-3 mEq/kg/day or correct hyperkalemia |
| Other complications | • Nephrocalcinosis<br>• Nephrolithiasis | • Rickets (children)<br>• Osteomalacia<br>• Osteopenia | • Hyperkalemia |

a: Response to **bicarbonate** (0.5-1.0 mEq/kg/hr infusion): Urine pH and fractional excretion of bicarbonate will remain constant in RTA type I, but will rise markedly in RTA type II

b: Response to **$NH_4Cl$** (0.1 g/kg): Urine pH in RTA type I should remain above 5.3 despite a 4-5 mEq/L fall in plasma $HCO_3$ within 4-6 hr

c: TTKG = trans-tubular $K^+$ gradient = $(U_{K+} \times P_{Osm}) \div (P_{K+} \times U_{Osm})$, valid only if $U_{osm} > P_{Osm}$

# Metabolic Alkalosis[6]

| Mechanism | Cause |
|---|---|
| Gastrointestinal $H^+$ loss | • Vomiting or nasogastric suction<br>• Antacids (in uremia or milk-alkali syndrome) |
| Renal $H^+$ loss | • 1° mineralocorticoid excess (including hyper-aldosteronism, Cushing's, licorice)<br>• Diuretics (loop or thiazide)<br>• Post-hypercapnia<br>• Hypercalcemia due to milk-alkali syndrome |
| Intracellular shift of $H^+$ | • Hypokalemia |
| Alkali administration | • Citrate (transfusions), acetate (parenteral nutrition), bicarbonate (sports doping) |
| Volume contraction | • Massive diuresis<br>• Vomiting or NG suction in achlorhydria<br>• Sweat losses in cystic fibrosis<br>• Villous adenoma or laxative abuse |

6 Rose BD, et al. Clinical physiology of acid-base and electrolyte disorders 5/e. NY McGraw-Hill; 2001; Adrogue HJ, et al. Management of life-threatening acid-base disorders. N Engl J Med 1998; 338: 26-34; Galla JH. Metabolic alkalosis. J Am Soc Nephrol 2000; 11: 369-375; Gluck SL. Acid-base. Lancet 1998; 352: 474-479.

## Urine chloride concentration in diagnostic evaluation

| < 10-25 mEq/L (→ Cl-depletion) | > 40 mEq/L (→ renal K-wasting) |
|---|---|
| Vomiting or NG suction | 1° mineralocorticoid excess |
| Diuretics (after administration) | Diuretics (while in effect) |
| Laxative abuse | Alkali load |
| Post-hypercapnia | Bartter's or Gitelman's syndrome |
| Cystic fibrosis | ($U_{K+}$ > 30 mEq/L) |
| Low chloride intake | Severe hypokalemia (serum K$^+$ ≤ 2.0 mEq/L) or hypomagnesemia |

## Consequences of severe alkalosis (pH > 7.60 or $HCO_3$ > 45 mEq/L)

- Reduced cerebral blood flow • Tetany, seizures, lethargy, delirium and stupor
- Reduced coronary blood flow • Predisposition to refractory arrhythmias
- Reduced threshold for angina • Hypoventilation • ↓ K, ↓ Mg, ↓ Ca, ↓ $PO_4$

### Treatment

- Treat underlying cause (*i.e.* suppress vomiting)
- Saline infusion if volume depleted
- KCl supplementation if hypokalemic or ongoing K$^+$ losses (*e.g.* diuretics)
- H$_2$-blocker or proton pump inhibitor if ongoing nasogastric suction
- Addition of potassium-sparing diuretics to diuretic regimen; as second-line alternative consider addition of acetazolamide (250-375 mg PO qd-bid) with caution regarding "overshoot" acidosis and excessive K$^+$-wasting
- Severe alkalosis (*e.g.* pH > 7.60 or $HCO_3$ > 45 mEq/L): Consider infusion of 0.1-0.2 N HCl (= 100-200 mEq H$^+$ per liter) via central line at rate ≤ 0.2 mEq/kg/hr
- Calculated HCl deficit (mEq) = $HCO_3$ excess/L x $V_D(HCO_3)$ = (actual $HCO_3$ - 40) x (lean body wt x 0.5)

**Note:** calculation is approximate, and actual change in pH should be re-assessed 30 min after completing infusion

- Consider hemodialysis for severe alkalosis in setting of cardiac or renal dysfunction

# *Hyponatremia*[7]

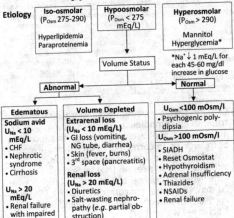

**Etiology**

| Iso-osmolar ($P_{Osm}$ 275–290) | Hypoosmolar ($P_{Osm}$ < 275 mEq/L) | Hyperosmolar ($P_{Osm}$ > 290) |
|---|---|---|
| Hyperlipidemia Paraproteinemia | | Mannitol Hyperglycemia* |

*$Na^+$ ↓ 1 mEq/L for each 45–60 mg/dl increase in glucose

Volume Status

**Abnormal** ← → **Normal**

**Edematous**

Sodium avid
$U_{Na}$ < 10 mEq/L
• CHF
• Nephrotic syndrome
• Cirrhosis

$U_{Na}$ > 20 mEq/L
• Renal failure with impaired $H_2O$ excretion

**Volume Depleted**

Extrarenal loss
($U_{Na}$ < 10 mEq/L)
• GI loss (vomiting, NG tube, diarrhea)
• Skin (fever, burns)
• 3rd space (pancreatitis)

Renal loss
($U_{Na}$ > 20 mEq/L)
• Diuretics
• Salt-wasting nephropathy (*e.g.* partial obstruction)
• ↓ Aldosterone

$U_{Osm}$ <100 mOsm/l
• Psychogenic poly-dipsia

$U_{Osm}$ >100 mOsm/l
• SIADH
• Reset Osmostat
• Hypothyroidism
• Adrenal insufficiency
• Thiazides
• NSAIDs
• Renal failure

[7] Adrogue HJ, *et al.* Management of life-threatening acid-base disorders. *N Engl J Med* 1998; 338: 26-34.

## Differentiating causes of chronic hyponatremia

| Etiology | $U_{Osm}$ (mOsm/l) | $U_{Na}$ (mEq/l) | Response to $H_2O$ restriction | Response to $H_2O$ challenge |
|---|---|---|---|---|
| SIADH | > 100 | > 20 | $U_{Osm}$ remains high $P_{Osm}$ rises slowly | Water retained ($U_{Osm}$ remains high, $P_{Na}$ & $P_{Osm}$ fall) |
| Reset Osmostat | Variable (often > 100) | > 20 | $U_{Osm}$ rises or remains high $P_{Osm}$ rises slowly | Water load excreted ($U_{Osm}$ falls, $P_{Na}$ stays at "set point") |
| Psychogenic polydipsia | < 100 | Variable | $U_{Osm}$ stays low $P_{Osm}$ rises rapidly | No change |

## Treatment:[8]

(1) Classify. <u>Severe</u> = vomiting, cardiorespiratory distress, deep somnolence, seizures, coma. <u>Moderately-severe</u> = nausea, confusion, headache. In both, risk of uncorrected brain edema exceeds risk of iatrogenic osmotic demyelination

(2) Immediately raise serum [Na] by 5mEq/L
• 3% hypertonic saline 150 mL (or 2mL/kg) IV over 20 min. {If severe, concurrently recheck [Na] during 2-3 subsequent cycles of 3% saline until target ↑ achieved within 1 hr}

(3) If symptoms are not improved: • IV saline 3% aiming for 1 mmol/h increase in serum [Na] according to formula:
• Predicted ↑ [Serum Na] after 1L 3% saline = {513 - [Serum Na]} ÷ {1 + estimated body water}, where estimated body water (L) = body weight (kg) x water fraction, and water fraction= Male: 0.5 elderly, 0.6 non-elderly; Female: 0.45 elderly, 0.5 non-elderly.

(4) Stop 3% saline when symptoms improve OR ↑ [Na] > 10 mEq/L or [Na] reaches 130 mEq/L.

(5) If symptoms only mild, treat precipitants and restrict fluid intake

(6) No clear role for demeclocycline, lithium, vasopressin receptor antagonists ('vaptans).

---

[8] Spasovski G, et al. Clinical practice guideline on diagnosis and treatment of hyponatraemia. Eur J Endocrinol 2014; 170: G1-47.

## Osmotic demyelination (pontine or extrapontine myelinolysis)

- Symptoms of lethargy (after initial improvement during treatment), then dysarthria, pseudobulbar palsy (chewing, swallowing, slurred speech), spastic quadriparesis
- Associated with too-rapid $Na^+$ correction > 12 mEq/L/24 hr, chronic hyponatremia
- MRI or CT edema may confirm diagnosis

# Syndrome of Inappropriate Antidiuretic Hormone (SIADH)[9]

### Diagnosis (all of following):
- Decreased serum osmolality (< 275 mOsm/L)
- Urine osmlolality > 100 mOsm/L during serum hypotonicity
- Euvolemia: No signs of volume depletion (orthostasis, tachycardia, dry membranes); No signs of excess extracellular fluid (edema, ascites)
- Urinary sodium > 40 mmol/L during normal salt intake
- Normal thyroid and adrenal function
- No recent diuretic use
- Additional features: • Plasma uric acid < 4 mg/dL; • BUN < 10 mg/dL; • $FE_{Na}$ < 1%; • $FE_{UN}$ > 55%; Failure to correct hyponatremia with 0.9% saline; Correction with fluid restriction; • Abnormal <u>water load test</u>: < 80% urination of 20 mL/kg water taken over 4 hr, or failure to dilute urine < 100 mOsm/L

- **Etiology of SIADH**
- Malignancy & ectopic ADH: lung small-cell & mesothelioma; oropharynx; GI; GU; thymoma; lymphoma; Ewing sarcoma
- Pulmonary: bacterial/viral pneumonia, abscess, TB, aspergillus, asthma, CF, positive-pressure ventilation

---

9 Ellison DH, *et al.* The syndrome of inappropriate antidiuresis. *N Engl J Med* 2007; 356: 2064-2072.

- CNS: meningitis, encephalitis, abscess, RMSF, AIDS; intracranial mass; stroke (caution not to confuse with "cerebral salt wasting" & volume depletion); trauma; hydrocephalis; multiple sclerosis; Guillain-Barre; delirium tremens;
- Drugs: antipsychotics; nicotine; narcotics; NMDA "ecstasy," chlorpropramide; SSRIs; tricyclics; carbamazepine; vincristine; ifosamide; cyclophosphamide; NSAID; exogenous AVP: desmopressin, oxytocin, vasopressin
- Other: general anesthesia, severe nausea, pain, stress; marathon runners; intentional water excess

# Hypernatremia[10]

## Etiology

| Mechanism | Cause |
|---|---|
| Inadequate $H_2O$ intake | • Lack of thirst • Poor intake or access to water |
| Renal losses of hypotonic fluid | • Central or nephrogenic diabetes insipidus (DI) <br> • Osmotic diuresis (glucose, urea, mannitol) <br> • Loop diuretics • Post-obstructive diuresis <br> • Polyuric phase of ATN • Intrinsic renal disease |
| Gastrointestinal losses of hypotonic fluid | • Vomiting • Nasogastric drainage <br> • Enterocutaneous fistula <br> • Osmotic diarrhea (e.g. lactulose, malabsorption) |
| Other loss | • Insensible (skin, respiratory) • Burns <br> • Excessive sweating |
| Hypertonic $Na^+$ gain ($U_{Na+} > 800$ mEq/L) | • Hypertonic saline or bicarbonate <br> • Hypertonic feedings (TPN, tube feeds) <br> • Ingestion of NaCl or sea water <br> • Hypertonic enemas or dialysis |

## Diabetes insipidus (DI)

- Most patients with DI have symptoms of polyuria (rather than hypernatremia) **unless** there is impaired thirst mechanism or access to free water

---

[10] Adrogue HJ, et al. Hypernatremia. N Engl J Med 2000; 342: 1493-1499; Rose BD, et al. Clinical physiology of acid-base and electrolyte disorders 5/e. McGraw-Hill; 2001.

- Diagnosis: low $U_{Osm}$ (< 300 mOsm/l) despite adequate stimulus to ADH secretion, *i.e.* ↑ serum osmolarity or sodium concentration after water deprivation
- After administration of ADH (10 mcg nasal ddAVP or 5 units vasopressin SQ) patients with **central** DI will appropriately increase $U_{Osm}$ by ≥ 50%, while patients with **nephrogenic** DI will have little or no response
- Hypernatremia with mid-range urine osmolality (300-800 mOsm/l) may be seen in: • Central DI with marked volume contraction • Partial DI (central or nephrogenic) • Osmotic diuresis, in which case daily solute excretion ($U_{Osm}$ x daily urine volume) is typically > 1000 mOsm

## Etiology of diabetes insipidus

| Central DI | Nephrogenic DI |
|---|---|
| • Idiopathic • After trauma or surgery<br>• Space-occupying sellar lesions: cysts, tumors, histiocytosis, TB, sarcoid<br>• Inflammatory lesions: encephalitis, meningitis, Guillain-Barré, Lyme<br>• Vascular: aneurysm, infarction, Sheehan syndrome | • Renal disease: medullary sponge kidney, amyloid, myeloma, Sjögren<br>• Electrolytes: hypercalcemia, hypokalemia<br>• Drugs: lithium, foscarnet, ampho B, methoxyflurane<br>• Congenital |

## Clinical manifestations

- Symptoms related to osmotic decrease in brain volume and include lethargy, confusion, and irritability. More advanced symptoms include seizures, coma, and intracerebral bleeding due to rupture of cerebral veins following brain shrinkage
- Symptoms are related to both rapidity of onset (acute >> chronic) and severity of hypernatremia (symptoms rare with [$Na^+$] < 160 mEq/L)
- High mortality with [$Na^+$] > 180 mEq/L, or [$Na^+$] > 160 mEq/L for > than 48 hr

## Treatment

- Free water deficit (in liters $H_2O$) = [($P_{Na+}$ ÷ 140) −1] x lean body weight (kg) x 0.4

- Actual fluid correction may need to account for ongoing losses
- Goal should be $[Na^+] \leq 145$ mEq/L
- If hypernatremia is chronic or of unclear duration, rate of correction should be $\leq 0.5$ mEq/L per hour, or $\leq 10\text{-}12$ mEq/L per day
- In acute hypernatremia *e.g.* accidental sodium loading occurring over several hours, $[Na^+]$ may be lowered at up to 1 mEq/L per hour
- Overly rapid correction may lead to cerebral edema producing seizures, irreversible neurologic damage or death
- May use D5W, ½ or ¼ normal saline as replacement fluid; normal saline generally ineffective unless profound volume depletion and should be avoided

# *Hypokalemia*[11]

## Etiology

| | |
|---|---|
| Trans-cellular shift | • Alkalosis<br>• Drugs: β-agonists (including pressors, bronchodilators, tocolytic agents and nasal decongestants), insulin over-dose, methylxanthines, verapamil or chloroquine overdose<br>• Correction of megaloblastic anemia<br>• Periodic paralysis (familial or thyrotoxic)<br>• Delirium tremens |
| Renal loss (TTKG* > 3) | • Drugs: diuretics, fludrocortisone, high-dose steroids, high-dose penicillins, drugs causing hypomagnesemia (ampho B, aminoglycosides, cisplatin, foscarnet)<br>• Metabolic alkalosis • Magnesium depletion<br>• Mineralocorticoid excess (1° aldosteronism, Cushing's, congenital adrenal hyperplasia, renovascular HTN, lico-rice)<br>• RTAs (type I > II) • Bartter, Gitelman & Liddle syndromes<br>• Acute myelogenous leukemia |
| Gastrointestinal loss | • Diarrhea (infectious or malabsorptive)<br>• Secretory tumors (villous adenoma, VIPoma, Zollinger-Ellison syndrome)<br>• Intestinal bypass or fistula |

* TTKG = trans-tubular $K^+$ gradient = $(U_{K+} \times P_{Osm}) \div (P_{K+} \times U_{Osm})$; valid only if $U_{osm} > P_{Osm}$

---

[11] Gennari FJ. Hypokalemia. *N Engl J Med* 1998; 339: 451-458.

## Clinical manifestations

- Symptoms rare if $[K^+] > 3.0$ mEq/L
- Early symptoms include weakness and constipation; as $[K^+]$ falls $< 2.0$ mEq/L may develop rhabdomyolysis or ascending paralysis with respiratory compromise
- Risk of lethal tachycardia, especially in setting of ischemia, CHF, LVH or digoxin
- ECG: U waves, T-wave flattening, and ST-segment changes

## Treatment

**Note:** Total body potassium deficit correlates poorly with serum levels (deficit is roughly 150-400 mEq per 1.0 mEq/L drop in serum $[K^+]$)

- Correct underlying disorders, especially low Mg, alkalosis & volume contraction
- For $[K^+] < 2.0$ mEq/L or $[K^+] < 3.0$ mEq/L associated with symptoms or ECG abnormalities, give IV supplementation (maximum 20-40 mEq/hour via central IV line) with continuous cardiac monitoring
- Otherwise, give oral supplementation in form of KCl 20-40 mEq PO q4-24 hr. [1 inch banana or 1 oz orange juice contains ~ 1.6 mEq $K^+$]
- In patients with ongoing diuretic use daily $K^+$ requirements are as high as 40-100 mEq; consider addition of $K^+$-sparing diuretic such as amiloride, triamterene or spironolactone

# Hyperkalemia

## Etiology

| Mechanism | Cause |
|-----------|-------|
| Spurious (plasma $K^+$ normal) | • Hemolysis (during or after phlebotomy)<br>• Thrombocytosis or leukocytosis |
| Trans-cellular shift | • Metabolic acidosis<br>• Diabetic ketoacidosis<br>• Hyperosmolar states<br>• Drugs: β-blockers, succinylcholine, digitalis<br>• Hyperkalemic periodic paralysis<br>• Tissue destruction: rhabdomyolysis, crush injuries, tumor lysis, hemolysis<br>• Cardiac surgery |
| Increased intake | • Dietary (rare as isolated cause unless associated renal disease)<br>• Potassium salt drugs, e.g. penicillin G potassium |
| Decreased renal excretion | • Type IV RTA* (see table, page 206)<br>• Acute or chronic renal failure<br>• Decreased renal perfusion (CHF, sepsis)<br>• Adrenal insufficiency • HIV<br>• Congenital adrenal hyperplasia<br>• Drugs: ACE inhibitors/receptor blockers, heparin, NSAIDs, cyclosporine, trimethoprim, pentamidine, $K^+$-sparing diuretics |

* In absence of apparent cause, Type IV RTA (hyporeninemic hypoaldosteronism) accounts for 50-75% of cases. Trans-tubular $K^+$ gradient (TTKG, see p. 214) is typically less than 5 when aldosterone is absent or inhibited.

## Clinical manifestations
• Cardiac arrhythmias, including idioventricular rhythm, sine-wave pattern VT, sinoventricular conduction and VF arrest
• ECG: peaked T waves, flattened P waves, prolonged P-R interval, widened QRS, and deepened S waves with merging into T waves
• Muscle weakness also seen with $[K^+] > 8$ mEq/L

## Emergency treatment

| Degree of hyperkalemia | Treatment |
|---|---|
| Mild (K⁺ < 6.0 mEq/L) | **Decrease total body K⁺ stores with**<br>• IV diuretic, e.g. furosemide 40-80 mg<br>• Kayexalate 30 g in 50 ml of 20% sorbitol, PO/PR<br>• Consider dialysis if renal failure |
| Moderate (K⁺ 6.0-7.0 mEq/L) | **Shift K⁺ into cells temporarily by adding**<br>• $NaHCO_3$ 50 mEq IV over 5 minutes (hypertonic; may exacerbate fluid overload or hypernatremia)<br>• D50 (50 g) plus insulin 10 units IV over 15 min<br>• Albuterol 10-20 mg nebulized over 15 min |
| Severe (K⁺ > 7.0 mEq/L or ECG Δs) | **Protect myocardium by adding**<br>• CaCl (central line) 5-10 ml 10% solution, or Ca gluconate (peripheral IV) 15-30 ml of 10% solution; either given IV over 2-5 min<br>**Avoid** in suspected digitalis toxicity. |

*Newer oral agents (patiromer, zirconium cyrosilicate) too slow for emergency use.*

# Hypomagnesemia

| Mechanism | Etiology |
|---|---|
| Gastrointestinal loss | • Malabsorption or small bowel bypass<br>• Acute or chronic diarrhea |
| Renal loss | • Diuretics (thiazide or loop)<br>• Alcohol<br>• Nephrotoxic drugs: aminoglycosides, amphotericin B, pentamidine, cyclosporine, cisplatin<br>• 1° aldosteronism<br>• Post-ATN or post-obstruction |
| Miscellaneous | • Poor intake/malnutrition<br>• Pancreatitis (sequestration)<br>• Diabetes (? mechanism)<br>• Post-operative or post-transfusion (citrate) |

## Clinical manifestations
• Secondary electrolyte disturbances: hypokalemia, hypocalcemia (↓ PTH secretion/action, ↓ 1-hydroxylation of 25-OH vitamin D)
• Neuromuscular: weakness, anorexia, tetany, convulsions

- Cardiac: widened QRS, peaked or inverted T-waves, prolonged QT and PR intervals, S-T segment depression; polymorphic ventricular tachycardia *(torsades de pointes)*; accentuation of digitalis toxicity

**Diagnosis**

- Poor correlation between serum and tissue levels; if patient has evidence of hypomagnesemia *(e.g. hypokalemia, torsades, etc.)* consider empiric treatment for "normomagnesemic magnesium depletion"
- Fractional magnesium excretion:
  - In presence of Mg depletion, FEMg < 1% suggests extrarenal losses or "normomagnesemic" depletion
  - FEMg > 4% suggests renal losses
  - After supplementation, FEMg increases substantially such that much of administered doses are renally wasted

$$FE_{Mg}(\%) = \frac{U_{Mg} \times P_{Cr}}{0.7 \times P_{Mg} \times U_{Cr}} \times 100$$

**Treatment**

- Symptomatic: Give $MgSO_4$, 1-2 grams IV slowly; may need daily replacement. *See* magnesium *on page 315.*
- Asymptomatic or mild: Oral Mg++ as gluconate, oxide, lactate or chloride. Typical dose 6-8 tabs PO daily in divided doses, or 2-4 tabs daily as maintenance in presence of ongoing losses *(e.g.* diuretics)

# Hypocalcemia

## Etiology

| | |
|---|---|
| Pseudo-hypocalcemia | • $Ca^{++}$ ↓ 0.8 mg/dl for each 1.0 g/dl ↓ in serum albumin<br>• Ionized (*i.e.* biologically active) calcium unaffected |
| Calcium sequestration | • ↑ $PO_4$ (renal failure, rhabdomyolysis, tumor lysis)<br>• Pancreatitis; • Widespread osteoblastic metastasis<br>• "Hungry bone" syndrome after correction of hyperparathyroidism, hyperthyroidism or prolonged metabolic acidosis<br>• Intravascular binding: citrate (blood transfusion), lactate or lactic acidosis, EDTA, resp. alkalosis (↑ albumin binding) |
| ↓ PTH secretion | • Post-surgical (parathyroidectomy, thyroidectomy, radical neck resection) or XRT<br>• Autoimmune; • HIV<br>• ↓ $Mg^{++}$ (< 0.8 mEq/L) or severe ↑ $Mg^{++}$ (> 5 mEq/L)<br>• Infiltrative disease (hemachromatosis, metastases) |
| ↓ PTH action | • Congenital (pseudohypoparathyroidism)<br>• ↓ $Mg^{++}$ (ethanol, diarrhea, diuretics, aminoglycosides) |
| ↓ 25-OH vitamin D | • Poor intake or malabsorption; • Inadequate sunlight;<br>• Liver disease; • Anticonvulsants |
| ↓ $1,25-(OH)_2$ vitamin D | • Kidney disease |
| Miscellaneous | • Sepsis or toxic shock syndrome; • Post-surgical<br>• Fluoride |

## Manifestations

• **Neuromuscular:** Generalized irritability (twitching, paresthesias) progressing to frank tetany (carpopedal spasm, laryngospasm); Chvostek sign (facial nerve stimulation causes ipsilateral facial muscle tetany), Trousseau sign (cuff occlusion of brachial artery causes hand/forearm tetany); Tetany exacerbated by alkalosis, ↓ $Mg^{++}$, ↓ $K^+$.

• **CNS:** Fatigue or lethargy; emotional irritability; generalized seizures; papilledema

• **Cardiac:** ECG QT prolongation (with narrow T); heart block; hypotension; myocardial dysfunction

**Treatment of acute symptomatic hypocalcemia**
*(page 270)*

(1) Confirm true hypocalcemia by checking ionized $Ca^{++}$ or correcting for albumin. Corrected [Ca] (mg/dL) ≈ 0.8 x (normal albumin (gm/dL) – measured albumin). Albumin is principal calcium buffer; use ionized calcium as index of serum [Ca].

(2) If etiology unclear draw pre-treatment creatinine, $PO_4$, albumin, PTH, 25-OH vitamin D (**not** 1,25-$(OH)_2$ vitamin D unless renal disease)

(3) In **symptomatic** hypocalcemia, give 1-2 amps 10% **calcium gluconate** (93 mg elemental $Ca^{++}$/10 ml) IV in 50-100 ml D5W. Then start drip of 10 amps Ca gluconate in 1 liter D5W at 50 ml/hour. Titrate drip to low-normal serum calcium. Calcium chloride IV used less frequently. Start oral calcium 500-1000 mg po qid when patient stable.

(4) If magnesium deficiency suspected, give empiric infusion of **magnesium sulfate** (2 grams IV over 1 hr) unless serum level elevated, *e.g.* renal failure

(5) If vitamin D deficiency, start 1,25-$(OH)_2$ vitamin D (calcitriol) 0.25 mcg po qd x 1 week, then switch to non-hydoxylated form for chronic therapy. Monitor 25(OH)-vitamin D levels.

(6) If inadequate 1-alpha hydroxylation (renal failure, PTH deficiency or resistance), start 1,25-$(OH)_2$ vitamin D (calcitriol) 0.25 mcg PO qd.

# *Hypercalcemia*[12]

**Etiology:** 90% of cases caused by **malignancy** (most common in inpatients) and **primary hyperparathyroidism** (most common in outpatients)

---

[12] Bilezikian JP. Management of acute hypercalcemia. *N Engl J Med* 1992; 326: 1196-1203; Ahmad S, *et al.* Hypercalcemic crisis. *Am J Med* 2015; 128: 239-245.

| Malignancy | • Usually clinically apparent primary (myeloma, breast, lung, head/neck, renal cell, bladder most common)<br>• Three mechanisms: (1) diffuse skeletal metastases • (2) ectopic production of PTH-like protein (PTH-rP) • (3) elevated vitamin D metabolites (lymphoma) |
|---|---|
| Hyperpara-thyroidism | • Primary (adenoma, MEN syndrome)<br>• Chronic renal failure with 3° hyperparathyroidism |
| ↑ Vitamin D | • 25-OH vitamin D: dietary supplements<br>• 1,25-$(OH)_2$ vitamin D: granulomatous disease (sarcoid, TB), lymphoma, meds (calcitriol) |
| Skeletal mobilization | • Immobilization; • Multiple fractures |
| Medications | • HCTZ • Lithium • Vitamin A intoxication<br>• Antacids (Milk-alkali syndrome) • tamoxifene |
| Miscella-neous | • Pheochromocytoma; • Adrenal insufficiency; • Thyrotoxicosis;• Rhabdomyolysis with renal failure; • Pseudohypercalcemia (normal ionized calcium but elevated bound fraction to albumin or paraproteins) |

## Manifestations
- **CNS:** confusion, lethargy, psychosis, coma
- **GI:** constipation, anorexia, nausea, pancreatitis
- **Cardiac:** ↓ QT, ↑ PR and QRS, ↑ QRS voltage, T-wave flattening and widening, notching of QRS, A-V block, cardiac arrest ($Ca^{++}$ > 15 mEq/L)
- **Renal:** volume depletion, renal insufficiency, stones, distal RTA, nephrogenic diabetes insipidus

## Treatment of acute symptomatic hypercalcemia
(1) Diagnostic studies: ionized calcium, $PO_4$, creatinine, intact PTH, 1,25-$(OH)_2$ and 25-OH vitamin D levels
(2) Promote urinary calcium excretion with aggressive **saline** infusion (NS 250 mL/hr IV); when volume deficit is repleted follow with loop diuretic (*e.g.* **furosemide** 20-40 mg IV q2-4 hr) to maintain euvolemia. Initial effect within 2-4 hr. Dialysis indicated if intolerance to fluids due to renal insufficiency or CHF.

**(3)** Inhibit bone resorption with **zoledronate** 4 mg IV over 15 min (*see page 357*) or **pamidronate** 60-90 mg IV infused over 4 hr (*See page 333*). Onset of action 1-2 d with maximum effect in 4-6 d.

**(4)** For severe hypercalcemia give **calcitonin** 4 units/kg IM/SQ q 12 hr x 4 doses; effective within 4-6 hr but tachyphylaxis usually develops over 2-3 d

**(5)** IV glucocorticoids (*e.g.* **prednisone** 20-40 mg qd) beneficial if hypercalcemia due to lymphoma or granulomatous disease

**(6)** Inhibit GI absorption of calcium with oral $PO_4$ 500 mg PO qid (but risk of ectopic calcification if serum $PO_4$ is raised in setting of hypercalcemia)

**(7)** Consider **gallium nitrate** for refractory hypercalcemia (effective but significant nephrotoxicity; avoid concurrent nephrotoxic drugs and in CRI)

# *Hypophosphatemia*

### Etiology

- Glucose loading (especially in malnourished); • Total parenteral nutrition; • Diabetic ketoacidosis especially after insulin therapy; • Respiratory alkalosis; • Inhaled β-agonists; • Phosphate-binding agents including sucralfate; • Pseudohypophosphatemia: mannitol; • Increased urinary excretion: carbonic anhydrase inhibitors, diuretics, bisphosphonates, acyclovir

### Note

Phosphorus 1 mmol = 31 mg; Intravenous phosphates contain Na or K. *See* phosphorus administration *on page 338.*

Symptoms are uncommon except in severe life-threatening hypophosphatemia (<1.0 mg/dL) including heart failure, rhabdomyolysis, encephalopathy, hematologic dysfunction

# $FE_{Na}$ [13]

- $FE_{Na}$ = fractional excretion of sodium, measures sodium avidity of the renal tubule (represents % of filtered sodium that is excreted in the urine)

$$FE_{Na}(\%) = \frac{U_{Na}}{P_{Na}} \times \frac{P_{Cr}}{U_{Cr}} \times 100$$

- Normal value varies with $Na^+$ intake, GFR and volume status but is typically $\leq 1\%$
- Useful in acute renal failure to differentiate pre-renal azotemia ($FE_{Na} < 1\%$) from acute tubular necrosis ($FE_{Na} > 2\%$). $FE_{Na}$ of 1-2% is indeterminate.

| FENa | Effective Intravascular Volume Status | |
|---|---|---|
| | Hypovolemic | Normal or Volume Overloaded |
| < 1% | • Pre-renal azotemia <br> • Cirrhosis or hepatorenal syndrome <br> • Congestive heart failure | • Non-oliguric ATN (10% of cases) <br> • ATN with underlying CHF or cirrhosis <br> • Drugs: ACE-I, NSAIDs <br> • Acute glomerulonephritis or vasculitis <br> • Acute interstitial nephritis * <br> • Acute renal allograft rejection <br> • Intratubular obstruction: myoglobin (rhabdomyolysis), contrast media <br> • Acute extrarenal obstruction * <br>   (FENa depends on duration/severity) |
| > 2% | • Diuretics <br> • Chronic renal failure | • Oliguric ATN <br> • Non-oliguric ATN (90% of cases) <br> • Obstruction |

\* Seen in only some cases     ATN: acute tubular necrosis

## Pearls
- $FE_{Na}$ is more useful in oliguric than in non-oliguric renal failure
- Variability of $FE_{Na}$ in non-oliguric patients without renal failure makes it a poor measure of volume status (unless **very** low, e.g. < 0.1-0.2 %)

---

[13] Zarich S, et al. Fractional excretion of sodium. Exceptions to its diagnostic value. Arch Intern Med 1985; 145: 108-112.

# FE-Urea[14]

- FE-Urea = fractional excretion of urea

$$FE_{Urea}(\%) = \frac{UUN}{BUN} \times \frac{P_{Cr}}{U_{Cr}} \times 100$$

- Unlike $FE_{Na}$, may be able to distinguish intrinsic from prerenal azotemia in patients treated with diuretics.
- FE-Urea < 35% suggests prerenal azotemia; FE-Urea > 35% suggests ATN

# Tumor Lysis Syndrome[15]

**Definition:** • Laboratory two or more concurrent (uric acid > 8 mg/dL, K > 6 mEq/dL, $PO_4$ > 4.5 mg/dL adults, Ca < 7mg/dL) or Δ25% or • Clinical (creatinine > 1.5ULN, seizure, arrhythmia/death) within -3 to +7d of chemotherapy.

**Predisposition:** Bulky, proliferative, chemosensitive, usually hematological tumor.

**Prevention:** • Prehydration 2-3L/$m^2$/d; • Loop diuretics; • Allopurinol (if low risk and uric acid < 7.5mg/dL) or • rasburicase (if high risk and no G6PD deficiency).

**Treatment:** • Uric acid: rasburicase (see page 350), volume, loop diuretics, renal replacement therapy; • Potassium: monitoring and polystyrene sulfonate or dialysis; • Calcium: replete after phosphorus correction; • Phosphorus: hydration; dialysis when calcium x phosphate product ≥ 60-70 mg$^2$/dL$^2$; • Renal: dialysis as needed for electrolytes

---

[14] Carvounis CP, et al. Significance of the fractional excretion of urea in the differential diagnosis of acute renal failure. *Kidney Int* 2002; 62: 2223-2229.

[15] Howard SC, et al. The tumor lysis syndrome. *N Engl J Med* 2011; 364: 1844-1854; Cairo MS, et al. Recommendations for the evaluation of risk and prophylaxis of TLS. *Br J Haematol* 2010; 149: 578-586.

# Rheumatology

## *Autoantibody Tests[1]*

**Pearls about antinuclear antibody (ANA)**
- Test for ANA in patients with symptoms of auto-immune disease, because of frequent false positives (women, > age). Generally order only once.
- Interpret ANA titers < 1:40 as negative, 1:40 – 1:80 low positive, > 1:160 positive
- Test for α-ds-DNA only in when ANA-positive and SLE is suspected
- Test for specific antibodies only if immunofluorescence ANA-screen positive, or specific diagnoses suspected, *e.g.* polymyositis or Sjögren syndrome
- ANA titers are not recommended for monitoring disease activity

**Recommended profile based on clinical question**

| Antibody | Disease | Sensitivity | Specificity |
|---|---|---|---|
| **Screening immunofluorescence** (usually HEp-2 cells) | | | |
| Immuno-fluores-cence ANA | SLE | 93 | 57 |
| | Sjögren Syndrome | 48 | 52 |
| | Systemic Sclerosis | 85 | 54 |
| | Polymyositis, Dermatomyositis | 61 | 63 |
| | Raynaud phenomenon | 64 | 41 |

*(Continued)*

---

[1] Moder KG. Use and interpretation of rheumatologic tests. *Mayo Clin Proc 1996; 71: 391-396;* Tozzoli R, *et al.* Guidelines for the laboratory use of autoantibody tests in the diagnosis and monitoring of autoimmune rheumatic diseases. *Am J Clin Pathol 2002; 117: 316-324;* Kumar Y, *et al.* Antinuclear antibodies and their detection methods in diagnosis of connective tissue diseases. *Diagn Pathol 2009; 4: 1.*

| Antibody | Disease | Sensitivity | Specificity |
|----------|---------|-------------|-------------|
| **Specific autoantibodies (extractable nuclear antigens)** | | | |
| α-dsDNA | SLE, correlates with disease activity | 57 | 97 |
| α-Sm | SLE, highly specific | 25-30 | High |
| α-SSA/Ro | Sjögren, subacute cutaneous SLE, neonatal lupus complete heart block, ↓ nephritis risk | 8-70 | 87 |
| α-SSB/La | Like α-Ro; ↓nephritis risk | 16-40 | 94 |
| α-histone | Drug-induced SLE (75%), SLE (50%) | 50-70 | 95 |
| α-Scl-70 (topoisomer-ase-1) | Diffuse scleroderma, predicts worse prognosis including pulmonary fibrosis. Mutually exclusive with centromere. | 20 | 100 |
| α-centromere | Limited scleroderma, frequent pulmonary hypertension, may predict Raynaud progression. Digital ischemic ulcers. | 65 | 99.9 |
| α-U3-RNP (fibrillarin) | Systemic Sclerosis, PA hypertension, interstitial lung disease, SS renal crisis | 12 | 96 |
| α-Jo-1 | Polymyositis, dermatomyositis, associated with interstitial lung disease, Raynaud. AKA α-tRNA synthetase. | 30 | 95 |
| Rheumatoid factor (RF) | RA 80%, Sjögren 50%. Nonspecific (in fever&arthritis, predicts endocarditis > RA). High titer in RA predicts aggressive course. | | |
| α-CCP | CCP = cyclic citrullinated peptides. RA 85%, improved specificity. High titers predict worse outcome. | | |
| α-phospho-lipid | Tests include cardiolipin, β2glycoprotein1. Antiphospholipid syndrome 80%. Positive ANA suggests APS from SLE. IgG confers highest risk. | | |
| c-ANCA (cytoplasmic) | Antineutrophil cytoplasm antibody (ANCA) against Proteinase-3. Granulomatosis with polyangiitis 80-95%. More specific than p-ANCA; 99% specific for vasculitis in autoimmune disease, nonspecific in general population (ie isolated sinusitis). | | |
| p-ANCA (perinuclear) | α-myeloperoxidase. Nonspecific for granulomatosis with polyangiitis (10%), other vasculitis, glomerulonephritis, mixed connective tissue disease, primary sclerosing cholangitis, ulcerative colitis, drug reactions, cystic fibrosis, inflammatory bowel disease, chronic infection, etc. | | |
| α-Mitrochon-drial | Primary biliary cirrhosis 90% | | |

## Immunofluorescence ANA patterns

| Pattern | Antigen | Associated disease |
|---------|---------|--------------------|
| Speckled | ENA, RNP, Sm, SSA/Ro, SSB/La, Scl-70, Jo-1, ribosomal-P | SLE, Mixed connective tissue disease, scleroderma, Sjögren syndrome, polymyositis |
| Homogenous | dsDNA, Histones | SLE, drug-induced SLE |
| Peripheral (rim) | RNP, Sm, SSA/Ro | SLE, scleroderma |
| Nucleolar | α-PM-Scl, α-RNA, α-U3-RNP, polymerase I-III | scleroderma, polymyositis |
| Centromere | CENP A-E | Limited scleroderma |
| Mitochondrial | Various | Primary biliary sclerosis |

# Vasculitis[2]

| | Vasculitis | Vessels affected | Diagnostic Features | Comments |
|---|------------|------------------|---------------------|----------|
| **L A R G E** | Takayasu arteritis | Aorta & 1° branches | Granulomas; arteriography | Age < 40 yr, 80% female. Non-specific symptoms (fever, weight loss) followed by vascular obstruction |
| | Giant cell (temporal) arteritis (GCA) | L, M | ↑ ESR; granulomas | Mean age 70 yr, 60% female. Headache, jaw claudication, visual loss, PMR common. |
| **M E D I U M** | Polyarteritis nodosa (PAN) | M, S | Hep B in 10%; arteriography | Mononeuritis multiplex, hypertension, abdominal pain |
| | Kawasaki disease | L, M, S | | Aneurysms of coronary arteries. Adult cases rare. |
| | Isolated CNS vasculitis | M, S | Arteriography | Diffuse vasculitis limited to CNS. Symptoms include confusion, headache, cranial nerve palsies. |
| **S M A L L** | Henoch-Schönlein purpura (HSP) | Capillaries, venules or arterioles | IgA deposits in vessels | Mean age < 20 yr. Often follows URI. Symptoms: purpura, arthralgias, abdominal pain. Renal involvement common but renal failure rare (5%). |

*(Continued)*

2 Hunder GG, *et al.* ACR 1990 criteria for the classification of vasculitis. *Arthritis Rheum* 1990; 33: 1065-1067. Jennette JC, *et al.* Small-vessel vasculitis. *N Engl J Med* 1997; 337: 1512-1523.

| | Vasculitis | Vessels affected | Diagnostic Features | Comments |
|---|---|---|---|---|
| **S M A L L** | Essential cryo-globulinemic vasculitis | | Cryoglobulin in serum & vessels; HCV Ab; ↓ C4, Normal C3 | 95% of cases caused by HCV. Symptoms: purpura, arthralgias, nephritis, neuropathy. Morbidity related to glomerulonephritis and chronic liver disease. |
| | Microscopic polyangiitis (MP) | | p-ANCA | Similar pathology to PAN but smaller vessels; features of GA without granuloma. Common cause of pulmonary-renal syndrome. |
| | Granulomatosis with angiitis (formerly Wegener) | Capillaries, venules, arterioles and arteries | c-ANCA; necrotizing granulomas | Predilection for respiratory tract including sinuses, trachea & lung. 80% develop glomerulonephritis although only 20% at presentation. |
| | Eosinophilic granulomatosis with polyangiitis (formerly Churg-Strauss) | | ANCA (p > c); eosinophilia; necrotizing granulomas | Asthma initially, followed by eosinophilic tissue infiltration and vasculitis (typically within 3 yr). Cardiac disease major cause of morbidity. |

**Abbreviations:** ANCA = anti-neutrophil cytoplasmic antibody; HCV = hepatitis C virus; PAN = polyarteritis nodosa; PMR = polymyalgia rheumatica; GA = granulomatosis with angiitis

## Differential diagnosis of vasculitis
• Primary vasculitis (*see table*); • Secondary vasculitis from connective tissue disease, SLE, rheumatoid arthritis, Sjögren, etc; • Fibromuscular dysplasia (mimics large vessel vasculitis); • Cholesterol emboli (especially after catheterization); • Endocarditis or atrial myxoma; • Mycotic aneurysm; • Thrombotic microangiopathy (thrombotic thrombocytopenic purpura, hemolytic-uremic syndrome, antiphospholipid antibody syndrome, eclampsia)

## Organ system involvement (%) in selected vasculitides

| Organ | Manifestations | HSP | Cryo | MP | GA | EGP |
|---|---|---|---|---|---|---|
| Skin | Purpura, livedo | 90 | 90 | 40 | 40 | 60 |
| Renal | GN, hematuria, ARF | 50 | 55 | 90 | 80 | 45 |
| Pulmonary | Infiltrates, hemoptysis | < 5 | < 5 | 50 | 90 | 70 |
| Upper airway | Sinusitis, ulcers | < 5 | < 5 | 35 | 90 | 50 |
| Musculoskeletal | Arthralgias/arthritis | 75 | 70 | 60 | 60 | 50 |
| Neurologic | Mononeuritis multiplex | 10 | 40 | 30 | 50 | 70 |
| GI | Abd pain, GI bleeding | 60 | 30 | 50 | 50 | 50 |

**Abbreviations:** ARF = acute renal failure; cryo = cryoglobulinemic; EGP = eosinophilic granulomatosis with polyangiitis; GA = granulomatosis with angiitis; GN = glomerulonephritis; HSP = Henoch-Schönlein purpura; MP = microscopic polyangiitis;

# *Systemic Lupus Erythematosus:*
## *ARA Criteria*[3]

### Four or more of the following criteria

(1) **Malar rash:** Fixed erythema, flat or raised, over malar eminences, tending to spare the nasolabial folds

(2) **Discoid rash:** Erythematous raised patches with adherent keratotic scaling and follicular plugging; atrophic scarring may occur in older lesions

(3) **Photosensitivity:** Skin rash as an unusual reaction to sunlight, by patient history or physician observation

(4) **Oral ulcers:** Oral or nasopharyngeal ulcers, usually painless, seen by MD

---

[3] Tan EM, *et al.* The 1982 revised criteria for the classification of SLE. *Arthritis Rheum* 1982; 25: 1271-1277; Hochberg MC. Updating the ACR revised criteria for the classification of SLE. *Arthritis Rheum* 1997; 40: 1725.

**(5) Arthritis:** Nonerosive arthritis involving ≥ 2 peripheral joints, characterized by tenderness, swelling, or effusion

**(6) Serositis**
- **Pleuritis:** Convincing history of pleuritic pain or rub heard by a physician or evidence of pleural effusion, *or*
- **Pericarditis:** By ECG or rub or evidence of pericardial effusion

**(7) Renal disorder:**
- Persistent proteinuria > 0.5 grams per day or greater than 3+, *or*
- Cellular casts of any type

**(8) Neurologic disorder**
- Seizures *or* psychosis (in absence of drugs or metabolic derangement, *e.g.* uremia, ketoacidosis, or electrolyte imbalance )

**(9) Hematologic disorder**
- Hemolytic anemia with reticulocytosis, *or*
- Leukopenia < 4000/mm$^3$ total on ≥ 2 occasions, *or*
- Lymphopenia < 1500/mm$^3$ on ≥ 2 occasions, *or*
- Thrombocytopenia < 100,000/mm$^3$ in absence of offending drugs

**(10) Immunologic disorder**
- Anti-ds-DNA antibody in abnormal titer *or*
- Anti-Sm antibody *or*
- Antiphospholipid antibodies based on IgG/IgM anticardiolipin antibodies *or* a positive test for lupus anticoagulant *or* a false-positive serologic test for syphilis (> 6 mo duration and confirmed by secondary testing)

**(11) Antinuclear antibody:** Without drugs typical of "drug-induced" lupus syndrome

Additional signs and symptoms suggestive of SLE but not included in classification criteria include: Raynaud's, hair loss, unexplained fever, unexplained lymphadenopathy or splenomegaly, and unexplained thromboembolic phenomena.

# Synovial Fluid Analysis[4]

- **Useful tests:** total WBC • percent PMNs • crystal exam • gram stain • culture
- **Not useful:** glucose • LDH • protein
- **Gram stain/culture:** high yield in bacterial infections **except** gonorrhea and Lyme/higher yield from direct inoculation of blood culture bottles. If gonorrhea is suspected, swabs for culture for gonorrhea should be taken from pharynx/cervix/urethra/anus. In the setting of (+) serum Lyme antibodies, PCR for Lyme from synovial fluid may be helpful.

- **Crystals:**
  - Uric acid: thin, needle-like, negatively birefringent (yellow when ∥, blue when ⊥ to polarized axis)
  - Calcium pyrophosphate (pseudogout): short rhomboid crystals, weakly positive birefringence (yellow when ⊥, blue when ∥ to polarized axis
  - Betamethasone (post-injection), calcium oxalate and lithium heparin (artifact from blood tube) can mimic uric acid

| Patterns * | Normal | Non-Inflammatory | Inflammatory | Purulent | Hemorrhagic |
|---|---|---|---|---|---|
| Appearance | Clear | Clear yellow | Cloudy yellow | Opaque | Opaque, red |
| Viscosity | High | High | Low | Low | Variable |
| WBC/mm³ | < 200 | < 2000 | 2000-50,000 | > 50,000 | Variable |
| PMNs | < 25% | < 25% | > 50% | > 75% | Variable |

* non-specific with considerable overlap

**Non-inflammatory pattern:** • trauma; • osteoarthritis; • chronic or subsiding crystal synovitis (gout, pseudogout); • SLE; • early rheumatoid arthritis (RA); • polyarteritis nodosa; • osteonecrosis; • scleroderma; • amyloidosis; • polymyalgia rheumatica;

4  Shmerling RH, *et al.* Synovial fluid tests. What should be ordered? *JAMA* 1990; 264: 1009; Pascual E, *et al.* Synovial fluid analysis. *Best Pract Res Clin Rheumatol* 2005; 19: 371; Margaretten ME, *et al.* Does this adult patient have septic arthritis? *JAMA* 2007; 297: 1478.

• endocrine arthropathy; • hypertrophic pulmonary osteoarthropathy; • avascular necrosis; • osteochondritis dessicans

**Inflammatory pattern:** • crystal synovitis (gout, pseudogout) ; • rheumatoid arthritis; • reactive arthritis (Reiter's syndrome) • psoriatic arthritis; • seronegative spondyloarthropathy (*e.g.* inflammatory bowel disease, ankylosing spondylitis, Behçet's); • juvenile chronic arthritis; • sarcoidosis; • some infectious arthritis (Lyme, gonococcal, viral, coagulase negative staph); • acute rheumatic fever

**Purulent pattern:** • infection: bacterial, fungal, TB; • rarely RA, pseudogout

**Hemorrhagic pattern:** • trauma or fracture; • Charcot joint; • sickle-cell disease; • coagulopathy (hemophilia, warfarin, thrombocytopenia, vWD); • tumor (especially pigmented villonodular synovitis)

# *Arthritis & Fever*[5]

| Causes | | Distinguishing features | |
|---|---|---|---|
| **Diagnosis** | **Confirmation** | **Symptom/ Sign** | **Possible Diagnosis** |
| **Infectious arthritis** | | T > 40°C | Still's disease; SLE Bacterial arthritis |
| Septic arthritis | Culture | | |
| Bacterial endocarditis | Blood cx | Antecedent fever | Viral; Lyme Reactive; Still's Bacterial endocarditis |
| Lyme disease | Serology | | |
| Mycobacteria/fungi | Culture, Bx | | |
| Viral arthritis (parvo) | Serology | | |
| **Postinfectious or reactive** | | Migratory arthritis | Rheumatic fever Gonococcal; Meningococcal; Viral arthritis SLE; Acute leukemia Whipple's disease |
| Enteric infection | Cx/serology | | |
| Reactive (Reiter's) | Genital cx | | |
| Rheumatic fever | Clinical | | |
| Inflammatory bowel | Clinical | | |

*(Continued)*

5  Pinals RS. Polyarthritis and fever. N Engl J Med 1994; 330: 769-774. Adapted with permission of *The New England Journal of Medicine*, Copyright 1994, Massachusetts Medical Society.

| Causes | |
| --- | --- |
| **Diagnosis** | **Confirmation** |
| **Systemic rheumatic disease** | Biopsy/ |
| Systemic vasculitis | angio |
| SLE | Serology |
| Rheumatoid arthritis | Clinical |
| Still's disease | Clinical |
| **Crystal-arthritis** | |
| Gout / pseudogout | Microscopy |
| **Other diseases** | |
| Familial Med. Fever | Clinical |
| Malignancy | Biopsy |
| Sarcoidosis | Biopsy |
| **Mucocutaneous syndromes** | |
| Dermatomyositis; | Clinical or |
| Behçet's disease; | Biopsy |
| Henoch-Schönlein purpura; | |
| Kawasaki disease; | |
| Erythema nodosum; | |
| Erythema multiforme; | |
| Pyoderma gangrenosum; | |
| Pustular psoriasis; | |

| Distinguishing features | |
| --- | --- |
| **Symptom/ Sign** | **Possible Diagnosis** |
| Effusion>> Pain | TB |
| | Bacterial endocarditis |
| | Inflamm bowel disease |
| | Giant-cell arteritis |
| | Lyme disease |
| Pain >> effusion | Rheumatic fever |
| | Fam Mediterran. fever |
| | Acute leukemia |
| | AIDS |
| (+) Rheumatoid factor | Rheumatoid arthritis |
| | Viral arthritis |
| | Tuberculous arthritis |
| | Bacterial endocarditis |
| | Sarcoidosis; SLE |
| | Systemic vasculitis |
| Morning stiffness | Rheumatoid arthritis |
| | Polymyalgia rheum. |
| | Still's disease |
| | Some viral/reactive |
| Symmetric small-joint synovitis | Rheumatoid arthritis |
| | SLE |
| | Viral arthritis (parvo) |
| WBC > 15k/mm$^3$ | Bacterial arthritis |
| | Bacterial endocarditis |
| | Still's disease |
| | Systemic vasculitis |
| | Acute leukemia |
| Leukopenia | SLE; Viral arthritis |
| Episodic | Crystal-induced |
| | Inflammatory bowel |
| | Lyme; Whipple |
| | Familial Med. fever |
| | Still's disease; SLE |

**Prompt arthrocentesis essential!**
- Gram stain 50-75% sensitive
- Culture > 90% sensitive for diagnosis of septic arthritis

# Toxicology

## *General Management*[1]

**Initial management: Treat the patient, not the poison**

- **A**irway, **B**reathing, **C**irculation; co-existing Trauma; Level of Consciousness
- Cardiac & hemodynamic monitoring & oximetry.
  - Manage hypothermia.
- Consider empiric treatment with:
  - **Oxygen**; • **Naloxone** 0.4 mg followed by 1-2 mg IM/IV (if suspected opiate ingestion); • **Thiamine** 100 mg IM/IV (alcoholism, malnutrition); • **Dextrose** 50% (if suspected hypoglycemia); • **Flumazenil** for isolated benzodiazepine ingestion; controversial in mixed overdose because of seizure risk
- Treat specific toxic syndromes: <u>National Poison Control Center</u> 1-800-222-1222
- Coma: *see* Coma, common reversible causes on page 159

**Laboratory tests**

- Electrolytes, BUN/creatinine, anion gap, ABG/VBG, osmolality; • Consider lactate, serum and urine toxicology screen including salicylate, acetaminophen, ethanol; • <u>Osmolal</u> gap (*see p 202*); • <u>Lactic acid</u> (*see p 204*)
- Pulse oximetry may **not** reveal methemoglobinemia or CO; use blood co-oximetry

---

[1] Mokhlesi B, *et al.* Adult toxicology in critical care: part I: general approach to the intoxicated patient. *Chest* 2003; 123: 577-592; Nelson LS, *et al.* Principles of managing the acutely poisoned or overdosed patient. In: Nelson LS, *et al.*, editors. Goldfrank's Toxicologic Emergencies, 9/e. 2010.

## Decontamination[2]

- Intubate trachea to protect airway if consciousness depressed, unable to speak or swallow secretions. Gag reflex is a poor indicator.
- **Decontaminate the skin** (*e.g.* radiation, insecticides, nerve agents). Consider using protective equipment.
- **Activated charcoal** (PO or NG): Indicated early after most oral poisonings; • Dose 0.5-1 g/kg within 1 hr of ingestion. Repeat q 4 hr for massive or life-threatening ingestions. *See page 271.* Especially effective for high MW compounds & ingestions known to delay GI transit. Avoid if aspiration risk or GI tract not functioning. Ineffective: Alcohols (ethylene glycol, methanol, ethanol); Iron, lithium; Acids & alkali; Hydrocarbons; Organophosphates, carbamates, DDT.
- **Whole bowel irrigation:** No clear evidence. Indications: Sustained-release drugs, evacuate illicit drug "cargo" from "body packers," failure or not suitable for charcoal. Dose: Polyethylene glycol electrolyte solution 20-30 mL/min or 1.5-2L/h via NG x 4-6 hr until effluent clear. May require antiemetic. Contraindicated: hemodynamic instability, GI tract not intact or functional, leaking cocaine packs. Reduces charcoal efficacy.
- **Orogastric lavage** (36-40 Fr OG tube, 250 mL NS x liters) reserved for < 1-2 hr since life-threatening ingestion, toxin still expected to be in stomach, not adsorbed by charcoal, serious toxicity expected and/or no specific antidote, comatose patients. Protect airway. Maintain L lateral decubitus position. Confirm gastric tube position. Contraindicated: corrosive or hydrocarbon ingestion; sharp object; coagulopathy; varices.

---

2 Gude AB, *et al.* Techniques used to prevent gastrointestinal absorption. In: Nelson LS, et al., editors. Goldfrank's Toxicologic Emergencies, 9/e. *2010;* Howland, MA. Activated Charcoal, Whole-bowel Irrigation. In Nelson LS, *et al.* editors, Goldfrank's Toxicologic Emergencies, 9/e. 2010.

**Enhanced elimination**[3]

<u>Forced alkaline diuresis</u>: salicylates, phenobarbital, chlorpropamide, methotrexate

<u>Hemodialysis</u>: methanol, ethylene glycol, metformin lactic acidosis, lithium, salicylate, valproic acid.

<u>Charcoal hemoperfusion</u> (overcomes protein binding): theophylline, carbamazepine, disopyramide, methotrexate, paraquat, phenobarbital, phenytoin

**Specific antidotes**

| Toxin or drug | Specific Antidote |
|---|---|
| Acetaminophen | N-acetylcysteine |
| Benzodiazepines | Flumazenil |
| β-blockers | Atropine, beta-agonists, calcium, glucagon, phosphodiesterase inhibitors |
| Calcium Channel blockers | Atropine, calcium, glucagon, beta-agonists |
| Carbon monoxide | Hyperbaric oxygen |
| Cholinesterase inhibitors | Atropine, pralidoxime |
| Crotalid Snakebite | Crotalidae Polyvalent Immune Fab |
| Cyanide | Amyl+sodium nitrite, thiosulfate, hydrocobalamin |
| Digitalis | Digoxin Fab |
| Ethylene glycol | Fomepizole, ethanol, pyridoxine, thiamine |
| Heparin | Protamine sulfate |
| Iron | Deferoxamine |
| Isoniazid | Pyridoxine |
| Methanol | Fomepizole, ethanol, folinic acid, folate |
| Methotrexate/anti-folates | Folinic acid |
| Methemoglobinemia | Methylene blue |
| Opioids | Naloxone |
| Oral hypoglycemic agents | Dextrose, glucagon |
| Organophosphates | Atropine, pralidoxime |
| Sulfonylureas | Octreotide |
| Sympathomimetics[#] | Phentolamine, benzodiazepines |
| Tricyclic antidepressants | Bicarbonate |
| Warfarin/ rodenticides | Vitamin K, plasma |

[#] *Including MAO inhibitor interactions, cocaine, epinephrine, ergotism*

---

[3] Goldfarb DS. Principles and techniques applied to enhance elimination. In: Nelson LS, *et al.*, editors. Goldfrank's Toxicologic Emergencies, 9/e. 2010.

# Common Toxic Syndromes[4]

### Anticholinergic syndromes
- **Common signs:** • delirium with mumbling speech • tachycardia • dry flushed skin • dilated pupils • myoclonus • slightly elevated temperature • urinary retention • decreased bowel sounds • seizures and dysrhythmia
- **Common causes:** • antihistamines • antiparkinsonians • atropine • scopolamine • amantadine • antipsychotics • antidepressants • antispasmodics • mydriatics • skeletal muscle relaxants • many plants (e.g. jimson weed, *Amanita muscaria*)

### Sympathomimetic syndromes
- **Common signs:** • delusions and paranoia • tachycardia (bradycardia if pure α-adrenergic agonist) • hypertension • hyperpyrexia • diaphoresis • piloerection • mydriasis • hyperreflexia • seizures, hypotension, and dysrhythmia
- **Common causes:** • cocaine • amphetamine, methamphetamine • NMDA (e.g. "ecstasy") • decongestants (ephedrine, pseudoephedrine) • herbal compounds including ephedra and ma huang • caffeine and theophylline causing catecholamine release

### Opiate, sedative, or ethanol intoxication
- **Common signs:** • coma • respiratory depression • miosis • hypotension • bradycardia • hypothermia • pulmonary edema • decreased bowel sounds • hyporeflexia • needle marks • seizures after some e.g. propoxyphene
- **Common causes:** • narcotics • barbiturates • benzodiazepines • ethanol • clonidine

### Cholinergic syndromes
- **Common signs:** • *Muscarinic:* "SLUDGE" (salivation, lacrimation, urination, defecation, GI cramps, emesis) • miosis • bradycardia • AV block • bron-

---

4 Kulig K. Initial management of ingestions of toxic substances. *N Engl J Med* 1992; 326: 1677-1681.

choconstriction • rhinorrhea and bronchial secretions **Nicotinic:** • fasciculation • cramps • weakness
• tachycardia, • mydriasis
- **Common causes:** • organophosphate and carba-
mate insecticides • nerve agents • cholinesterase
inhibitors (physostigmine, neostigmine, pyridostigmine, edrophonium) • some mushrooms

# *Tricyclic antidepressant toxicity*[5]

## Pharmacologic characteristics
- Class Ia antiarrhythmic (sodium blocker prolongs
QRS and QT); • Muscarinic anticholinergic;
• Peripheral $\alpha$-adrenergic blocker; • Lipophilic with
large volume of distribution; • Highly protein bound
except in acidosis; • Enterohepatic circulation

## Clinical manifestations
- <u>Sinus tachycardia</u> most common sign of toxicity.
- Refractory <u>myocardial depression</u> with <u>hypotension</u>
most common cause of death.
- <u>ECG signs</u> of toxicity and adverse outcome: (1) QRS >
100 ms predicts serious adverse events including seizure; QRS > 160 ms predicts ventricular arrhythmia;
(2) RV conduction delay characteristics ($R_{AVR}$ > 3 mm,
$R/S_{AVR}$ > 0.7); "Brugada" morphology *(see page 27)*:
may represent Ia-agent unmasking of Brugada
syndrome or may represent unique TCA toxicity.
- <u>Ventricular tachycardia</u> and ventricular fibrillation;
*torsades* is unusual
- Agitation, delirium, hyperthermia, ileus, coma from
<u>anticholinergic</u> effects

## Management
- Consider orogastric lavage (with endotracheal
inubation) in symptomatic intoxication because
of highly toxic residual drug. **Note** anticholinergic
effect delays gastric emptying. • GI decontamination with activated charcoal.

5 Liebelt EL. Cyclic antidepressants. In: Nelson LS, *et al.*, editors.
Goldfrank's Toxicologic Emergencies, 9/e. NY: *McGraw-Hill; 2010.*

- **Sodium bicarbonate**, increases serum protein binding and counteracts Na-channel blockade. Indicated in any hemodynamic instability, seizure, or ECG alteration (other than isolated sinus tachycardia or prolonged QT interval)
- Goal serum pH 7.50-7.55; • Bolus 1-2 mEq/kg bicarbonate followed by "normal bicarbonate" (3 x 50 mEq ampules + 0.85 L D5W) at 150-200 mL/hr until 12-24 hr after ECG abnormalities and hypotension reverse; • Recheck pH often to maintain > 7.50;
- **Hyperventilation** for seizing or arresting patients (maintain pH > 7.50);
- **Treat seizures** aggressively with benzodiazepines (acidosis exacerbates toxicity);
- **Hypotension** usually responds to volume; give bicarbonate or vasopressors (norepinephrine preferred) if non-responsive;
- **Extracorporeal circulation** (ECMO) for <u>refractory hypotension</u>;
- **Antiarrhythmic agents:** Unclear benefit from any agent. If refractory VT/VF despite alkalinization, consider magnesium or lidocaine
- Intravenous lipid emulsion (*Intralipid*) , may be helpful (*See page 315*).
- Avoid physostigmine (exacerbates rhythm instability); flumazenil (↑ seizure threshold); procainamide (exacerbate rhythm instability)

**Disposition**
- All known/suspected ingestions warrant observation & serial ECGs/telemetry. • If asymptomatic after GI decontamination and ≥ 6 hr observation, may transfer for psychiatric evaluation or outpatient care. • If persistent sinus tachycardia or isolated $QT_c$ prolongation, observe 24 hr. • Otherwise treat aggressively.

# *Beta-adrenergic blocker & calcium-channel blocker toxicity*[6]

**Manifestations**

Hypotension, bradycardia. With β-blockers: repolarization abnormalities (Brugada-like susceptibility to ventricular arrhythmia especially membrane-stabilizing β-blockers such as propranolol and acebutolol; Torsades, from sotalol)

**Treatment:** escalating in sequence

<u>Gastric decontamination</u> using orogastric lavage, activated charcoal (for water-soluble agents), polyethylene glycol for lipid-soluble & sustained release agents

<u>Atropine</u>: For bradycardia.

<u>Glucagon</u>: stimulates adenyl cyclase through non-β-adrenergic receptor pathway. Restores chronotropy and inotropy better than vascular tone. Often not successful as monotherapy. *See glucagon on page 292.*

<u>Calcium</u>,: Chloride 1 g of 10% central IV or 3 g gluconate 10% peripheral IV; may repeat 3 times total. Treats hypotension not bradycardia in animal models.

<u>Insulin-euglycemic therapy</u>: *see insulin on page 304.*

<u>Catecholamines</u>: Epinephrine may be preferred for beta blocker.

<u>Intravenous lipid emulsion</u>: May be helpful for lipid-soluble agents (*e.g.* propranolol). *See page 315.*

<u>Bicarbonate</u>: IV may ameliorate Brugada-like arrhythmia.

---

[6] Graudins A, *et al.* Calcium channel antagonist and beta-blocker overdose. Br J Clin Pharmacol 2015; Brubacher JR. Beta-adrenergic antagonists. In: Nelson L, *et al.*, editors. Goldfrank's Toxicologic Emergencies, 9/e. *2010;* DeRoos FJ. Calcium channel blockers. In: Nelson L, *et al.*, editors. Goldfrank's Toxicologic Emergencies, 9/e. *2010.*

# Neuroleptic Malignant Syndrome[7]

**Drug Precipitants**
- <u>Typical antipsychotics</u>: chlorpromazine; droperidol; fluphenazine; haloperidol; loxapine; molindone; mesoridazine; perphenazine; pimozide; thioridazine; thiothixene; trifluoperazine;
- <u>Atypical antipsychotics</u>: ariprazole; clozapine; olanzapine; quetiapine; risperidone; ziprasidone
- <u>Other dopamine Blockers</u>: metoclopramide; prochlorperazine; promethazine

**Diagnosis**
- Autonomic instability, drooling, pallor, variable mental status changes ranging from alert to mute/catatonic to stuporous, rigidity.
- Differential diagnosis: Serotonin syndrome, anticholinergic syndrome, malignant hyperthermia, drug withdrawal, encephalitis
- <u>Distinguishing feature from serotonin syndrome</u>: hyporeflexia, normal or decreased bowel sounds, normal pupils

**Treatment, escalating**
- Discontinue offending agents (all dopamine blockers)
- Supportive care including hydration, electrolytes, external cooling
- <u>Benzodiazepines</u> for mild symptoms especially catatonia and immobility
- Consider <u>dopamine agonists</u> to treat rigidity: bromocriptine 2.5-5 mg q 8 h; amantadine 100 mg q 8 h.
- Consider <u>dantrolene</u> for extreme hyperthermia & rigidity. Benefit still controversial
- Electroconvulsive therapy has been suggested for otherwise refractory NMS

---

[7] Guze BH, *et al.* Current concepts. Neuroleptic malignant syndrome. *N Engl J Med* 1985; 313: 163-166; Strawn JR, *et al.* Neuroleptic malignant syndrome. Am J Psychiatry 2007; 164: 870-876.

# Serotonin Syndromes[8]

**Drug Precipitants**

Usually a combination of one or more: selective serotonin reuptake inhibitors (SSRI) and to a lesser extent cyclic antidepressants, monoamine oxidase inhibitors (MAOI), triptans, L-tryptophan, linezolid, fentanyl, meperidine, mirtazapine, amphetamines especially MDMA, lithium, tramadol, methylene blue

**Diagnosis**

- Hunter Serotonin Toxicity Criteria[9] present IF Serotonergic agent + (Spontaneous clonus) OR (inducible or ocular clonus + agitation or diaphrosis) OR (tremor + hyperreflexia) OR (hypertonic + T > 38°C + ocular or inducible clonus)
- Manifestations: <u>autonomic instability</u> (hyperthermia, HR and BP fluctuation, arrhythmia, flushing, diaphoresis, diarrhea, vomiting), <u>altered sensorium</u> (delirium, agitation, hallucination, anxiety, stupor), <u>neuromuscular</u> (<u>myoclonus</u>, rigidity, akathisia, mydriasis, hyper-reflexia, shivering ~ "wet dog shakes"). Severe outcomes: seizure, rhabdomyolysis, DIC.
- Differential diagnosis: neuroleptic malignant syndrome, malignant hyperthermia, cholinergic syndrome.

**Treatment**

- Withdraw offending agent. Typically resolves in 24 hr.
- Focus on reducing muscle rigidity, which is thought to contribute to hyperthermia and death. Care includes • external cooling • muscle relaxation with benzodiazepines (neuromuscular blockers & mechanical ventilation if needed)

---

[8] Stork CM. Serotonin reuptake inhibitors and atypical antidepressants. In: Nelson LS, *et al.*, editors. Goldfrank's Toxicologic Emergencies, 9/e: *2010*; Boyer EW, *et al.* The serotonin syndrome. *N Engl J Med 2005; 352:* 1112-1120.

[9] Dunkley EJ, *et al.* The Hunter Serotonin Toxicity Criteria. *QJM 2003; 96:* 635-642.

- Data supporting cyproheptadine (serotonergic antagonist, 8-16 mg po) are sparse
- Dantrolene probably not effective

## Ethylene Glycol & Methanol Toxicity[10]

**Mechanism**

Liver metabolism leading to production of glycolic acid (ethylene glycol) and formic acid (methanol), resulting in anion-gap acidosis and multi-system effects

**Clinical manifestations**

- **Ethylene glycol:** Onset 4-12 hr after ingestion • Intoxication → coma • Nausea/vomiting • Seizures or brain herniation • Cardiogenic or non-cardiogenic pulmonary edema • Oliguric renal failure with flank pain (oxaluria) • Hypocalcemia
- **Methanol:** Onset of symptoms may be delayed up to 30 hr • Headache → lethargy → coma and seizures • Visual changes or loss (optic disc & nerve & putamen toxin: sluggish or fixed/dilated pupils, papilledema) • Gastritis or pancreatitis • Bradycardia • Respiratory failure
- Presentation with either toxin may be delayed by ethanol co-ingestion

**Diagnostic evaluation**

- Suspect if unexplained anion gap acidosis *(see pages 201, 203)*
- Osmolal gap (> 10) often present but absence does not exclude serious ingestion
- Serial urine microscopy for calcium oxalate crystalluria (ethylene glycol only)
- Ethylene glycol and methanol levels may be measured directly, but if ingestion is suspected, start treatment before confirmatory testing

[10] Brent J. Fomepizole for ethylene glycol and methanol poisoning. *N Engl J Med* 2009; 360: 2216-2223; Barceloux DG, *et al.* AACT practice guidelines on the treatment of methanol poisoning. *J Toxicol Clin Toxicol* 2002; 40: 415-446; Barceloux DG, *et al.* AACT practice guidelines on the treatment of ethylene glycol poisoning. *J Toxicol Clin Toxicol* 1999; 37: 537-560.

- Toxicity correlates best with degree of acidosis rather than EG or methanol level
- CT/MRI may show putamen or caudate lesions in severe methanol neurotoxicity

**Management goals - General**

- Gastric suctioning if recent ingestion (use charcoal only for mixed ingestion)
- IV fluids to maintain urine output
- Sodium bicarbonate to correct acidosis. High doses may be require d to reach goal pH 7.35-7.45. Correction of acidosis also limits tissue penetration of toxic metabolites and increases urinary excretion of acid metabolites.
- Calcium for *symptomatic* hypocalcemia
- Magnesium, thiamine and multivitamin in chronic alcohol abusers
- Lorazepam or diazepam for seizures. Hyperventilation, mannitol and intracranial pressure monitoring warranted if cerebral edema develops.
- Co-factors: glycolate clearance increased by pyridoxine (50 mg IM qid) and thiamine (100 mg IM qid); for methanol add leucovorin or folate (50 mg IV q4-6 hr)

**Antidote therapy**

- **Indications**

  - Methanol or ethylene glycol level ≥ 20 mg/dl (regardless of symptoms or acidosis)
  - Recent ingestion, serum levels not available and osmolal gap > 10 mOsm/l
  - Suspected ingestion and pH < 7.3, $HCO_3$ < 20 mEq/L or Osm gap > 10 (2 of 3)
  - Anion gap acidosis with ocular signs or urinary oxalate crystals

| **Dialysis** indicated for |
|---|
| • Refractory acidosis (pH < 7.2) |
| • Deteriorating clini-cal status despite treatment |
| • Renal failure |
| • Visual symptoms or signs (methanol) |
| • Methanol or ethylene glycol levels > 50 mg/dl (relative indication if fomepizole used, pH is normal and patient is asymptomatic) |

- **Treatment**
  - Begin fomepizole (*page 290*) or ethanol (*page 283*) as soon as possible
  - Continue until ethylene glycol/methanol levels are undetectable (or < 20 mg/dl), pH is normal and patient is asymptomatic
  - If ethanol used, monitor levels frequently to assure therapeutic levels of 100-150 mg/dl

# Acetaminophen (APAP) Toxicity [11]

## Clinical manifestations

- Toxic insult (1-24 hr): anorexia, N/V; may be asymptomatic
- Hepatic injury (24-72 hr): mild RUQ pain, asymptomatic increase in LFTs
- Hepatic failure (72-96 hr): sequelae of hepatic necrosis including jaundice, renal failure, coagulopathy, encephalopathy, coma. Fatal multiorgan failure 3-5 d.

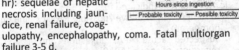

## Initial lab assessment

- Serum APAP level • AST
- PT/INR, lytes, glucose, renal function if patient is ill-appearing or AST is elevated

## Hepatic toxicity

- Toxicity increased by chronic ethanol, anticonvulsants, INH, malnourishment

---

[11] Hendrickson RG. Acetaminophen. In: Nelson LS, *et al.*, editors. Goldfrank's Toxicologic Emergencies, 9/e: 2010; Heard KJ. Acetylcysteine for acetaminophen poisoning. *N Engl J Med* 2008; 359: 285-292.

- Rumack-Matthews nomogram[12] (*see figure on previous page*) has high sensitivity but low specificity for toxicity. Initial level should be checked ≥ 4 hr after ingestion (although level < 50 mcg/ml between 1-4 hr suggests non-toxic dose).
  - **Probable** toxicity if log[level] ≥ 2.6 − (0.075 x hr since ingestion)
  - **Possible** toxicity (*i.e.* treatment indicated) if log[level] ≥ 2.48 − (0.075 x hr)
  - Use conservative time estimate to assure appropriate treatment
- Toxic effects generally ingestions ≥ 150 mg/kg; however, severe hepatitis or fulminant hepatic failure may occur after single doses of 7.5 g in normal adults or less than 4 g in alcoholics
- For ingestion of extended release formulations, acetaminophen level should be re-checked in 4 hr if initial determination is below treatment line

**Treatment**
- **Decontamination** with activated charcoal
- **N-acetylcysteine** (*p. 258*) blocks production of toxic metabolites. Indicated for:
  - APAP level on or above "possible toxicity" line on nomogram
  - Suspected acute APAP ingestion and ↑ AST, regardless of serum [APAP]
  - Serum level > 10 mcg/ml and time since acute ingestion completely unknown
  - Chronic/repeated APAP ingestion at excessive doses *and*
    - AST > 2x normal, *or*
    - AST > normal and symptoms or APAP level > 10 mcg/ml, *or*
    - APAP level above expected for appropriate dose (> 30 mcg/ml at 1 hr or > 10 mcg/ml at 4-6 hr after dose)
  - Prompt treatment for suspected ingestions ≥ 4 g

---

[12] Adapted from Rumack, BH, Matthew H. Acetaminophen poisoning and toxicity. *Pediatrics. 1975; 55:871.*

(with completion of treatment pending serum APAP level). Acetylcysteine most effective ≤ 8 hr of ingestion, but delayed administration (*i.e.* 24 hr post-ingestion) remains beneficial.

- **Standard dose:** 140 mg/kg PO load then 70 mg/kg q 4 hr x 17 doses
- Prolonged administration warranted in severe toxicity; continue drug until encephalopathy resolved and INR < 2
- IV for **(1)** fulminant hepatic failure **(2)** patient unable to take POs and high serum levels at or beyond 8 hr post-ingestion **(3)** pregnant (higher placental delivery prior to first pass metabolism).

**Prognosis**
- Patients who survive through liver failure ~ 5 days generally recover completely
- Patients at high risk for death without liver transplant:
  - Persistent acidosis (pH < 7.30) after fluid and hemodynamic resuscitation
  - Combination of PT > 1.8 x control, creatinine > 3.3 mg/dl and grade III/IV encephalopathy
  - Abnormal INR that is rising on 4th day after overdose
  - Prothrombin time (sec) > hours since ingestion

# *Salicylate Toxicity*[13]

**Epidemiology**
- 2nd most common cause of analgesic-related death, after acetaminophen
- Intentional overdose of ASA vs. accidental overdose of salicylate-containing compounds including ASA-narcotic combos, Pepto Bismol and oil of wintergreen

---

[13] Flomenbaum NE. Salicylates. In: Nelson LS, *et al.*, editors. Gold-frank's Toxicologic Emergencies, 9/e. NY: *McGraw-Hill; 2010*; Mokhlesi B, *et al.* General approach to the intoxicated patient. *Chest 2003; 123: 577-592.*

## Pharmacokinetics
- Rapidly absorbed from GI tract, though peak serum levels delayed 4-6 hr
- Normal $T_{1/2}$ of 2-4 hr increases to 20 hr at toxic levels
- Lethal dose 10-30 g (> 35 tablets ASA) or 150 mg/kg
- Therapeutic levels 15-30 mg/dl; toxicity usually at levels > 40 mg/dl, although severe poisoning may occur at lower levels, especially in elderly

## Pathophysiology
- Mixed respiratory alkalosis (central respiratory stimulation → hyperventilation) and metabolic acidosis (uncoupled oxidative phosphorylation → lactic acidosis)
- Hypoglycemia caused by hepatic damage, including low CSF glucose levels
- Acute lung injury (pulmonary edema) caused by unknown mechanism

## Presentation
- **Acute intoxication:** Nausea/vomiting, hyperventilation, tinnitus, lethargy, delirium
- **Severe toxicity:** Coma, seizures, hypoglycemia, fever, pulmonary edema. Signs may progress rapidly. Death occurs from cerebral edema and cardiovascular collapse due to acidosis.
- **Chronic intoxication:** More common in elderly (accidental or iatrogenic). Frequently unrecognized or misdiagnosed. Hearing loss, tinnitus, hyperventilation, non-specific confusion or agitation, dehydration, metabolic acidosis. Cerebral and pulmonary edema more common than in acute intoxication.

## Diagnosis
- Based on signs and symptoms, serum pH and salicylate levels (though serum levels correlate inexactly with toxicity). Levels 30-40 mg/dl without symptoms or acidosis do not require treatment.
- Delayed absorption common; measure serial levels after acute ingestion

- Acidosis drives drug into tissues and thereby lowers serum levels; falling serum level reassuring **only** if pH stable or rising

**Treatment**

- Multi-dose activated charcoal (acute ingestions only)
- Replace fluid deficits to promote renal clearance, but avoid overcorrection in light of risk of pulmonary edema. Forced diuresis not helpful.
- Bicarbonate (*see page 268*) to correct acidosis, enhance urinary elimination and prevent CSF penetration (serum pH goal 7.45-7.50, urinary pH $\geq$ 8)
- Correct hypokalemia to facilitate urinary alkalinization
- **Hemodialysis** indicated for • Renal failure; • CHF or non-cardiogenic pulmonary edema; • Coma or seizures; • Progressive deterioration in vital signs; • Severe acidosis or electrolyte imbalance despite treatment; • Hepatic dysfunction with coagulopathy; • Salicylate level > 100mg/dL (or > 60 mg/dL in chronic ingestion)

# Cyanide Poisoning[14]

**Overview**

Inhibits cytochrome oxidase and interrupts oxidative phosphorylation. Sources: Industrial; Smoke inhalation; Nitriles (nail & glue remover); Nitroprusside prolonged infusion. Lethal Dose 50-200 mg. Death within minutes from hypoxia and acidosis. "Cherry red" usually postmortem; acutely retinal arteries & veins equally red.

Nitrites therapy is intended to induce methemoglobinemia. MetHb binds cyanide at expense of hemoglobin oxygen-carrying capacity.

---

[14] Gracia R, *et al.* Cyanide poisoning and its treatment. Pharmacotherapy 2004; 24: 1358-1365; Shepherd G, *et al.* Role of hydroxocobalamin in acute cyanide poisoning. Ann Pharmacother 2008; 42: 661-669; Hall AH, *et al.* Which cyanide antidote? *Crit Rev Toxicol 2009; 39: 541-552.*

Thiosulfate combines with extracellular cyanide to form thiocyanate, which is excreted renally. Few side-effects, but small volume of distribution and slow acting, therefore usually used along with faster-acting, less-well tolerated nitrites.

Hydroxocabalamin preferentially binds cyanide over cytochrome oxidase.

**Treatment**

• Oxygen

• Cyanide antidote kit includes all of the following three agents:

(1) Amyl Nitrite (1 ampule crushed and inhaled over 15-30 sec); repeat q 3-5 min until sodium nitrite available. Each ampule generates ~ 5% methemoglobinemia. Induces hypotension and methemoglobinemia.

(2) Sodium Nitrite 300 mg (10 mL of 3%) or 4-6 mg/kg IV over 2-4 min, may repeat 50% dose if response after 2 hr. Induces hypotension and methemoglobinemia. Generates 15-20% methemoglobinemia. Avoid when carboxyhemoglobin is expected to be elevated.

(3) Sodium thiosulfate 150-200 mg/kg (typically 50 mL of 25% solution) IV over 10 min. Can be used without nitrites in smoke inhalation.

**Alternative and Adjunctive Treatments**

(4) Hydroxocabalamin 5 g IV over 15 min, repeat 2.5-5 g if needed. Requires dedicated IV line. Few side effects.

(5) Hemodialysis for severe thiocyanate toxicity

(6) Methylene blue for methemoglobinemia

# Methemoglobinemia, acquired[15]

**Drugs commonly causing methemoglobinemia**
- Anesthetic agents: Lidocaine, benzocaine, cetocaine (classic exposure before endoscopy); • Nitrates: nitroglycerin, nitric oxide after prolonged exposure; • Nitrites: amyl nitrite, sodium nitrite (used to generate MetHb in cyanide poisoning); • Methylene blue: in high doses (paradoxically) or G6PD deficiency; • Sulfa drugs; • Metoclopramide; • Dapsone; • Chloroquine; • Primaquine

**Diagnosis**
- "Cyanosis" in setting of normal $PaO_2$. • "Chocolate-brown" color arterial blood. • "Oximetry gap:" Conventional pulse-oximetry values higher than arterial blood gas. • Co-oximetry identifies methhemoglobinemia. Often manifest in setting of anemia.
- MetHb > 20% causes symptoms: headache, dizziness, altered sensorium, etc
- MetHb > 50% imminently life-threatening

**Treatment**
- Methylene blue (*see page 316*). • Exchange transfusion if in shock.

[15] Cortazzo JA, *et al.* Methemoglobinemia: a review and recommendations for management. *J Cardiothorac Vasc Anesth* 2014; 28: 1043-1047; Ash-Bernal R, *et al.* Acquired methemoglobinemia. *Medicine (Baltimore)* 2004; 83: 265-273.

# *Nerve Agents*[16]

**Tabun (GA), Sarin (GB), Soman (GD), VX**

- Highly toxic, irreversible acetylcholinesterases used as chemical warfare agents
- Chemically similar to organophosphate pesticides, similar pathophysiology
- G agents are water-soluble, highly volatile, colorless, tasteless liquids that may have slight odor
- VX is an amber-colored, oily, odorless liquid that is less volatile (more persistent) and 10-fold more potent than G agents
- All are readily absorbed via inhalation, exposure to skin or eyes, or ingestion. Vapors are not toxic except via respiratory tract.

## Symptoms

- Usually start within 20-30 min of inhalation, but dermal exposure may cause insidious progression after delay of up to 18 hr
- Eye: Lacrimation, injection, miosis, pain, diminished vision
- Neurologic: CNS irritability, impaired judgment. Flaccid paralysis, coma, seizures, apnea at higher doses. Extensive muscarinic & nicotinic effects (*see cholinergic syndrome, page 237*)
- Respiratory: Major cause of mortality. Rhinorrhea, bronchial secretions, dyspnea, bronchoconstriction. Respiratory muscle paralysis, decreased central drive.
- Cardiac: Arrhythmias, bradycardia, hypertension
- GI: Abdominal pain, nausea/vomiting (early marker of severe toxicity)

---

[16] Lee EC. Clinical manifestations of sarin nerve gas exposure. *JAMA* 2003; 290: 659-662; Newmark J. Therapy for nerve agent poisoning. *Arch Neurol* 2004; 61: 649-652; Suchard JR. Chemical weapons. In: Nelson LS, *et al.*, editors. Goldfrank's Toxicologic Emergencies, 9/e. 2010; Agency for Toxic Substances & Disease Registry. Medical management guidelines for nerve agents. 2015. http://www.atsdr.cdc.gov/MMG/MMG.asp?id=523&tid=93

- Other: Twitching, cramping, profuse sweating, drooling

**Triage of exposed patients**

- <u>Immediate treatment</u> for symptomatic patients. Conscious patients with full muscular control will need minimal care.
- <u>Observation</u> for ≥ 18 hr for those who may have had topical exposure to liquid. Carefully decontaminate hair and clothes.
- <u>No treatment</u> if possible exposure to vapor only but no symptoms at medical facility – patient unlikely to have been exposed and can be discharged safely

**Diagnosis**

- RBC cholinesterase activity < 30% normal may aid in diagnosing unconfirmed cases. Do not withhold treatment awaiting results.

**Management**

- Decontaminate patients by removing clothes and washing exposed skin with water or 0.5% hypochlorite (bleach). **Patients' skin and clothing can contaminate medical personnel by direct contact or vapor.** "Level A" biohazard gear preferred. Purifying respirators and latex gloves do not provide protection.
- Early airway management in patients with respiratory compromise or excessive secretions. Intubation and extensive suctioning may be needed. Avoid depolarizing paralytic agents (*e.g.* succinylcholine), which may cause prolonged neuromuscular blockade due to cholinesterase inhibition.
- Irrigate eyes with water or saline for 5 to 10 min

## Antidotes for Nerve Agents

|  | Mild-mod symptoms sweating fasciculations, N/V, dyspnea | Severe symptoms coma, seizures, apnea, flaccid paralysis |
|---|---|---|
| Normal adult | Atropine 2 mg IV/IM<br>2-PAM* 15 mg/kg IV slowly | Atropine 6 mg IV/IM<br>2-PAM* 15 mg/kg IV slowly |
| Frail or elderly adult | Atropine 1 mg IV/IM<br>2-PAM* 5-10 mg/kg IV slowly | Atropine 2 mg IV/IM<br>2-PAM* 5-10 mg/kg IV slowly |

\* 2-PAM: pralidoxime HCl

- Repeat atropine 2 mg IV/IM q 2-5 min until symptoms resolved (**Note:** Atropine may not reverse miosis and nicotinic effects, including skeletal muscle weakness – do not use as clinical endpoints). Typical total dose is 20 mg but some cases may require cumulative doses approaching 100 mg. Administer via endotracheal tube if needed.
- Diazepam or lorazepam for seizures
- Phentolamine 5 mg IV for pralidoxime-induced hypertension
- Topical atropine, tropicamide or homatropine for eye-related symptoms
- IM atropine (2 mg) for severe rhinorrhea
- Activated charcoal for possible ingestion. **Do not induce emesis**

tochrome P450 (CYP)  
  interactions...................................256  
ociximab (ReoPro) ......................258  
cetylcysteine  
 (Mucomyst, Acetadote) ............258  
denosine  
 (Adenocard, Adenoscan)............258  
minophylline ...............................259  
miodarone (Cordarone) .............260  
nticholinesterases ......................262  
nticoagulants..............................263  
rgatroban ...................................264  
tropine .......................................265  
eta-Adrenergic Blockers ............266  
carbonate ...................................268  
valirudin (Angiomax)..................269  
alcium .........................................270  
alcium channel blockers ............270  
harcoal, activated ......................271  
hlorothiazide (Diuril) .................271  
levidipine (Cleviprex) .................272  
lonidine (Catapres) ....................272  
orticosteroids .............................273  
abigatran (Pradaxa) ...................273  
antrolene ...................................274  
esmopressin (ddAVP, Stimate) ...274  
exmedetomidine (Precedex) ......275  
igoxin .........................................276  
igoxin Immune Fab (Digifab) ......277  
iltiazem IV ...................................278  
iuretics, Loop .............................279  
obutamine ..................................279  
opamine .....................................280  
pinephrine (Adrenalin) ..............281  
smolol (Brevibloc) ......................282  
thanol ........................................283  
tomidate (Amidate) ...................284  
ibrinolytic Agents  
 (aka thrombolytics) ..................285  
lumazenil (Romazicon) ..............289  
omepizole (Antizol) ...................290  
ondaparinux (Arixtra) ................291  
lucagon .....................................292  
lycoprotein II$_b$III$_a$ Inhibitors ........293  
aloperidol (Haldol) .....................295  
eparin (Unfractionated,  
 UFH)..........................................296  
eparin, Low Molecular Weight  
 (LMWH): Enoxaparin  
 (Lovenox) ..................................298  
ydralazine (Apresoline) .............300  
ydroxocobalamin (Cyanokit) ....301  
ypoglycemic agents  
 other than insulin ......................301  
butilide (Convert) .......................306  

Idarucizumab (Praxbind)  
 reversal of dabigatran ...............307  
Insulin .........................................304  
Iron intravenous ........................308  
Isoproterenol (Isuprel)................310  
Ketamine (Ketalar) .....................310  
Labetalol .....................................311  
Levothyroxine (T4) .....................313  
Levetiracetem (Keppra) ..............312  
Lidocaine ....................................313  
Liothyronine (T3; Triostat IV) .....314  
Lipid or fat emulsion (Intralipid) ..315  
Magnesium .................................315  
Mannitol .....................................316  
Methylene Blue ...........................316  
Methylnaltrexone (Relistor) ........317  
Midazolam (Versed) ....................317  
Milrinone (Primacor) ..................318  
Naloxone (Narcan) ......................319  
Neuromuscular blockers .............320  
Nicardipine IV (Cardene) ............323  
Nimodipine .................................324  
Nitroglycerin...............................325  
Nitroprusside (Nipride)...............325  
Norepinephrine (Levophed) ........327  
Novel Oral Anticoagulants  
 (NOACs) ....................................328  
Octreotide (Sandostatin)............331  
Ondansetron (Zofran).................331  
Opiate analgesics .......................332  
Pamidronate (Aredia) .................333  
Pentobarbital (Nembutal) ..........334  
Phenobarbital sodium ................334  
Phentolamine (Regitine) .............335  
Phenylephrine (Neo-Synephrine) ..336  
Phenytoin (Dilantin) ...................336  
Phosphorus .................................338  
Platelet P2Y$_{12}$ Inhibitors .............339  
Pralidoxime (2-PAM, Protopam) ...340  
Procainamide ..............................341  
Propofol (Diprivan).....................343  
Propylene Glycol Diluent ............344  
Protamine....................................344  
Prothrombin complex concentrate  
 (4-factor PCC; Kcentra) .............345  
Pulmonary Vasodilators ..............346  
Rasburicase (Elitek) ....................350  
Remifentanil (Ultiva) ..................351  
Sodium polystyrene sulfonate  
 (Kayexalate) ..............................351  
Vasopressin ................................352  
Verapamil ...................................354  
Warfarin (Coumadin) ..................354  
Zoledronic acid (Zometa) ............357  

GROOVY DRUGS

## Cytochrome P450 (CYP) interactions[1]

| | | |
|---|---|---|
| 1A2 | | paclitaxel, torsemide, amodia-quine, cerivastatin, repaglinide |
| 2B6 | | artemisinin, bupropion, cyclophos-phamide, efavirenz, ifosfamide, ketamine, meperidine, methadone, nevirapine, propofol, selegiline |
| 2C8 | | paclitaxel, torsemide, amodiaquine, cerivastatin, repaglinide |
| 2C9 | | celecoxib, diclofenac, fluvastatin, glipizide, glyburide, ibuprofen, irbesartan, losartan, naproxen, phenytoin, piroxicam, rosiglitazone, tolbutamide, torsemide, valproic acid, warfarin, zafirlukast |
| 2C19 | CYP substrates | amitriptyline, carisoprodol, citalopram, clomipramine, clopidogrel, cyclophosphamide, diazepam, esomeprazole, imipramine, labetalol, lansoprazole, omeprazole, pantoprazole, phenobarbitone, phenytoin, proguanil, voriconazole |
| 2D6 | | amitriptyline, aripiprazole, atomoxetine, carvedilol, clomipramine, codeine, desipramine, dextromethorphan, doxepine, duloxetine, flecainide, fluoxetine, haloperidol, imipramine, mexiletine, ondansetron, oxycodone, paroxetine, propafenone, risperidone, risperidone, tamoxifen, thioridazine, timolol, tramadol, venlafaxine |
| 2E1 | | acetaminophen → NAPQI, chlorzoxazone, enflurane, ethanol, halothane, isoflurane, methoxyflurane, sevoflurane, theophylline → 8-OH |
| 3A4,5,7 | | alfentanyl, alprazolam, amlodipine, aripiprazole, astemizole, atorvastatin, boceprevir, buspirone, carbamazepine, chlorpheniramine, cisapride, clarithromycin, cyclosporine, diazepam → 3OH, diltiazem, erythromycin (not 3A5), felodipine, gleevec, haloperidol, indinavir, lovastatin, midazolam, nevirapine, nifedipine, nisoldipine, nitrendipine, pimozide, quinidine → 3-OH (not 3A5), quinine, ritonavir, saquinavir, sildenafil, simvastatin, sirolimus, tacrolimus, tadalafil, tamoxifen, telaprevir, trazodone, triazolam, vardenafil, verapamil, vincristine |

---

[1] Flockhart DA. Drug Interactions: Cytochrome P450 Drug Interaction Table. Bloomington, IN: *Indiana U School of Medicine 2009.* http://medicine.iupui.edu/clinpharm/ddis/

| | | CYP inhibitors (W=weak; M=moderate, ↑ plasma 1.25-2x; S=strong, ↑ plasma >2x; ↑ plasma > 5x) | CYP inducers | |
|---|---|---|---|---|
| **1A2** | | amiodarone, cimetidine(W), efavirenz, fluoroquinolones, fluvoxamine1, ticlopidine | carbamazepine, Chargrilled Meat, rifampin, tobacco | |
| **2B6** | | clopidogrel, thiotepa, voriconazole | artemisinin, carbamazepine, efavirenz, nevirapine, phenobarbital, phenytoin, rifampin | |
| **2C8** | | gemfibrozil(S), montelukast | | |
| **2C9** | | amiodarone(M), efavirenz, fluconazole(S), isoniazid, metronidazole, paroxetine, sulfamethoxazole, voriconazole | carbamazepine, nevirapine, phenobarbital, rifampin, St.John's Wort | |
| **2C19** | | cimetidine, ésomeprazole, felbamate, fluoxetine, fluvox-amine, isoniazid, ketoconazole, lansoprazole, omeprazole, oral contraceptives, pantoprazole, ticlopidine2, voriconazole | efavirenz, rifampin, ritonavir, St.John'sWort | |
| **2D6** | | bupropion(S), amiodarone(W), aripiprazole, chlorpheniramine, cimetidine(W), clomipramine, diphenhydramine, doxepin, duloxetine(M), fluoxetine(S), aloperidol, methadone, paroxetine(S), quinidine(S), ritonavir, terbinafine | | |
| **2E1** | | disulfiram | ethanol, isoniazid | |
| **3A4,5,7** | | indinavir(S), suboxone, amioda-rone, cimetidine(W), clarithro-mycin(S), diltiazem, erythromy-cin(M), fluvoxamine, Grape-fruitJuice(M), itraconazole(S), ketoconazole(S), nefazodone(S), nelfinavir(S), ritonavir(S), troleandomycin, verapamil(M), voriconazole | carbamazepine, efavirenz, nevirapine, phenobarbital, phenytoin, pioglitazone, rifabutin, rifampin, St.John'sWort | |

## Abciximab *(ReoPro)*
*See* Glycoprotein II$_b$III$_a$ inhibitors, *page 293*

## Acetylcysteine[1] *(Mucomyst, Acetadote)*
<u>Action</u>: Treats acetaminophen overdose (*see page 245*) by repleting hepatic reducing capacity. Best given < 8 hr of ingestion, but beneficial up to 24 hr. Likely unable to prevent contrast nephropathy.

<u>PO</u>: Load 140 mg/kg, then 70 mg/kg q 4 hr x 17 doses. Dilute to 5% in cola or juice; serve chilled. Repeat dose if patient vomits within 1 hr of administration; use anti-emetic or nasogastric tube if recurrent vomiting.

<u>IV</u>:   Load 150 mg/kg IV over 15-60 min, then 50 mg/kg IV over 4 hr, then 100 mg/kg IV over 16 hr. PO remains preferred. Premedicate with ondansetron 4 mg. Shortened UK regimen[2]: 100 mg/kg in 200 mL over 2h, then 50 mg/kg in 1L over 10 hr; avoid in late presentation. <u>Prevention of radiocontrast nephropathy</u>: Prophylactic (600 mg PO q 12 hr x 4 before OR 150 mg/kg over 30 min before contrast, followed by 50 mg/kg over 4 hr) in conjunction with saline loading. Benefit disproven.

<u>Kinetics</u>:   Elimination T$_\frac{1}{2}$ 5.6 hr, prolonged in liver disease. Hepatic elimination.

<u>Side-effects</u>: N/V, diarrhea (PO); anaphylaxis, rash, bronchospasm, hypotension (IV). Treat as anaphylactoid if reaction involves more than skin flushing & erythema.

<u>Interactions</u>:   Charcoal prevents oral absorption; stagger other medications by 1-2 hr.

## Adenosine *(Adenocard, Adenoscan)*
<u>Action:</u> Slows AV node conduction. Locally acting coronary vasodilator. T$_\frac{1}{2}$ < 10 sec, metabolized by

---

[1] Heard KJ. Acetylcysteine for acetaminophen poisoning. *N Engl J Med* 2008; 359: 285-292.

[2] Bateman DN, *et al.* Reduction of adverse effects from intravenous acetylcysteine treatment for paracetamol poisoning. *Lancet* 2014; 383: 697-704.

red blood cells. Use to interrupt reentrant tachycardias involving AV node, or to diagnose wide complex tachycardias. Also used as coronary vasodilator (*e.g.* perfusion imaging, rotational atherectomy, fractional flow reserve).

<u>IV:</u> 6 mg IV **rapid push and flush** within 3 sec, repeat 12 mg after one min and may repeat 12mg if needed. Give via central venous line if possible.

<u>Myocardial perfusion imaging:</u> 140 mcg/kg/min x 6 min, consider reduced dose in heart transplant.

<u>Warnings:</u> Causes transient 1°-3° heart block or asystole. May cause bronchospasm. Prolonged effect in denervated (transplanted) hearts.

<u>Interactions:</u> Competitively antagonized by theophylline and caffeine (larger adenosine doses required); potentiated by dipyridamole (lower doses of adenosine required) and carbamazepine.

<u>Side effects:</u> Transient flushing, lightheadedness, dyspnea, nausea, angina.

## Alteplase *(tPA; Activase)*
*See* Fibrinolytic Agents on *page 284*

## Aminophylline

<u>Action:</u> Phosphodiesterase inhibitor and nonspecific adenosine antagonist. Used as bronchodilator in acute and chronic bronchospasm; may also augment respiratory muscle action. Therapeutic window is narrow and efficacy controversial. Not recommended for acute asthma exacerbations because of no benefit but increase toxicity over beta agonists[3]. Other uses include reversal of intravenous dipyridamole. Dose equals theophylline ÷ 0.8.

<u>Kinetics:</u> $T_{1/2}$ 3-15 hr in healthy nonsmokers; typically shorter in smokers, longer in elderly and cirrhosis. Hepatic metabolism.

---

[3] NHLBI Expert Panel Report 3. Guidelines for the Diagnosis and Management of Asthma
*https://www.nhlbi.nih.gov/files/docs/guidelines/asthgdln.pdf.*
*2007.*

**IV: Loading dose:** Naïve: 5.7mg/kg IV over 30 min. Already using methylxanthines: Loading dose = [desired-measured plasma level (mg/L)] x 0.45 L/kg. Each 0.5 mg/kg of aminophylline increases theophylline levels by 1 mcg/mL; if respiratory distress and levels unavailable, empirically load 2.5 mg/kg. Maximum rate 25 mg/min IV, or 17 mg/min if cor pulmonale, heart failure, drugs reducing clearance.

| Maintenance Dose | 1st 12 hr | Max without levels |
|---|---|---|
| Smokers | 0.88 mg/kg/h | 0.8mg/kg/h |
| Nonsmokers 16-60yr | 0.5 mg/kg/h | 1125 mg/d |
| > 60 yr old | 0.38 mg/kg/h | 500 mg/d |
| R or L heart failure or liver disease | 0.25mg/kg/h | 400 mg/d |

**Reversal** of 0.4mg regadenoson (after 1 min): 100 mg slow IV over 1 min.

**Levels:** Therapeutic: 5-15 mcg/mL; Toxic: > 20 mcg/mL (risk of seizure, arrhythmia). Measure levels 15-30 min after IV load; 4-8 hr after maintenance infusion.

**Renal failure:** No adjustment. Supplement ½ dose after hemodialysis.

**Interactions:** $T_{1/2}$ shortened by phenytoin, barbiturates, tobacco, marijuana. $T_{1/2}$ lengthened by CHF or cirrhosis (20-30 hr), macrolide and quinolone antibiotics, cimetidine, propranolol, allopurinol, thyroid hormones

**Pregnancy:** Category C. Neonates may show signs of theophylline toxicity. Nursing infants may receive up to 10% maternal dose.

# Amiodarone *(Cordarone)*

**Action:** Complex antiarrhythmic with sodium, potassium, calcium, and beta-blocking activity. Unlike oral formulation, IV administration prolongs AV nodal refractoriness without short-term effect on SA node, intraventricular conduction, or QT interval. Increases short-term survival in cardiac arrest.

<u>Indications:</u> **(1)** Antiarrhythmic of choice in VF/VT arrest **(2)** Treatment of hemodynamically stable or unstable VT, polymorphic VT or wide-QRS tachycardia of unclear etiology <u>Off-label:</u> **(3)** Control of ventricular rate in rapid atrial arrhythmias or accessory pathway conduction in pre-excitation syndromes **(4)** Pharmacological cardioversion of atrial fibrillation, or as an adjunct to electrical cardioversion in supraventricular tachycardias. Preferred to other antiarrhythmics especially in impaired LV function.

<u>Kinetics:</u> Rapid effect attributed to high peak serum concentration. Subsequent distribution results in fall of serum levels to 10% of peak concentration within 30-45 min of infusion. $T_{1/2}$ of parent compound is approximately 53 d, metabolite $T_{1/2}$ approximately 61 d. Hepatic elimination, CYP3A4 & CYP2C8.

<u>IV:</u> Best administered through central vein. <u>VF/VT arrest:</u> 300 mg rapid infusion in 20-30 mL NS or D5W. <u>Stable arrhythmia:</u> Load 150 mg over 10 min; then 900 mg at 1 mg/min x 6 hr (360 mg) then 0.5 mg/min x 18 hr (540 mg). **Breakthrough events:** Bolus 150mg/100mL over 10 min. **Maintenance:** 0.5 mg/min. **Maximum daily dose:** 2.2 g.

<u>Oral loading:</u> 800-1600 mg PO qd (divide daily doses >1000 mg) x 1-3 wk, reduce to 400-800 mg qd x 1 mo when arrhythmia controlled, then to 200-400 mg QD maintenance. Bioavailability approximately 50%.

<u>Renal failure, liver failure:</u> No dose-adjustment thought warranted.

<u>Side effects:</u> <u>Acute:</u> Hypotension, CHF, *torsades* (rare), profound bradycardia, phlebitis, nausea, confusion, biochemical hepatitis, thrombocytopenia, fever. <u>Chronic:</u> pulmonary and thyroid toxicity, hepatitis, corneal deposits, optic neuritis, photosensitivity, *etc.*

<u>Warning (Black Box):</u> Amiodarone has several fatal toxicities, including hypersensitivity pneumonitis or interstitial/alveolar pneumonitis, liver injury. Load during inpatient monitoring. Can exacerbate underlying arrhythmia.

Interactions: Precipitates with aminophylline, heparin, acetic acid or acetate, cefazolin. Potentiates warfarin effect and increases digoxin levels (decrease usual doses by 50%). Avoid grapefruit juice.

# Anticholinesterases

Neostigmine, Physostigmine, Pyridostigmine. *Also see pralidoxime on page 340.*

Action: Reversible acetylcholinesterase inhibitors, increase acetylcholine concentration by blocking degradation. Restore muscle contraction. Decrease intraocular pressure. Action resembles organophosphates (which are irreversible anticholinesterases).

Indications: (1) Reversal of nondepolarizing neuromuscular blockade (2) myasthenia gravis (3) anticholinergic neurotoxicity (culprit drugs include atropine, belladonna alkaloids, tricyclics, phenothiazines, neuromuscular blockers, antihistamines) (4) colonic pseudo-obstruction (5) open-angle glaucoma (6) post-op urinary retention.

Warning: When reversing neuromuscular blockade co-administer atropine or glycopyrrolate to avoid muscarinic effects *e.g.* bradycardia/asystole, salivation, etc. Use cautiously in setting of asthma, diabetes, obstructed viscus.

Side effects: Cholinergic "crisis": bradycardia, seizures (esp. if given too rapidly); bronchospasm; excessive salivation, emesis, urination, defecation.

Interactions: Prolong effects of succinylcholine. Antagonized by Class 1a anti-arrhythmics, magnesium, corticosteroids. Cause severe hypotension when used with ganglionic blockers.

## Neostigmine

Indication: Reversal of nondepolarizing neuromuscular blocker; myasthenia gravis; colonic pseudo-obstruction (Ogilvie syndrome)[4]; prevention of post-operative urinary retention.

---

[4] Ponec RJ, *et al.* Neostigmine for the treatment of acute colonic pseudo-obstruction. *N Engl J Med* 1999; 341: 137-141.

<u>Kinetics:</u> Onset 4-8 min IV, duration 2-4 hr. $T_{1/2}$ 1.3 hr (ESRD 3h)

<u>IV:</u> 0.5-2.0 mg (not to exceed 5 mg total dose) preceded by atropine 0.6-1.2 mg IV or with glycopyrrolate 0.2 mg per each 1 mg neostigmine. For colonic pseudo-obstruction: 2.0 mg IV.

<u>Renal failure:</u> CrCl 10-50 mL/min: 50% usual dose; CrCl <10 mL/min: 25% usual dose.

## Physostigmine

<u>Indication:</u> Anticholinergic drug toxicity. Tertiary amine crosses blood-brain barrier unlike neostigmine.

<u>Kinetics:</u> Onset 1-5 min. Duration 45-60 min.

<u>IV:</u> 0.5-2mg IV at rate ≤ 1mg/min. Repeat q 10-30 min or prn. <u>Anticholinergic syndrome:</u> 1-2 mg IV over 5 min. May repeat in 5-10 min if needed and cholinergic effects not noted.

## Pyridostigmine

<u>Indication:</u> Reversal of nondepolarizing neuromuscular blockade; myasthenia gravis.

<u>Kinetics:</u> Onset 2-5 min IV, duration 2-4 hr. $T_{1/2}$ 1.5-2h (ESRD 6h).

<u>IV:</u> 0.1-0.25 mg/kg (usual 10-20 mg) preceded by atropine 0.6-1.2 mg or glycopyrrolate 0.2 mg per each 5 mg pyridostigmine.

<u>Renal failure:</u> CrCl >50 mL/min: 50% usual dose; CrCl 10-50 mL/min: 35% usual dose; CrCl <10 mL/min: 20% usual dose.

# Anticoagulants

<u>Direct thrombin inhibitors:</u> *see* argatroban (next page), bivalirudin *(page 269)*, dabigatran *(page 329)*

<u>Factor Xa inhibitors:</u> *see* apixaban *(page 328)*, fondaparinux *(page 291)*, rivaroxaban *(page 330)*

<u>Heparins:</u> see heparin unfractionated *(page 296)*, enoxaparin *(page 298)*

# Argatroban[5]

Indication: Prevention and treatment of thrombosis in heparin-induced thrombocytopenia (HIT), including those undergoing percutaneous coronary intervention (PCI).

Action: Direct selective reversible thrombin inhibitor, does not require antithrombin III. Synthetic derivative of L-arginine. Prolongs PT (additively with warfarin) & aPTT. Does not interact with heparin-induced antibodies.

Kinetics: Hepatic metabolism; fecal excretion. $T_{1/2}$ = 40-50 min.

IV:Heparin Induced Thrombocytopenia (HIT) treatment or prophylaxis: 2 mcg/kg/min infusion. Check aPTT 2 hr after starting infusion. Adjust dose (up to 10 mcg/kg/min) q 2 hr until aPTT is 1.5-3 times baseline (but not > 100 sec). ACCP recommends reduced initial infusion 0.5-1.2 mcg/kg/min in patients with heart failure, multi-organ failure, anasarca, moderate livery dysfunction, and early after cardiac surgery. Percutaneous coronary intervention with HIT: Bolus 350 mcg/kg IV over 3-5 min and infuse 25 mcg/kg/min. Check activated clotting time (ACT) 5-10 min after bolus with goal > 300 sec. For ACT < 300: rebolus 150 mcg/kg, ↑ infusion to 30 mcg/kg/min, recheck ACT in 5-10 min. For ACT > 450: ↓ infusion to 15 mcg/kg/min, recheck ACT in 5-10 min.

Overlap with warfarin: Initiate warfarin once platelet count > 100-150 k/mL. Argatroban interferes with INR measurement; ACCP recommends checking factor X levels < 45% indicate warfarin INR < 2. Argatroban dose ≤ 2 mcg/kg/min: Stop infusion when INR > 4 on combined treatment and repeat INR in 4-6 hr. If INR is low, reinstitute infusion and repeat until desired INR is reached on warfarin alone. Argatroban dose > 2 mcg/kg/min: Reduce

5  Linkins LA, et al. Treatment and prevention of heparin-induced thrombocytopenia. 9/e ACCP. Chest 2012; 141: e495S-530S.

dose to 2 mcg/kg/min and follow previous procedure.

<u>Renal failure</u>: No dosage adjustment necessary.

<u>Hepatic dysfunction</u>: 4-fold decrease in drug clearance. Reduce initial dose to 0.5 mcg/kg/min for moderate liver impairment and HIT.

<u>Interactions</u>: Increased bleeding risk with antiplatelet drugs, fibrinolytics, warfarin.

<u>Adverse effects</u>: Major bleeding, hypotension, fever, diarrhea, allergic reaction.

## Atracurium (*Tracrium*)
*See Neuromuscular blockers, page 320*

## Atropine
<u>Action</u>: Muscarinic acetylcholine receptor antagonist. Blocks vagal influence on SA and AV nodes reversing functional bradycardia and AV block. Inhaled bronchodilator in severe bronchospasm, with significant systemic absorption (unlike ipratropium). Reduces oropharyngeal secretions for endotracheal intubation. Also used to counteract organophosphate and anticholinesterase drugs/toxicity.

<u>Kinetics</u>: Hepatic metabolism. Onset 1-2 min; $T_{\frac{1}{2}}$ 2 hr initially then 12 hr.

<u>IV</u>: <u>Bradycardia</u>: 0.5-1.0 mg q 3-5 min to max 0.04 mg/kg or 3 mg. May be administered via endotracheal tube at 2-3 times normal dose (diluted to 10 mL NS). <u>Asystole or "slow" pulseless electrical activity (PEA)</u>: Unlikely to have benefit[6]. 1.0 mg IV, may be repeated in 3-5 min to total dose 3mg.

<u>Anticholinesterase poisoning</u>: 2-4 mg IV/IM q 20 min until muscarinic symptoms disappear, max 6 mg/hr. (*See* Pralidoxime (*page 340*), Nerve Agents (*page 252*).

---

[6] Link MS, *et al.* Adult ACLS: 2015 AHA Guidelines Update. *Circulation* 2015; 132: S444-464.

Adverse effects: Paradoxical bradycardia for dose < 0.5 mg. Tachycardia may cause myocardial ischemia. Delirium, mydriasis, urinary retention. May exacerbate intestinal ileus or obstruction, myasthenia gravis.

## Beta-Adrenergic Blockers[7]

See individual entries for **Esmolol** and **Labetalol**

Action and indications: Antagonize circulating catecholamines. $\beta 1$-adrenergic activity: cardiac inotropy, chronotropy, dromotropy, lusitropy, vasoconstriction; $\beta 2$ effect: visceral smooth muscle relaxation including pulmonary bronchioles. Used to suppress angina, tachycardia, hypertension, anxiety, tremor, thyrotoxicosis, aortic dissection, pheochromocytoma crisis, reduce MI size, postinfarction cardiac death, and adverse neurohormonal response to CHF. Significant interindividual variability in dose-response; titrate dose to target heart rate or blood pressure. Reduced heart rate may increase pulse pressure and attenuate purported benefit in hypertension. Utility after revascularization may be exaggerated.

Adverse effects: Bronchospasm, bradycardia, AV block, hypotension, CHF, blunts manifestations of hypoglycemia in diabetes (especially in ESRD), depression, fatigue.

Relative contraindications: Decompensated CHF, hypotension/shock, AV block or PR > 260 ms, COPD or asthma, diabetes with severe or frequent hypoglycemia (masks symptoms), Raynaud's phenomenon, allergic rhinitis.

Caution: Additive AV block with diltiazem, verapamil, digoxin, amiodarone. Use cautiously in ischemic LV dysfunction, myasthenia gravis or if MAO inhibitors given within past 2 wk. Avoid agents with intrinsic sympathomimetic activity (ISA) in acute cor-

---

[7] Westfall TC, *et al.* Adrenergic Agonists and Antagonists. In: Brunton LL, *et al.*, editors. Goodman & Gilman's The Pharmacological Basis of Therapeutics, 11/e: *McGraw-Hill; 2006.*

onary syndromes and post-MI care. Sudden discontinuation can exacerbate angina or ischemia. Pre-treat with α-blocker in suspected sympathomimetic crises, *e.g.* pheochromocytoma or severe cocaine toxicity. Treat β-blocker-induced CHF with beta-agonists, phosphodiesterase inhibitors, glucagon, atropine.

<u>Acute MI:</u> **Caution:** Early IV beta-blockers increase risk of cardiogenic shock when used routinely in acute myocardial infarction[8]. Use with caution. **Metoprolol:** 5 mg IV q 5 min x 3 doses; after 15 min start 50 mg PO q 12 hr x 24 hr, then increase to 100 mg PO bid. **Atenolol:** 5 mg IV over 5 min, repeat once after 10 min if tolerated; follow by 50 mg PO bid or 100 mg PO qd. **Propranolol:** 0.1 mg/kg by slow IV push divided into 3 equal doses at 2-3 min intervals (max 1 mg/min), may repeat after 2 hr if necessary; follow with 40 mg PO after 2 hr, then 40 mg PO q 4 hr x 7 doses; then start long-term therapy with 180-240 mg/d in divided doses.

## Comparative properties:

| Name | T½ (h) (normal/ ESRD) | Typical Dose (mg) | Comments |
|------|------|------|------|
| Acebutolol | 7-9 / 7 | 200-600 bid | β1, ISA |
| Atenolol | 7 / 15-35 | 25-200 qd | β1, Low lipid solubility |
| Betaxolol | 14-22 / ? | 10-40 qd | β1, Low lipid solubility |
| Bisoprolol | 10-12/24 | 2.5-20 qd | β1, CHF, Low lipid solubility |
| Carvedilol | 6-10/ n/a | 3.125-25 bid | α1β1β2, CHF |
| Carteolol | 7/ 33 | 2.5-10 qd | β1β2, ISA, Low lipid solubility |
| Esmolol | 0.13 / 0.13 | IV only | β1, Low lipid solubility |
| Labetalol | 3-9 / 3-9 | 100-1200 bid | α1β1β2, low lipid solubility, used in pregnancy |
| Metoprolol | 3.5/2.5-4.5 | 12.5-200 bid | β1, CHF |
| Nadolol | 19 / 45 | 20-240 qd | β1β2, Low lipid solubility |
| Nebivolol | 10-12 / 19-32 | 2.5-10 qd | β1, Low lipid solubility |

*(continued)*

---

8 Chen ZM, *et al.* Early intravenous then oral metoprolol in 45,852 patients with acute myocardial infarction. *Lancet* 2005; 366: 1622-1632.

| Name | T½ (h) (normal/ ESRD) | Typical Dose (mg) | Comments |
|------|------------------------|-------------------|----------|
| Penbutolol | 17-26/100 | 20-80 qd | β1β2, ISA |
| Pindolol | 3-4 / 3-4 | 5-30 bid | β1β2, ISA, Low lipid solubility |
| Propranolol | 2-6 / 1-6 | 10-160 qid | β1β |
| Timolol | 2.7 / 4 | 10-20 bid | β1β2 |

β1 = β1 specificity   β1β2 = non-specific β-blocker   α1β1β2 = non-specific α and β-blocker   CHF = studied in compensated CHF   ISA = intrinsic sympathomimetic activity (partial β1 agonism), may cause less bradycardia and negative inotropy, but **no** survival benefit in post-MI patients (unlike agents without ISA)

## Bicarbonate

<u>Action</u>: Systemic and urinary alkalinizing agent. Used in hyperkalemia (transiently shifts potassium intracellularly), severe metabolic acidosis (*see page 203*), intoxications (tricyclic antidepressants, ethylene glycol, methanol, phenobarbital, cocaine), diuresis of drugs (salicylates) and nephrotoxic agents (uric acid, myoglobin, radiocontrast). **Note**: Ventilation is the primary therapy of respiratory acidosis; restoring adequate perfusion is the primary therapy of lactic acidosis from tissue hypoperfusion[9].

<u>Caution</u>: **Multiple adverse effects:** may induce paradoxical intracellular acidosis by liberating $CO_2$ which crosses cell membrane more freely than $HCO_3$; shifts oxyhemoglobin saturation curve and reduces $O_2$ delivery; induces hypernatremia and hyperosmolarity; may cause IV catecholamines to precipitate in IV line.

<u>IV</u>: Dilute in sterile water or dextrose. <u>Hyperkalemia or urgent intractable acidosis</u>: $NaHCO_3$ 1 mEq/kg bolus (1 amp = 50 mEq) then 0.5mEq/kg q 10 min as guided by arterial blood gas analysis. **Note**: Bicarbonate is distributed in total body water = 0.5-0.6 x body weight. Typical desired bicarbonate ≈ 8-10 mEq/L. Bicarbonate deficit (mEq) = (desired mi-

---

9 Forsythe SM, *et al.* Sodium bicarbonate for the treatment of lactic acidosis. Chest 2000; 117: 260-267.

nus actual $HCO_3$ mEq/L) x 0.5 L/kg x body weight (kg). <u>Urinary alkalinization:</u> 2-5 mEq/kg IV over 4-8 hr (mix 3.5 amps [150 mEq] $NaHCO_3$ in 850 mL D5W = 150 mEq/L).

<u>Adverse effects:</u> (See "Caution") volume overload, hypercapnia, alkalemia, hyperosmolarity, hypocalcemia, hypokalemia.

## Bivalirudin (*Angiomax*)

<u>Action:</u> Reversible direct thrombin inhibitor, inhibits free- and clot-bound thrombin, not neutralized by products of platelet activation. 20-peptide analogue of hirudin. Effect manifest in activated clotting time. Indicated as anticoagulant for percutaneous coronary intervention, including heparin-induced thrombocytopenia. May reduce bleeding compared with unfractionated heparin + $GPII_bIII_a$ inhibitors at expense of more thrombotic events. Monitor aPTT or ACT.

<u>Kinetics:</u> $T_{1/2}$ 25 min in normal renal function, 57 min if GFR 10-20, 3.4 hr if ESRD. Time-to-peak 2 min after IV bolus.

<u>IV:</u> PCI or PCI with heparin-induced thrombocytopenia (HIT): 0.75 mg/kg bolus followed by 1.75 mg/kg/hr during PCI. Measure activated clotting time 5 min after bolus, and rebolus 0.3 mg/kg as needed. Infusion typically discontinued at conclusion of procedure. <u>HIT (off-label)</u>[10]: Initial infusion rate, 0.15-0.20 mg/kg/h, target 1.5-2.5 x aPTT.

<u>Renal insufficiency:</u> PCI infusion reduced for renal impairment: GFR < 30 mL/min infuse 1.0 mg/kg/hr; hemodialysis infuse 0.25 mg/kg/hr.

<u>Hepatic insufficiency:</u> No adjustment.

<u>Caution:</u> No known antidote.

<u>Pregnancy:</u> Category B.

## Bumetanide (*Bumex*)
*See Diuretics on page 279*

---

[10] Linkins LA, *et al.* Treatment and prevention of heparin-induced thrombocytopenia. 9/e ACCP. Chest 2012; 141: e495S-530S.

## Calcium

Indications: Symptomatic hypocalcemia; reverse calcium channel blocker mediated hypotension; prophylaxis against hyperkalemic arrhythmias. No benefit used routinely in pulseless electrical activity.

IV: 20 mg elemental $Ca^{++}$= 1 mmol = 2 mEq. **Calcium chloride**: 1amp = 1 g/10 mL (10% solution) = 272 mg or 13.6 mEq elemental $Ca^{++}$. Severe desiccant; should be given via central line. **Calcium gluconate**: 1 amp = 1g/10mL (10% solution) = 93 mg or 4.65 mEq elemental $Ca^{++}$. Gluconate form is less irritating (may be given via peripheral IV) but contains 1/3 elemental $Ca^{++}$ per unit volume compared to CaCl. Hypocalcemia: See regimen on page 220. Or simplified: 10mL of 10% $CaCl_2$ (or 30 mL gluconate) in 500 mL over 6 hr. Acute hyperkalemia: 5-10 mL of 10% $CaCl_2$ (or 15-30 mL gluconate) IV over 1-5 min. Tetany: 10 mL of 10% CaCl (or 30 mL gluconate) IV over 10 min. Calcium antagonist toxicity: 10-20 mL of 10% $CaCl_2$, infuse 0.5 mEq/kg/hr.

Caution: May augment digoxin toxicity. Causes bradycardia, paresthesias, hypercalcemia. Incompatible IV with phosphate, sulfate, carbonates. Correct hypokalemia before hypocalcemia. **Note:** Hypomagnesemia common in hypocalcemia.

## Calcium channel blockers

See clevidipine on page 272; diltiazem on page 278; nicardipine on page 323; nimodipine on page 324; verapamil on page 354; Calcium blockers as pulmonary vasodilators on page 346.

# Charcoal, activated[11]

Action: Nonspecific adsorbant for toxin or overdose exposure when benefit thought to exceed risk of vomiting and aspiration. Not routinely indicated in all poisoning. Multidose may act as "GI dialysis" in prolonged absorption or elimination agents. Especially useful for high MW compounds & ingestions known to slow GI transit.

PO/NG: **Single dose:** Minimum 1 g/kg or 10:1 charcoal:toxin. Usually 1:8 slurry in water or cola. **Multiple dose:** 0.5 g/kg q 4-6 hr up to 12-24 hr.

Caution: Assure airway is controlled. Assure bowel function will not predispose to aspiration or obstruction. Concurrent cathartics may not add value. hortened transit time from cathartics or lavage may reduce efficacy. May cause diarrhea or constipation.

Contraindication: Presumed GI perforation, need for GI endoscopic examination.

# Chlorothiazide (Diuril)

Action: Parenteral thiazide diuretic. Used in combination with loop diuretic to prevent distal sodium reabsorption; effective in overcoming diuretic "resistance" in refractory edema or heart failure.

Kinetics: Onset 15 min, peak 30 min. $T_{1/2}$ 45-120 min, renal excretion.

IV: 500-1000 mg IV qd or bid.

Caution: $K^+$ and $Mg^{++}$ wasting, monitor levels closely. May exacerbate hyponatremia or hypercalcemia.

# Cisatracurium (Nimbex)

*See* Neuromuscular Blockers on *page 320*

---

11 Howland, MA. Activated Charcoal. In Nelson LS, *et al.* editors, Goldfrank's Toxicologic Emergencies, 9/e. NY: McGraw-Hill; 2010

## Clevidipine (*Cleviprex*)

*See* nicardipine on *page 323*.

<u>Action</u>: Parenteral dihydropyridine calcium channel blocker. Used as parenteral antihypertensive as alternative to nitroprusside.

<u>Kinetics</u>: Initial $T_{1/2}$ 1 min; terminal $T_{1/2}$ 15 min. Onset 2-4 min, offset 5-15 min. Hydrolyzed by blood esterases.

<u>IV</u>: Begin infusion at 1-2 mg/hr. Titrate by doubling each 90 sec. As target blood pressure approaches, reduce increments and intervals. Dose increases of 1-2 mg are expected to lower systolic BP 2-4 mm Hg. Maximum 16-32 mg/hr.

<u>Renal & hepatic insufficiency</u>: No dosage adjustment.

<u>Warning</u>: Emulsion contraindicated in soy or egg allergy, severe hypertriglyceridemia, may support microbial growth. Consider clevidipine calories (2 fat kcal/mL) in nutritional calculations. Limited experience with infusions > 72 hr.

<u>Pregnancy</u>: Category C.

## Clonidine (*Catapres*)

<u>Action</u>: Central $\alpha2$ adrenergic agonist reduces peripheral sympathetic activity, causes vasodilation and vagal mediated bradycardia, decreased renin-angiotensin-aldosterone activity without reduction of renal blood flow. Used as antihypertensive; also in management of opiate and ethanol withdrawal. No benefit and possible harm in reducing perioperative risk[12]. Epidural treats neuropathic pain.

<u>Kinetics</u>: Onset 30-60 min after PO dose, max effect 3-5 hr. Elimination $T_{1/2}$ 6-24 hr, 39-42 hr in ESRD. 50% liver metabolism, remainder excreted unchanged. Highly lipid soluble.

<u>PO</u>: <u>Urgent HTN</u>: 0.1-0.2 mg then 0.1 mg hourly (until max 0.6 mg or target BP). <u>Reduction of drug withdrawal symptoms (off-label)</u>: 0.3-0.6 mg PO q 6 hr.

---

[12] Devereaux PJ, *et al.* Clonidine in patients undergoing noncardiac surgery. *N Engl J Med* 2014; 370: 1504-1513.

<u>Renal failure:</u> No adjustment.
<u>Caution:</u> Withdrawal syndrome (uncommon) 24-72 hr after stopping; usually sympathetic hyperactivity signs, rarely hypertension. Discontinue by gradual dose reduction over 2-4 d. Use cautiously in angina or with β-blockers (withdraw β-blockers first). Convert to transdermal by dose reduction 50% day 2 and 75% day 3.
<u>Side effects:</u> Dry mouth, sedation, postural hypotension, constipation, urinary retention.
<u>Interactions:</u> Decreased efficacy with tricyclics, prazosin, MAO inhibitors. β-blockers may reverse antihypertensive effects. Exacerbates sedation from other drugs.

# Corticosteroids[13]

| Drug | Approximate equivalent dose (mg) | Relative anti-inflammatory potency | Relative mineralo-corticoid potency | Biological half-life[†] |
|---|---|---|---|---|
| Betamethasone | 0.6-0.75 | 25 | 0 | Long |
| Cortisone | 25 | 0.8 | 0.8 | Short |
| Dexamethasone | 0.75 | 25 | 0 | Long |
| Fludrocortisone* | n/a | 10 | 125 | Medium |
| Hydrocortisone | 20 | 1 | 1 | Short |
| Methylprednisolone | 4 | 5 | 0.5 | Medium |
| Prednisolone | 5 | 4 | 0.8 | Medium |
| Prednisone | 5 | 4 | 0.8 | Medium |
| Triamcinolone | 4 | 5 | 0 | Medium |

\* Not used for glucocorticoid effects
[†] Short = 8-12 hr, Intermediate = 12-36 hr, Long = 36-72 hr

# Dabigatran (*Pradaxa*)
*See novel oral anticoagulants on page 328.*

---

[13] Adapted from Schimmer BP, *et al*. Adrenocorticotropic Hormone; Adrenocortical Steroids and Their Synthetic Analogs. In: Brunton LL, et al., editors. Goodman & Gilman's The Pharmacological Basis of Therapeutics, 11/e. NY: *McGraw-Hill; 2006.*

# Dantrolene[14]

Action: Selective skeletal muscle relaxation; interferes with calcium release from sarcoplasmic reticulum probably blocking ryanodine receptor. Indicated for "fulminant skeletal muscle hypermetabolism" of malignant hyperthermia, along with oxygen, cooling, and correction of acidosis. Possible role in neuroleptic malignant syndrome[15] (see page 241) although benefit remains controversial.

Kinetics: Onset rapid. $T_{1/2}$ 4-8 hr after IV.

Dose: 1 mg/kg rapid IV. Repeat rapidly as necessary until reversal of process (usually 2.5mg/kg) or maximum dose of 10 mg/kg. Follow with 1-2 mg/kg PO qid x 1-3 d.

Interactions: Causes marked cardiac depression when combined with calcium channel blockers such as verapamil. Potentiates non-depolarizing neuromuscular blockers.

# Desmopressin (ddAVP, *Stimate*)[16]

See also Vasopressin on page 352

Action: Synthetic vasopressin analog. Induces release of endothelial von Willebrand factor and hepatic factor VIII. Used to replace ADH; also to control hemorrhage in uremia, hemophilia A (when factor VIII activity > 5%) and von Willebrand disease.

Kinetics: Bleeding time minimized in 1-2 hr.

Dosage: Hemorrhage including uremic (off-label): 0.3-0.4 mcg/kg SQ or IV (mixed in 10-50 mL NS) over 15-30 min. Nasal spray: Use 150 mcg/0.1 mL formulation only, one spray per nostril. Administer 30-120 min before surgery. Central diabetes insipi-

---

[14] Krause T, *et al.* Dantrolene. *Anaesthesia* 2004; 59: 364-373.

[15] Guze BH, *et al.* Neuroleptic malignant syndrome. *N Engl J Med* 1985; 313: 163-166; Strawn JR, et al. Neuroleptic malignant syndrome. Am J Psychiatry 2007; 164: 870-876.

[16] Mannucci PM, *et al.* Deamino-8-D-arginine vasopressin shortens the bleeding time in uremia. *N Engl J Med* 1983; 308: 8-12. Hedges SJ, *et al.* Evidence-based treatment recommendations for uremic bleeding. *Nat Clin Pract Nephrol* 2007; 3: 138-153.

dus: 2 mcg IV/SQ qd-bid, or nasal spray (1-4 sprays of 10 mcg/0.1 mL formulation qd-tid); titrate to urine output, serum sodium and osmolality. Oral: Total 0.1-1.2 mg divided 2-3 times per day.

Caution: Avoid water intoxication, hyponatremia. Tachyphylaxis after one or more doses. After 2-3 doses for hemorrhage, must wait 3-4 d to rebuild von Willebrand factor stores.

Side effects: **IV:** Water intoxication, platelet-aggregation and thrombosis, myocardial ischemia, hypotension with rapid infusion, abdominal distress. **Nasal:** Water intoxication, flushing, headache, congestion.

## Dexmedotomidine (*Precedex*)

Action: Selective α2-adrenergic receptor agonist, acts at the locus ceruleus & spinal cord to produce sedation and analgesia, alternative to benzodiazepines.

IV: **ICU Sedation hrs:** Initiate 1 mcg/kg over 10 min, then 0.2-0.7 mcg/kg/hr. **Procedural sedation:** Initiate 1 mcg/kg over 10 min, then 0.6 mcg/kg/hr titrated to effect from 0.2-1.0 mcg/kg/hr. **Patients > 65 years or hepatic impairment:** reduced loading dose 0.5 mcg/kg over 10 minutes and reduced infusion. **Alcohol withdrawal:** (Off-label) Titrated up to 7mcg/kg/hr.

Kinetics: Distribution $T_{1/2}$ = 6 min, terminal elimination $T_{1/2}$ = 2 hrs. Hepatic elimination.

Renal failure: No dose adjustment.

Side-effects: Hypotension (especially volume depleted, elderly), augmented vagal tone, bradycardia, sinus arrest, transient hypertension during loading.

Warning: Arousability and alertness when stimulated are expected, and should not be interpreted alone as lack of efficacy. Withdrawal syndrome after prolonged (> 24 hr) infusion.

Pregnancy: Category C.

# Digoxin

<u>Action</u>: Inhibitor of sarcolemmal $Na^+$–$K^+$-ATPase, increases cytosolic calcium, increases inotropy. Increases vagal tone and suppresses atrioventricular nodal conduction. Indicated in symptomatic CHF with reduced LV function (reduces symptoms and hospital admissions without mortality benefit[17]). Indicated in control of atrial fibrillation ventricular response, especially persistent atrial fibrillation with congestive heart failure, mostly through vagal tone.

<u>Kinetics</u>: $T_{1/2}$ 36-44 hr, ESRD 80-120 hr. Cleared primarily by kidneys, 18-28% cleared via stool, liver. Loading dose saturates skeletal muscle receptors; without a loading dose, therapeutic effect delayed for 1-3 weeks, depending on renal function. Onset 20-30 min IV; 2 hr PO (once steady state is reached). Oral bioavailability 60-80%.

<u>Dose</u>: <u>Heart failure</u>: 0.125-0.25 mg/d po. Reduce dose to 0.125 daily or q.o.d. if age > 70, kidney disease, low body mass. No loading dose. <u>Atrial fibrillation</u> 0.25 mg IV q 2 hr until rate control or total 1.5 mg IV. Oral loading dose 0.5 mg if not urgent.

<u>Serum digoxin levels</u>: Target serum level 0.5-0.9 ng/mL. Measure at least 8-12 hr after last dose. Steady-state levels measured after one week. Levels less helpful in atrial fibrillation (endpoints: heart rate and toxicity). Measure column-separated digoxin levels in ESRD.

<u>Renal failure</u>: Halve load. CrCl > 50 mL/min: 100% q 24h; CrCl 10-50 mL/min: 25-75% q 36 hr; CrCl < 10 mL/min: 10-25% dose q 48 hr. CAVH supplement 24-75% Q36 hr.

<u>Warning</u>: Avoid in advanced AV conduction block, pre-excitation syndromes, hypertrophic or restrictive or amyloid cardiomyopathy or cor pulmonale. Withdraw for several days before electrical

---

[17] Digitalis Investigation Group. The effect of digoxin on mortality and morbidity in patients with heart failure. *N Engl J Med* 1997; 336: 525-533.

cardioversion.

<u>Digoxin Toxicity:</u> Arrhythmias (↑ automaticity, ↑ A-V block; many arrhythmias possible but most common serious include high-grade A-V block ± junctional escape and VT/VF); hyperkalemia; anorexia, nausea, vomiting, malaise, fatigue, confusion, insomnia, depression, vertigo, green/yellow halo around lights. Increased risk for toxicity with renal insufficiency, underlying cardiac disease, electrolyte abnormalities (esp. ↓ $K^+$, ↓ $Mg^{++}$, ↑ $Ca^{++}$), hypothyroidism, advanced pulmonary disease, drug interactions, concomitant use with sympathomimetics.

<u>Interactions:</u> Diuretic-induced hypokalemia and hypomagnesemia increase arrhythmic toxicity. **Drugs that increase digoxin level:** Quinidine, verapamil, diltiazem, amiodarone, propafenone, flecainide (↓ clearance), broad-spectrum antibiotics (↓ enteric bacterial breakdown), ↓ renal blood flow (beta-blockers, CHF), anticholinergics, omeprazole ↑ absorption) **Drugs that lower digoxin level:** ↓ absorption (GI edema, antacids, cholestyramine, metoclopramide, sulfasalazine, neomycin); ↑ clearance (ACE inhibitors, nitroprusside, hydralazine, phenytoin, rifampin; St. John's wort).

# Digoxin Immune Fab *(Digifab)*

<u>Action:</u> Ovine monovalent Fab binds digoxin with high affinity, blocks binding to Na,K-ATPase.

<u>Indication:</u> **Life-threatening** digoxin toxicity, typically arrhythmia or hyperkalemia or digoxin level > 10 ng/mL.

<u>IV:</u> **Steady-state digoxin levels:** Dose (# of 40 mg vials) = [(serum digoxin level in ng/mL) x (weight in kg) ÷100]. **Empirical dosing for chronic digoxin:** 6 x 40 mg vials usually adequate. **Empirical dosing for acute ingestion of unknown amount:** 20 vials, or 10 vials x 1-2 doses; latter reduces febrile reactions. Infuse over 30 min.

Caution: $K^+$ levels may drop precipitously after administration. May precipitate acute CHF. Correct electrolytes. Other adjuncts include potassium repletion, (lidocaine,) (phenytoin,) atropine, enteral activated charcoal. Renal failure may cause spuriously elevated digoxin levels by certain assays. Therapeutic calcium, transvenous pacing and beta-adrenergic blockers are purportedly contraindicated but controversial.

Contraindications: History of sensitivity to sheep products (package insert describes skin hypersensitivity testing methodology), previous Fab.

## Diltiazem IV

*See* verapamil on *page 354*

Action: Slow calcium-channel antagonist. Prolongs AV nodal refractoriness. Used IV to slow ventricular response to atrial fibrillation or flutter, to interrupt SVTs involving AV node, and to control rest angina. Lowers BP by relaxing vascular smooth muscle without significant reflex tachycardia. Negative inotrope.

Kinetics: IV response time 5 min, peak 11 min. Plasma elimination $T_{\frac{1}{2}}$ 3.4-4.9 hr. Hepatic metabolism via P450.

IV: Tachycardia: 0.25 mg/kg (15-20 mg) given over 2 min. If unsatisfactory response after 15 min give additional 0.35 mg/kg (20-25 mg). **Continuous infusion:** 5-15 mg/hr. Change to po after 3 hr.

Renal failure: No adjustment.

Contraindications: Undiagnosed wide-complex tachycardia, WPW, 2° AV block or higher, sick-sinus syndrome, hypotension, concurrent β-blockers.

Side-effects: Hepatitis, edema, blurred vision, flushing, injection site reaction.

Pregnancy: Category C.

# Diuretics, Loop[18]

Action: Cause natriuresis and obligate diuresis via inhibition of renal Na-K-2Cl cotransporter at luminal surface of thick ascending limb of loop of Henle.

| Kinetics and dosing | Furosemide (*Lasix*) | Bumetanide (*Bumex*) | Torsemide (*Demadex*) |
|---|---|---|---|
| Oral bioavailability | 10-80 % (typically 50%) | 70-100 % | 80-100 % |
| $T_{1/2}$ (normal) | 1.5-2 hr | 1 hr | 3-4 hr |
| $T_{1/2}$ (ESRD, cirrhosis, CHF) | 2.5-2.8 hr | 1.3-2.3 hr | 4-8 hr |
| **Bolus dosing** | | | |
| Starting dose (IV) | 20-40 mg | 0.5-1 mg | 10-20 mg |
| Maximum dose* | 500 mg | 10 mg | 200 mg |
| **Continuous infusion** | | | |
| Loading dose | 40 mg | 1 mg | 20 mg |
| Infusion rate | | | |
|   Normal renal function | 10-20 mg/h | 0.5-1 mg/h | 5-10 mg/h |
|   Renal insufficiency | 20-40 mg/h | 1-2 mg/h | 10- 20 mg/h |

* "Typical" maximum effective dose in renal insufficiency, lower doses usually needed with normal renal function. Doses of up to 2000 mg. furosemide per day have been administered without major adverse effects.

Adverse effects: Hearing loss (reversible or permanent), electrolyte wasting ($Mg^{++}$, $K^{+}$, $Cl^{-}$), rash, interstitial nephritis.

# Dobutamine

Uses: Inotrope for circulatory failure from decreased myocardial contractility, *e.g.* MI, de-compensated CHF, cardiac surgery. Increases cardiac output in right ventricular infarction unresponsive to volume. Action: Racemic mixture: L-isomer is α-1 agonist, D-isomer is nonspecific β-agonist. Reduces SVR as it increases inotropy. No dopaminergic activity. Hemodynamic effect comparable to dopamine + nitroprusside. Less chronotropy than isoproterenol. Onset 1-2 min, peak effect 5-10min, $T_{1/2}$ 2.4 min. Renal failure: No dose adjustment.

---

[18] Brater DC. Diuretic therapy. *N Engl J Med* 1998; 339: 387-395.

**IV**: Usual range 2-20 mcg/kg/min, maximum 40 mcg/kg/min.

Caution: Chronotropy exacerbates myocardial ischemia. Enhances AV conduction especially in atrial fibrillation. May precipitate or exacerbate ventricular arrhythmias. Caution with MAO inhibitors.

Contraindications: Hypertrophic cardiomyopathy. Incompatible IV with alkali (theophylline, bicarbonate).

# Dopamine

Indications: • Vasopressor for hypotension refractory to fluids; • Increases cardiac contractility (inotropy) in circulatory failure; • First-line catecholamine for bradycardia refractory to atropine (preferred over isoproterenol); • May improve renal blood flow, especially at low doses along with a vasopressor, but does not improve azotemia or outcome[19]. More arrhythmia compared with norepinephrine in shock[20].

Action: Low doses (1-5 mcg/kg/min) dilate renal, mesenteric, cerebral arteries via DA receptors with minimal cardiac effect. Intermediate range (5-10 mcg/kg/min) stimulates β1 and α-adrenergic receptors, acts as inotrope and vasopressor. High doses (>10 mcg/kg/min) act mostly as α-agonist vasopressor. Significant interindividual variability in dosage ranges and overlap of hemodynamic effects (*i.e.* titrate to achieve effect). Onset < 5 min, duration < 10 min.

IV: Typical starting dose 5-10 mcg/kg/min.

Caution: Start with 10% of dose in patients with circulating MAO inhibitors. Avoid cyclopropane or halogenated hydrocarbon anesthetics. Enhances AV conduction especially in atrial fibrillation. May exacerbate psychoses. Treat extravasation aggressively (*see* phentolamine, *page 335*). Spuriously elevates LV filling pressures (via constriction of pulmonary veins).

---

[19] Bellomo R, *et al.* Low-dose dopamine in patients with early renal dysfunction. *Lancet* 2000; 356: 2139-2143.

[20] De Backer D, *et al.* Comparison of dopamine and norepinephrine in the treatment of shock. *N Engl J Med* 2010; 362: 779-789.

Incompatibility: Alkali (bicarbonate, theophylline) inactivate dopamine. Interaction is slow enough that drugs may co-infuse in a single catheter.

Pregnancy: Category C.

## Enoxaparin *(Lovenox)*
See Heparin, Low Molecular Weight on *page 298*

## Epinephrine *(Adrenalin)*

Action: Nonspecific adrenergic agonist; has β-2 activity unlike norepinephrine (NE). Twice as potent inotrope and chronotrope compared to NE, but equipotent vasopressor. At low doses (< 4 mcg/kg/min) α effects less prominent; β-2 mediated vasodilator with compensatory increase in cardiac output. Potent bronchodilator. May be added to NE.

Indications: Cardiac arrest, anaphylaxis, severe bronchospasm and laryngospasm, cardiogenic shock especially after cardiac surgery.

IV: Cardiac arrest: Bolus 1 mg (10 mL of 1:10,000) q 3-5 min IV followed by 20 mL flush; or **endotracheal** 2-2.5 mg diluted to 10 mL with NS q 3-5 min. Data do not support higher bolus doses. Shock: _infusion 1 mg (1 ml of 1:1000) in 500 mL, initial 0.1-0.5 mcg/kg/min titrated to hemodynamic response. **Note:** α-effects predominate > 4 mcg/min. Anaphylaxis with cardiac arrest[21]: 1-3 mg IV (1:10,000 over 3 min), 3-5 mg IV (3 min), then 4-10 mcg/min infusion.

Intramuscular/Subcutaneous: Bronchospasm: 0.1 mg SQ (1:1000) q 15-20 min. Local vasoconstriction reduces absorption. Anaphylaxis[21]: 0.2-0.5 mg (1:1000) IM anterolateral thigh vastus lateralis (not SQ, not deltoid) repeat q 5-10 min if no improvement.

Adverse effects: Increased myocardial oxygen demand, tachyarrhythmias, decreased splanchnic perfusion, hypertension, hyperglycemia, hypokalemia, CNS

---

[21] Lieberman P, *et al.* The diagnosis and management of anaphylaxis. *J Allergy Clin Immunol* 2010; *126*: 477.

activation

Interactions: MAO inhibitors and tricyclics dramatically potentiate activity. Halothane anesthetics sensitize myocardium to arrhythmias.

## Epoprostenol (Prostacyclin)
See Pulmonary Vasodilators on page 346

## Eptifibatide (Integrilin)
See Glycoprotein $II_b III_a$ inhibitors on page 293

## Esmolol (Brevibloc)
Action: Intravenous cardioselective $\beta 1$-blocker. Slows AV node conduction in atrial fibrillation and flutter. Combine with nitroprusside for aortic dissection; combine with phentolamine for pheochromocytoma crisis. Reduces myocardial ischemia but more hypotensive than other $\beta$-blockers.[22] May be used to test tolerability of $\beta$-blockers in patients with strong relative contraindications.

Kinetics: $T_{1/2}$ 9 min, distribution time 2 min. Steady-state 5 min with load, 30 min without. $\beta$-blockade remits 10-30 min after stopping, longer after prolonged or higher dose infusion. Esterified in RBCs.

IV: Load 500 mcg/kg over one min then 50 mcg/kg/min. Titrate q 4 min by increasing infusion 50 mcg/kg/min and re-loading each time (skip load as target effect approaches). Maximum 300 mcg/kg/min.

Renal failure: No dose adjustment.

Transition to alternative agent: Decrease infusion by 50%, 30 min after 1st dose of oral agent (digoxin, calcium or $\beta$-blocker). Discontinue infusion 60min after 2nd dose of oral agent if response is satisfactory.

Caution: Bronchospasm, A-V block. IV irritant; avoid extravasation. $NaHCO_3$ incompatible. Propylene

---

[22] Deegan R, et al. Beta-receptor antagonism does not fully explain esmolol-induced hypotension. Clin Pharmacol Ther 1994; 56: 223-228.

glycol excipient.

<u>Side effects</u>: Pallor, nausea, flushing, bradycardia or asystole, pulmonary edema.

# Ethanol[23]

<u>Action</u>:  Second line treatment (after fomepizole) for ethylene glycol and methanol poisoning. Prevents build-up of toxic metabolites by competitively binding to alcohol dehydrogenase. Target levels 100-200 mg/dL, must be checked frequently (q 1-2 hr initially) along with glucose. Specific gravity = 0.79. Inferior to benzodiazepines for alcohol withdrawal syndromes. *See page 166.*

<u>IV</u>: (Off-label): Ethanol 10% 10 mL/kg IV then 1-2 mL/kg/hr IV. Double infusion during dialysis. *See table*. Continue infusion until acidosis corrected and symptoms resolve.

<u>PO</u>: For severe poisoning in which medical care will be delayed several hours, give 4 x 1 oz doses of ~ 86 proof alcohol (whiskey). Double dose if charcoal has been given.

|  | Absolute ethanol | Volume 86-proof whiskey po | Volume 10% ethanol IV |
|---|---|---|---|
| Loading dose | 600 mg/kg | 1.8 mL/kg | 7.6 mL/kg |
| Maintenance dose non-drinker | 66 mg/kg/h | 0.2 mL/kg/h | 0.83 mL/kg/h |
| Maintenance dose ethanol drinker | 154 mg/kg/h | 0.46 mL/kg/h | 1.96 mL/kg/h |
| During hemodialysis, non-drinker | 169 mg/kg/h | 0.5 mL/kg/h | 2.12 mL/kg/h |
| During hemodialysis, drinker | 257 mg/kg/h | 0.77 mL/kg/h | 3.26 mL/kg/h |

<u>Hemodialysis</u>:  Double infusion rate or supplement dialysis bath with 200 mg/dL ethanol.

<u>Caution</u>: Hypoglycemia and folate depletion may

---

[23] Barceloux DG, *et al.* AACT practice guidelines on the treatment of methanol poisoning. *J Toxicol Clin Toxicol* 2002; 40: 415-446; Barceloux DG, *et al.* AACT practice guidelines on the treatment of ethylene glycol poisoning. *J Toxicol Clin Toxicol* 1999; 37: 537-560.

occur during prolonged infusion. Administer through central line.

## Etomidate (*Amidate*)

<u>Action</u>: Sedative hypnotic with no analgesic properties, may enhance central GABA activity. Minimal hemodynamic effects, mild respiratory depressant. Useful in hypovolemia, cardiovascular instability, myocardial dysfunction. Not suitable for prolonged infusion or sepsis because of adrenocortical suppression.

<u>Kinetics</u>: Elimination $T_{1/2}$ 75 min. Rapid liver metabolism. Onset 30-60 sec, peak effect 1 min, duration 3-5 min by redistribution

<u>Renal failure</u>: No data.

<u>IV</u>: <u>Induction of general anesthesia</u>: 0.2-0.6 mg/kg, typically 0.3mg/kg over 30-60 sec. Maintenance 0.01 to 0.02 mg/kg/min. <u>Procedural sedation</u>: (off-label): 0.1-0.2 mg/kg over 30-60 sec, then 0.05 mg/kg q 3-5 min as needed.

<u>Caution</u>: Reduces cortisol levels, probably inhibits adrenal 11-β-hydroxylation, persists for 6-8 hr.

<u>Side effects</u>: Transient venous infusion site pain common. Transient skeletal movements are common. High incidence of postoperative nausea.

<u>Pregnancy</u>: Category C.

## Fibrinolytic Agents (aka thrombolytics)

<u>Action</u>: Convert plasminogen to plasmin, which degrades fibrin clots. Reduce mortality and preserve LV function in acute MI; reduce disability in acute stroke at expense of mortality; and reduce clinical deterioration in sub-massive pulmonary embolism. Benefit in all indications offset by significant incidence of serious bleeding including intracranial hemorrhage (ICH).

| Indications | Contraindications |
|---|---|
| **Acute MI (AMI)[24]**<br>• New ST ↑ at J-point in at least 2 contiguous leads ≥2 mm (0.2 mV) in men or ≥1.5 mm in women in leads V2-V3 and/or ≥ 1 mm in other contiguous chest leads or limb leads; time to therapy ≤ 12 hr; and age < 75 *or* LBBB and history suggesting AMI<br>• ST elevation and age > 75 (IIa)<br>• STEMI but time to therapy 12-24 hr (less benefit)<br>• STEMI but BP > 180/110 and high-risk MI (greater risk)<br><br>**Note:** Benefit greatest with early therapy (< 3 hr); anterior > inferior MI (unless posterior or RV involvement); diabetes; hypotension or tachycardia. | **Absolute:**<br>• Previous hemorrhagic stroke (ever)<br>• Structural cerebral vascular lesion (AVM)<br>• Known malignant intracranial neoplasm, primary or metastatic<br>• Ischemic stroke within 3 mo, except acute ischemic stroke within 4.5 hr<br>• Suspected aortic dissection<br>• Active bleeding or diathesis (excluding menses)<br>• Significant closed head or facial trauma within 3 mo<br>• Severe uncontrolled HTN unresponsive to emergency therapy<br>• For streptokinase, prior treatment within 6 mo<br>**Relative:**<br>• Ready availability of PCI center < 120 min for STEMI<br>• Chronic, severe, poorly controlled hypertension<br>• SBP > 180 or DBP > 110mmHg on presentation<br>• Prior ischemic stroke > 3mo<br>• Dementia<br>• Other known intracranial pathology<br>• Trauma or prolonged CPR > 10min<br>• Major surgery < 3wk<br>• Internal bleeding within 2-4 wk<br>• Noncompressible vascular punctures<br>• Pregnancy<br>• Active peptic ulcer<br>• Oral anticoagulation |

*(continued)*

---

[24] O'Gara PT, *et al.* 2013 ACCF/AHA guideline for the management of ST-elevation MI. *J Am Coll Cardiol* 2013; 61: e78-140.

| Indications | Contraindications |
|---|---|
| **Acute Ischemic Stroke**[25] <br> •Diagnosis of ischemic stroke causing measurable neurological deficit <br> • Onset < 3 hr before beginning treatment. Additional criteria if used onset 3-4.5 hr. <br> • Age > 18 yr <br><br> **Notes:** <br> •tPA is only approved agent <br> •Heparin/antiplatelet agents should be held for 24 hr after treatment <br><br> *See page 155* | <u>As contraindicated for AMI, with following modifications:</u> <br> • CT evidence of intracranial hemorrhage <br> • Head trauma or prior stroke < 3 mo; <br> • Symptoms suggest subarachnoid hemorrhage; <br> • SBP > 185 or DBP > 110 mmHg; <br> • Platelet < 100 k/mm$^3$ (discontinue tPA infusion if already started when this is discovered); <br> • Heparin < 48 hr causing aPTT > ULN; <br> • Anticoagulant with INR > 1.7 or PT > 15s; <br> • Direct thrombin or Xa inhibitors with elevated sensitive tests (aPTT, INR, ECG, TT, Xa activity); <br> • Glucose < 50 mg/dL; <br> • CT evidence of multilobar infarction (hypodensity > 1/3 of a cerebral hemisphere) <br> <u>Relative exclusion criteria (tPA may be tolerated despite 1 or more of these)</u> <br> • Only minor or rapidly improving stroke symptoms (clearing spontaneously); <br> • Pregnancy; <br> • Seizure at onset with postictal residual neurological impairments; <br> • Major surgery or serious trauma < 14 d; <br> • Recent GI or urinary tract hemorrhage < 21d; <br> • Recent acute MI < 3 mo; <br> <u>Additional exclusions if used 3-4.5 hr after symptom onset</u> <br> • Age > 80 yr; <br> • Severe stroke (NIHSS > 25); <br> • Oral anticoagulant regardless of INR; <br> • Diabetes mellitus and prior ischemic stroke |

*(continued)*

---

[25] Albers GW, *et al.* Antithrombotic and thrombolytic therapy for ischemic stroke: ACCP Guidelines. *Chest 2008; 133: 630S-669S.*

| Indications | Contraindications |
|---|---|
| **Pulmonary Thromboembolism (PE)**<br>• Hypotension related to PE<br>• Severe hypoxemia<br>• Moderate-severe right ventricular dysfunction from PE<br>• Free-floating right ventricular clot<br>• Extensive deep vein thrombosis | Same as acute myocardial infarction |

<u>Adverse effects:</u> Major hemorrhage, especially intracranial. **Increased risk with age > 65, body weight < 70 kg, and hypertension on presentation.** Risk of intracranial hemorrhage much higher in acute ischemic stroke compared to myocardial infarction.

<u>Reversal for hemorrhage</u>[26]: FFP, prothrombin complex concentrates, activated factor VII, cryoprecipitate, ε-aminocaproic acid.

## Alteplase[27] (tPA; *Activase*)

<u>Action:</u> Recombinant human tissue plasminogen activator

<u>Kinetics:</u> Plasma $T_{1/2}$ 5-10 min, prolonged in liver failure.

<u>IV:</u> **Acute MI**: 15 mg IV bolus followed by 0.75 mg/kg infusion over 30 min (maximum 50 mg) and then 0.50 mg/kg over 60 min (maximum 35 mg), maximum total 100 mg. Combine with antiplatelet and anticoagulants, *see STEMI on page 52).*

---

26 Sane DC, *et al.* Bleeding during thrombolytic therapy for acute myocardial infarction. *Ann Intern Med* 1989; 111: 1010; Broderick J, *et al.* Guidelines for the management of spontaneous intracerebral hemorrhage in adults. Stroke 2007; 38: 2001.

27 O'Gara PT, *et al.* 2013 ACCF/AHA guideline for the management of ST-elevation MI. J Am Coll Cardiol 2013; 61: e78; Jauch EC, *et al.* Guidelines for the early management of patients with acute ischemic stroke. Stroke 2013; 44: 870; Konstantinides SV, *et al.* 2014 ESC guidelines on the diagnosis and management of acute pulmonary embolism. *Eur Heart J* 2014; 35: 3033.

**PE:** 100 mg infusion over 2 hr followed by standard heparin therapy after aPTT returns to twice normal. **Acute ischemic stroke:** [28] 0.9 mg/kg total (up to 90 mg), give 10% as bolus over 1 min followed by 90% of the dose infused over 60 min. Discontinue infusion if severe headache, acute hypertension, N/V, worsening neuro exam. Control BP (goal less than 180/105) with labetalol, nicardipine, nitroprusside required after fibrinolytics. No anticoagulants or antiplatelet drugs for 24 hr. *See page 155.*

## Reteplase (rPA; *Retavase*)

Action: Recombinant derivative of tissue plasminogen activator (tPA) with longer $T_{1/2}$. Simplified dosing regimen with equivalent efficacy and side-effect profile. May be useful for pre-hospital thrombolysis.

Kinetics: Elimination $T_{1/2}$ 13 - 16 min, prolonged in renal and liver failure.

IV: **Acute MI:** 10 unit IV bolus over two min, given twice, 30 min apart. Combine with antiplatelet and anticoagulants, as for tPA above.

Incompatibility: Cannot be given in same line as heparin.

## Tenecteplase (TNK-tPA; *TNKase*)

Action: Mutant of wild-type tissue plasminogen activator with longer $T_{1/2}$; can be administered as single bolus. Less effect on systemic coagulation parameters *in vivo;* when compared to tPA has similar efficacy and major outcomes in MI.

Kinetics: $T_{1/2}$ 20-24 min.

IV: **Acute MI:** Single IV bolus dose over 5 sec based on body weight: < 60 kg, 30 mg; 60-69 kg, 35 mg; 70-79 kg, 40 mg; 80-89 kg, 45 mg; ≥ 90kg, 50 mg. Combine with antiplatelet and anticoagulants as per tPA above. **Pulmonary Embolism** (Off-

---

[28] Jauch EC, *et al.* Guidelines for the early management of patients with acute ischemic stroke. *Stroke* 2013; 44: 870-947.

label): PEITHO trial submassive PE, same dose acute MI; UFH was co-administered; hemodynamic decompensation reduced at expense of bleeding[29].

# Flumazenil[30] *(Romazicon)*

Action: Competitive antagonist of benzodiazepines at the GABA$_A$ receptor. Used to reverse sedation and respiratory depression from benzodiazepines, and to treat suspected benzodiazepine overdose. Contraindicated in mixed overdose.

IV: Known isolated benzodiazepine overdose: 0.2 mg over 30 sec. If still lethargic give 0.3 mg over 30 sec. May repeat 0.5 mg over 30 sec q min to maximum cumulative dose of 3 mg. May re-bolus 0.5 mg/h to maintain wakefulness. Benzodiazepine intoxication is unlikely if no response after 5 mg. Reversal of procedural sedation: 0.2-1.0 mg at 0.2mg/min, maximum 1.0mg at one time and maximum 3.0 mg/hr. Most respond to 0.6-1.0mg.

Kinetics: Onset of reversal 1-2 min, peak 6-10 min. Distribution T$_{1/2}$ 4-10 min. Metabolized by liver. Elimination half-time ~ 50-60 min if liver normal.

Caution: May provoke withdrawal syndrome including seizures in chronic benzodiazepine users and in concurrent tricyclic antidepressant overdose. T$_{1/2}$ of benzodiazepine may exceed that of flumazenil. Sedation may be reversed earlier than is respiratory depression. Monitor for re-sedation. Caution in head injury.

Side-effects: Agitation, myoclonus, nausea, vomiting, dizziness. Associated with panic attacks in patients with panic disorder.

---

29 Meyer G, *et al.* Fibrinolysis for patients with intermediate-risk pulmonary embolism. *N Engl J Med* 2014; 370: 1402-1411.
30 Hoffman RS, *et al.* The poisoned patient with altered consciousness. Controversies in the use of a 'coma cocktail'. *JAMA* 1995; 274: 562-569.

# Fomepizole[31] (*Antizol*)

Action: Competitive inhibitor of alcohol dehydrogenase with stronger binding affinity than ethanol, blocks formation of glycolate and oxalate (from ethylene glycol) and formaldehyde (from methanol). Indicated for ethylene glycol and methanol poisoning. Preferred over ethanol because **(1)** does not cause inebriation and **(2)** no need to monitor levels. Possible (unproven) benefit in isopropanol and diethylene glycol ingestions, and alcohol-disulfiram reactions. Hemodialysis is an essential part of treatment. *See page 243.*

Pharmacokinetics: Acidosis resolution begins within 4 hr of initial dose. Typical duration of treatment 30-60 hr. Hepatic metabolism. Significant clearance during hemodialysis.

IV: Load 15 mg/kg, then 10 mg/kg q 12 hr x 4 doses, then 15 mg/kg q 12 hr. Dilute > 100 mL and infuse slowly over 30 min. Continue infusion until pH normalizes and ethylene glycol or methanol levels < 20 mg/dL and asymptomatic.

Dialysis dosing: At beginning of dialysis, administer fomepizole only if ≥ 6 hr since last dose. During dialysis, administer fomepizol q 4 hr. At conclusion of hemodialysis, if 1-3 hrs since last dose, administer ½ dose fomepizole. If > 3 hr since last dose, administer full dose of fomepizole.

Toxicity: Generally well-tolerated. Hypertriglyceridemia, nausea, dizziness, headache.

Contraindications: None

Pregnancy: Category C.

---

[31] Brent J. Fomepizole for ethylene glycol and methanol poisoning. *N Engl J Med* 2009; 360: 2216-2223.

# Fondaparinux (*Arixtra*)[32]

<u>Action</u>: Pentasaccharide sequence of heparin that binds antithrombin to inactivate factor Xa. Inhibits thrombin formation. Does not inactivate thrombin and has no effect on platelets. Heparin-induced thrombocytopenia (HIT) and osteoporosis unlikely mechanistically. No monitoring required.

<u>Kinetics</u>: Primarily eliminated via kidney; $T_{1/2}$ 17-21 hr.

<u>SQ</u>: <u>Pulmonary embolism or DVT</u>: 5.0 mg qd (body weight < 50kg), 7.5 mg qd (weight 50-75kg), 10 mg qd (weight > 100 kg) for ≥ 5 days. <u>DVT prophylaxis</u>: 2.5 mg qd starting 6-8 hr post-op (giving earlier increases risk of bleeding) for up to 11 days; halve dose (off-label) or use alternative if Crcl 30-50 mL/min. <u>Acute coronary syndromes (off-label)</u>[33]: 2.5 mg SQ qd. <u>ACS+PCI (off-label)</u>[34]: SQ fondaparinux within 24 hr + UFH 85 unit/kg bolus (65 unit/kg if GPII$_b$III$_a$) + supplement UFH to achieve ACT 300-350 s (hemochron) or 250-300 (hemotec). <u>ST-elevation MI</u>: 2.5 mg IV followed in 24h by 2.5 mg SQ qd for duration of hospital stay up to 8 d. <u>Heparin-induced thrombocytopenia (HIT, off-label)</u>[35]: 5.0 mg qd (body weight < 50kg), 7.5 mg qd (weight 50-75 kg), 10 mg qd (weight > 100 kg).

<u>Renal dysfunction</u>: Caution if CrCl 30-50 mL/min, contraindicated if CrCl <30 mL/min.

<u>Hepatic dysfunction</u>: No adjustment for mild-moderate impairment.

<u>Contraindications</u>: Severe renal impairment, weight < 50 kg, active bleeding, thrombocytopenia with

[32] Garcia DA, *et al.* Parenteral anticoagulants: ACCP Guidelines. *Chest* 2012; 141: e24S-43S.

[33] Anderson JL, *et al.* Updated Guidelines for the Management of Patients With Unstable Angina/Non-ST-Elevation Myocardial Infarction. *Circulation*, 2011; 123:e426.

[34] Simoons, ML, *et al.* Effect of glycoprotein IIb/IIIa receptor blocker abciximab on outcome in patients with ACS without early coronary revascularization: GUSTO IV-ACS. *Lancet* 2001; 357:1915.

[35] Linkins LA, *et al.* Treatment and prevention of heparin-induced thrombocytopenia. 9/e ACCP. *Chest* 2012; 141: e495S-530S.

anti-platelet antibody in presence of fondaparinux.

Monitor: Anti-X$_a$ activity calibrated with fondaparinux. Mild aPTT ↑ at higher doses.

Interactions: Increased bleeding risk when used with ASA, NSAIDs, antiplatelet agents, warfarin and other anticoagulants.

Adverse Effects: Major bleeding (especially in elderly, low body weight, or renal dysfunction) and thrombocytopenia (rare). Spinal/epidural hematomas associated with neuraxial anesthesia or spinal punctures before and during treatment. Transient transaminase ↑. Protamine ineffective for reversal; recombinant factor VIIa may be effective[36].

Pregnancy: Category B.

## Fosphenytoin (Cerebyx IV)
See Phenytoin on page 336

## Furosemide (Lasix)
See Loop diuretics on page 279

## Glucagon[37]

Action: Peptide hormone. Counter-regulator of insulin useful in hypoglycemia. Transiently decreases GI motility via relaxation of smooth muscle. Positive inotrope in supraphysiologic doses (activates cAMP independently of adrenergic receptors); used in hypotension or bradycardia unresponsive to catecholamines, especially after calcium-channel or β-blocker overdose. Acts more as an inotrope than a chronotrope.

Kinetics: T½ 8-18 min. Onset 1-5 min, comparable to insulin.

IV: Hypoglycemia: Reserve for patients who cannot

---

[36] Bijsterveld NR, et al. Ability of recombinant factor VIIa to reverse the anticoagulant effect of the pentasaccharide fondaparinux in healthy volunteers. Circulation 2002; 106: 2550-2554.

[37] Howland, MA. Glucagon. In Nelson LS, et al. editors, Goldfrank's Toxicologic Emergencies, 9/e. 2010.

receive immediate glucose. Give 1mg IV/IM/SQ, may repeat q 15 min 1-2 times. <u>Bradycardia due to calcium channel or β-blocker toxicity (off-label)</u>: 50 mcg/kg bolus (max 10mg) over 1 min then infusion 2-10 mg/hr. <u>Anaphylaxis unresponsive to epinephrine (off-label)</u>: 1-5 mg IV/IM q 5 min or infuse 5-15 mcg/min. May be given <u>intranasal</u> especially via atomizer.

<u>Caution</u>: Hepatic glucose stores are rapidly depleted in fasting/starved patients or those with liver disease or adrenal insufficiency; use glucose instead. Promotes insulin release in insulinoma with resultant hypoglycemia. Elicits catecholamine release by pheochromocytoma.

# Glycoprotein II$_b$III$_a$ Inhibitors

<u>Indications</u>: Treatment of acute coronary syndromes and myocardial infarction, and as adjunct to non-elective percutaneous coronary interventions (PCI). See specific agents below. Routinely used along with ASA and antithrombins. Benefit mitigated in dual-antiplatelet therapy (e.g. with clopidogrel).

<u>Action</u>: Inhibit platelet cross-linking and aggregation by blocking of fibrinogen and vWF. Prolong bleeding time but do not directly affect PT or aPTT in absence of concurrent heparin treatment.

<u>Contraindications</u>: Active bleeding with 30 d, or GI/GU bleeding within 6 wk; history of thrombotic stroke within 3 mo; history of any hemorrhagic stroke; bleeding diathesis; warfarin with INR > 1.5; platelet count < 100-150 K; major surgery or trauma within 4-6 wk; intracranial neoplasm; severe, uncontrolled hypertension; suspected aortic dissection; acute pericarditis.

<u>Caution</u>: Weight < 50 kg and recent use of fibrinolytics increase risk of bleeding.

<u>Toxicity</u>: Major bleeding, thrombocytopenia (0.5-1 %).

<u>Overdose</u>: Platelet transfusion for serious bleeding (may be more effective for abciximab than for eptifibatide or tirofiban).

## Abciximab (*ReoPro*)

$F_{ab}$ of humanized murine monoclonal antibody to $GPII_bIII_a$ receptor.

Pharmacokinetics: > 90% platelet inhibition within 2 hr of bolus. Short plasma $T_{1/2}$ (25 min), since it binds platelets tightly/irreversibly. Unbound remainder undergoes proteolysis.

IV: PCI: Bolus 0.25 mg/kg 10-60 min prior to intervention, then infuse 0.125 mcg/kg/min (10 mcg/min max) x 12 hr. Acute coronary syndromes with planned PCI: Bolus 0.25 mg/kg, then infuse 10 mcg/min x 18-24 hr before PCI and 1 hr post-PCI.

Contraindicated as initial treatment of ACS without planned PCI (no benefit but increased bleeding)[38].

Antidote: Platelet dysfunction can be corrected with platelet transfusion. Transfusion should be offered only for bleeding and not prophylaxis.

Renal insufficiency: No dosage adjustment.

Pregnancy: Category C

## Eptifibatide (*Integrilin*)

Peptide inhibitor of $GPII_bIII_a$ receptor

Pharmacokinetics: Platelet function inhibited within 1 hr. Bleeding time normalizes within 15 min of discontinuation; platelet function recovers by 4 hr. Clearance is primarily renal.

IV: PCI: Bolus 180 mcg/kg, then infuse 2.0 mcg/kg/min for 18-24 hr (minimum 12 hr recommended). Give a second bolus 180 mcg/kg ten min following first. Acute coronary syndromes: Bolus 180 mcg/kg, then infuse 2.0 mcg/kg/min for up to 72 hr.

Renal insufficiency: Avoid if Cr > 4 mg/dL, or consider tirofiban. For creatinine clearance < 50 mL/min, use same bolus but infusion rate 1 mcg/kg/min.

---

[38] Simoons, ML. Effect of glycoprotein IIb/IIIa receptor blocker abciximab on outcome in patients with acute coronary syndromes without early coronary revascularisation: the GUSTO IV-ACS randomised trial. *Lancet.* 2001 Jun 16;357(9272):1915-24.

<u>Antidote</u>: Largely futile. Eptifibatide readily dissociates from platelets and "poisons" transfused platelets. Best to wait until agent clears ~ 4 hr.
<u>Incompatibility</u>: Do not give in same IV line as furosemide.
<u>Pregnancy</u>: Category B

## Tirofiban (*Aggrastat*)

Non-peptide inhibitor of GP $IIb_IIII_a$ receptor
<u>Pharmacokinetics</u>: Platelet function inhibited within 5 min. Platelet function recovers within 4-8 hr of discontinuation. Clearance is primarily renal.
<u>Dose</u>: Bolus 0.4 mcg/kg/min x 30 min, then infuse 0.1 mcg/kg/min for 48-108 hr.
<u>Renal insufficiency</u>: Reduce infusion rate by 50% if CrCl < 30 mL/min.
<u>Antidote</u>: Largely futile. Tirofiban readily dissociates from platelets and "poisons" transfused platelets. Best to wait until agent clears ~ 4 hr.
<u>Incompatibility</u>: Do not give in same IV line as diazepam.
<u>Pregnancy</u>: Category B

## Haloperidol[39] (*Haldol*)

<u>Action</u>: Antipsychotic and sedative via dopaminergic blockade.   Does not depress respiratory drive. Controversial in treatment of delirium in acutely ill elderly, probably not helpful in prevention.
<u>Kinetics</u>: $T_{1/2}$ 10-38 hr (average 20 hr). Liver metabolism.
<u>IV/IM</u>: Acute psychosis and severe agitation (off-label, not FDA-approved IV): 2-10 mg q 15-20 min until symptoms abate, then 25% of initial dose q 6 hr. Total dose usually < 10-15 mg/d.   May give IV over 2-3 min; has also been given as IV infusion at 3-25 mg/hr in delirious ICU patients. Start with 0.5 mg in elderly or debilitated.

---

[39] Barr J, *et al*. Clinical practice guidelines for the management of pain, agitation, and delirium in adult patients in ICU. *Crit Care Med* 2013; 41: 263-306.

<u>Renal failure</u>: T$_{1/2}$ unknown. No dosage adjustment. Not dialyzed.

<u>Caution</u>: Reduce dose in liver (extreme care) and renal failure. Thyrotoxicosis exacerbates extrapyramidal effects. High doses may cause QT$_c$ prolongation and polymorphic ventricular tachycardia. Black box warning increased mortality in elderly patients with dementia-related psychosis.

<u>Side-effects</u>: Anticholinergic, extrapyramidal, orthostatic hypotension. Neuroleptic malignant syndrome, tardive dyskinesia (risk greater in elderly with prolonged higher-dose therapy), leukopenia, rash, hyperprolactinemia.

<u>Pregnancy</u>: Suspected teratogen in 1st trimester.

# Heparin[40] (Unfractionated, UFH)

<u>Action</u>: Variable-length glycosaminoglycans MW 3k-30 k, one third containing antithrombin-binding pentasaccharide sequence. Accelerates antithrombin inhibition of factors II (thrombin), IXa, and Xa, thereby inhibiting thrombin-induced activation of factors V and VIII. Anticoagulant in treatment & prophylaxis of thrombosis, thromboembolism, coronary syndromes, cardiovascular procedures.

<u>Kinetics</u>: Anticoagulation increases disproportionately with increasing dose. Biological T$_{1/2}$ 30 min after 25 unit/kg bolus, but T$_{1/2}$ 60 min after 75 unit/kg.

<u>IV</u>: <u>Treatment of venous thromboembolism</u>: 80 units/kg IV then 18 units/kg/h. Adjust 6 hr afterwards for aPTT 1.5-2.5 x control. <u>Prevention of venous thromboembolism</u>: 5000 units SQ q 8-12 hr. High-risk patients should have dose adjusted to increase aPTT to upper-normal limits. <u>Acute coronary syndrome and non-ST-elevation myocardial infarction</u>: 60-70 units/kg (maximum 5000 IV then 12-15 units/kg/h (maximum initial 1000). Adjust 6 hr afterwards for aPTT 1.5-2.5 x control. <u>Myocardial</u>

---

[40] Garcia DA, *et al.* Parenteral anticoagulants: ACCP Guidelines. *Chest* 2012; 141: e24S-43S.

infarction with fibrinolytics: 60 units/kg IV bolus then 12 units/kg/h (max 4000 unit bolus and 1000 units/h for patients > 70 kg), targeting aPTT 1.5-2.0 x control. Adjust dose per nomograms below. Monitor aPTT q6h during first 24h of therapy and 6h after each heparin dosage adjustment. Frequency of aPTT monitoring can be reduced to daily when aPTT is stable within therapeutic range. Monitor platelet count at least every other day. Do not infuse > 48 hr because of risk of heparin-induced thrombocytopenia.

<u>Renal failure:</u> $T_{1/2}$ unchanged. No dosage adjustment.

<u>Dosage adjustment, Raschke[41]:</u>

| aPTT | Re-bolus | Suspend | Δ infusion | Next aPTT |
|------|----------|---------|-----------|-----------|
| < 35 sec<br>(< 1.2 x control) | 80 units/kg | - | 4 units/kg/h | 6 hr |
| 35-45 sec<br>(1.2-1.5 x control) | 40 units/kg | - | 2 units/kg/h | 6 hr |
| 46-70 sec<br>(1.5-2.3 x control) | - | - | - | Next AM |
| 71-90 sec<br>(2.3-3 x control) | - | - | ↓ 2 units/kg/h | Next AM |
| >90 sec (> 3 x control) | - | 60 min | ↓ 3 units/kg/h | 6 hr |

In the above table, aPTT 46-70s corresponds to anti-Xa level of 0.3-0.7 units/mL.

<u>Dosage adjustment, Cruickshank[42]</u>

| aPTT | Re-bolus | Suspend | Δ infusion | Next aPTT |
|------|----------|---------|-----------|-----------|
| < 50 sec | 5000 units | 0 | ↑ 120 unit/hr | + 6 hr |
| 50-59 | | 0 | ↑ 120 unit/hr | + 6 hr |
| 60-85 | | 0 | — | Next AM |
| 86-95 | | 0 | ↓ 80 unit/hr | Next AM |
| 96-120 | | 30 min | ↓ 80 unit/hr | + 6 hr |
| > 120 | | 60 min | ↓ 160 unit/hr | + 6 hr |

<u>Alternate anti-Xa monitoring:</u> May be useful in lupus anticoagulant, liver disease: aPTT range 1.5-2.5 x normal corresponds to 0.3-0.7 units anti-Xa or 0.2-

[41] Raschke RA, *et al*. The weight-based heparin dosing nomogram compared with a "standard care" nomogram. *Ann Intern Med* 1993; 119: 874-881.
[42] Cruickshank MK, *et al*. A standard heparin nomogram for the management of heparin therapy. *Arch Intern Med* 1991; 151: 333-337.

0.4 units by protamine titration, but should be calibrated to the local laboratory.

**Adverse effects**: Hemorrhage, especially in seriously ill, alcohol abusers, use with other anticoagulants or antiplatelet agents. Thrombocytopenia and thromboembolic complications (*see* Heparin-induced Thrombocytopenia, *page 121*). Osteoporosis after chronic use. Hyperkalemia (Type IV RTA) especially in renal insufficiency and diabetes.

**Interactions**: Increased bleeding with ASA, GPII$_b$III$_a$ inhibitors, NSAIDs, other antiplatelet agents, warfarin, dipyridamole.

**Caution**: Rebound thrombosis may occur when discontinuing heparin in acute coronary syndromes without revascularization; consider tapering over 4-8 hr.

**Reversal**: *see* Protamine, p 344.

**Pregnancy**: Category C. Does not cross placenta; anticoagulant of choice though has been reported to cause premature/still births.

# Heparin, Low Molecular Weight (LMWH): Enoxaparin (*Lovenox*)[43]

*Also see* alternative antithrombins including **Argatroban** (*page 264*) and **Fondaparinux** (*page 291*).

**General Indications**: **(1)** Prevention and treatment of deep vein thrombosis **(2)** Acute coronary syndromes and percutaneous coronary interventions (enoxaparin) **(3)** Pulmonary embolism **(4)** Acute stroke

**Action**: See unfractionated heparin (UFH). Have more targeted effects on factor Xa and less anti-thrombin (IIa) activity compared to UFH. Better subcutaneous bioavailability and more predictable dose-response compared to UFH, allowing fixed dosages without monitoring or dose adjustment in most patients. Preferred agent in cancer-associated thrombosis.

**Kinetics**: Peak effect 3-5 hr after SQ administration.

---

[43] Garcia DA, *et al*. Parenteral anticoagulants: ACCP Guidelines. *Chest* 2012; 141: e24S-43S. Kearon C, *et al*. Antithrombotic Therapy for VTE Disease: CHEST Guideline. *Chest*, 2016; 159: 315-352.

$T_{1/2}$ = 3- 4.5 hr SQ. Excreted renally, with doubling of $T_{1/2}$ in renal failure.
**Dose:** Treatment of venous thromboembolism: 1 mg/kg SQ q12 hr or 1.5 mg/kg SQ q 24h. Continue at least 5 d after warfarin initiated. If GFR < 30 mL/min: reduce dose to 1 mg/kg qd. Prevention of venous thromboembolism: Medical patients at risk: 40 mg SQ qd; orthopedic surgery: 30 mg SQ bid; abdominal surgery: 40 mg SQ qd, start 2 hr prior to surgery if no epidural. If GFR < 30mL/min use 30 mg QA qd. Acute coronary syndromes/non-ST-elevation MI: 1 mg/kg SQ q 12 hr x 2-8 d, combine with ASA. If GFR < 30mL/min use 1 mg/kg SQ qd. ST-elevation MI with fibrinolytics: 30 mg IV bolus followed in 15 min by 1 mg/kg (maximum 100 mg for first two doses) SQ q 12 hr. If age > 75, avoid bolus and use 0.75 mg/kg (maximum 75 mg for first two doses) SQ q 12 hr. If GFR < 30 mL/min, after bolus use 1 mg/kg SQ q 24 hr. Initiate within 15 min before to 30 min after fibrinolytic. Percutaneous coronary intervention: If last dose of enoxaparin ≤ 8 hrs, no additional anticoagulant. If last dose 8-12 hr before PCI, give 0.3 mg/kg IV "boost." Because of kinetics of absorption after SQ enoxaparin, some evidence also supports[44] 0.3 mg/kg "boost" IV when PCI is performed after < 3 consecutive SQ doses were used, < 30 min since last SQ dose. Cross-over to unfractionated heparin is not recommended because of increased bleeding. If no prior enoxaparin (off-label), give 0.5-0.75 mg/kg IV with or without GPII$_b$III$_a$ inhibitor. Arterial Sheath Removal: 6 hr after last

---

[44] Ferguson JJ, et al. Enoxaparin vs unfractionated heparin in high-risk patients with non-ST-segment elevation acute coronary syndromes managed with an intended early invasive strategy. *JAMA* 2004; 292: 45-54; Antman EM, et al. Enoxaparin versus unfractionated heparin with fibrinolysis for ST-elevation myocardial infarction. *N Engl J Med* 2006; 354: 1477-1488.

IV/SQ dose, or (off-label[45]) immediately after 0.5 mg/kg IV dose.

Monitoring: Usually unnecessary. Minimal effect on aPTT or thrombin time. Consider monitoring plasma anti-factor Xa concentration ("heparin level") in patients with renal insufficiency or weight < 50 kg or > 80 kg. Draw anti-$X_a$ level 3-6 hr after dose; target 0.4-1.0 units/mL for active thrombosis, 0.6-1.0 IU/mL for prosthetic heart valves, 0.1-0.2 units/mL for prophylaxis, > 0.5 units/mL and < 0.9-1.8 units/mL for PCI (can be drawn 5 min after IV dose, upper limit controversial). Consider monitoring platelets q 2-3 d x 14 d in post-operative patients treated with LMWH.

Adverse effects: Hemorrhage, especially if used in combination with anti-platelet drugs or NSAIDs. Particular risk for epidural hematoma after spinal/epidural anesthesia or lumbar puncture. May cause less osteopenia than unfractionated heparin.

Caution: Anticoagulation of prosthetic heart valves, especially during pregnancy, is challenging and controversial[46]. Use caution and monitor anti-$X_a$ levels frequently.

Interactions: Increased bleeding with ASA, antiplatelet drugs, NSAIDs, warfarin, dipyridamole.

Reversal: Protamine is relatively ineffective, but *see page 344* for dosing.

Pregnancy: Category B. See Caution (above).

## Hydralazine *(Apresoline)*

Action: Predominantly arteriolar vasodilator. Reflex tachycardia in healthy subjects, blunted tachycardia in patients with CHF. Used for CHF in combination with nitrates; hypertension in combination with diuretic or β-blocker; hypertensive emergencies (especially in pregnancy).

Kinetics: Peak hypotensive effect 10-80 min.

---

[45] Montalescot G, *et al.* Enoxaparin versus unfractionated heparin in elective percutaneous coronary intervention. *N Engl J Med* 2006; 355: 1006-1017.

[46] Bates SM, *et al.* VTE, thrombophilia, antithrombotic therapy, and pregnancy: ACCP Guidelines. *Chest* 2012; 141: e691S-736S.

Elimination $T_{1/2}$ 3-7 hr; 7-16 hr in renal failure. Liver metabolism; fast-acetylators need 25% more; slow-acetylators more susceptible to lupus-like syndrome.

<u>IV:</u> 10-20 mg q 20 min up to max 40 mg (25 mg in pregnancy) repeated prn to target BP. Transfer to oral in 24-48 hr.

<u>PO:</u> Begin 10 mg qid, titrate up to 300 mg/day in divided doses bid-qid. Give q 8-16h for CrCl < 10 mL/min.

<u>Caution:</u> Slow-acetylators should probably not receive > 200 mg/d.

<u>Side-effects:</u> Lupus syndrome rare < 200 mg/day. Fluid retention from renin release. Reflex tachycardia (contraindicated in angina). Polyneuropathy, drug fever rare.

<u>Pregnancy:</u> Category C.

## Hydroxocobalamin (Cyanokit)[47]

<u>Action:</u> Cyanide binds to hydroxocobalamin preferentially over cytochrome oxidase. Used in cyanide poisoning (See page 249).

<u>IV:</u> 5 g IV over 15 min, may repeat 2.5-5 g as needed.

<u>Caution:</u> Requires separate infusion line because of numerous incompatibilities. Dilute with 0.9% NS. Interferes with numerous colorimetric lab tests.

<u>Pregnancy:</u> Category C.

## Hypoglycemic agents other than insulin[48]

### Biguanides (Metformin)

<u>Mechanism & action:</u> Activates AMP-kinase; ↓ Hepatic glucose production + intestinal glucose absorption, ↑ insulin action. $HbA_{1c}$ reduction: 1-2%

<u>Advantages:</u> No weight gain, hypoglycemia; cardiovascular events ↓

[47] Shepherd G, et al. Role of hydroxocobalamin in acute cyanide poisoning. *Ann Pharmacother* 2008; 42: 661-669.

[48] ADA. Standards of medical care in diabetes 2012. *Diabetes Care* 2012; 35 Suppl 1: S11-63.

<u>Disadvantages</u>: GI diarrhea & cramping; Lactic acidosis (rare); Contraindicated in CKD
<u>Cost</u>: Low

## Sulfonylureas *(Glyburide, Glipizide, Gliclazide, Glimepiride)*

<u>Mechanism & action</u>: Closes βcell $K_{ATP}$ channels; ↑ insulin secretion. $HbA_{1c}$ reduction: 1-2%
<u>Advantages</u>: Well tolerated; cardiovascular events ↓
<u>Disadvantages</u>: Hypoglycemia even fatal; ↑ Weight; Low "durability"; may blunt cardiac ischemia preconditioning
<u>Cost</u>: Low

## Meglitinides *(Repaglinide, Nateglinide)*

<u>Mechanism & action</u>: Closes βcell $K_{ATP}$ channels; ↑ insulin secretion. $HbA_{1c}$ reduction: 0.5-1%
<u>Advantages</u>: Accentuated effects around meals
<u>Disadvantages</u>: Hypoglycemia; ↑ Weight; may blunt cardiac ischemia preconditioning;
<u>Cost</u>: Medium

## Thiazolidinediones *(Pioglitazone, Rosiglitazone)*

<u>Mechanism & action</u>: Activates PPAR-γ; ↑peripheral insulin sensitivity. $HbA_{1c}$ reduction: 0.5-1.4%
<u>Advantages</u>: No hypoglycemia; Pio: ↑ HDL, ↓ Triglycerides
<u>Disadvantages</u>: ↑ Weight; Edema & CHF; Bone fracture; ↑ LDL; Rosi: FDA warning contraindicated heart dz
<u>Cost</u>: High

## α-glucosidase inhibitors *(Acarbose, Miglitol)*

<u>Mechanism & action</u>: Inhibits intestinal α-glucosidase; slows digestion & absorption. $HbA_{1c}$ reduction: 0.5-0.8%
<u>Advantages</u>: Not systemic drug; ↓ Postprandial glucose
<u>Disadvantages</u>: GI gas, flatulence, diarrhea; Frequent dosing

Cost: Medium

## GLP-1 receptor agonists *(Exenatide, Liraglutide)*
<u>Mechanism & action</u>: Incretin mimetics. Activates GLP-1 receptors; ↑ insulin secretion; ↓ glucagon secretion; slows gastric emptying; ↑ satiety. <u>HbA$_{1c}$ reduction</u>: 0.5-1%

<u>Advantages</u>: ↑ Weight; Possible ↑ βcell mass or function

<u>Disadvantages</u>: GI N/V/D; occasional pancreatitis; injected; medullary thyroid tumor in animals; unknown long-term safety

Cost: High

## DPP-4 inhibitors *(Sitagliptin, Vildagliptin, Sax-agliptin, Linagliptin)*
<u>Mechanism & action</u>: prolonged ↑ urinary glucose excretion. HbA$_{1c}$ reduction: 0.5-0.8%

<u>Advantages</u>: Independent of insulin secretion and action.

<u>Disadvantages</u>: Risk of bone fractures and of ketoacidosis. Urinary & vaginal mycosis. Hyperkalemia.

Cost: High

## Sodium-glucose co-transporter 2 inhibitors *(cangliflozin, dapagliflozin, empagliflozin)*
<u>Mechanism & action</u>: Binds bile acids and cholesterol; hypoglycemic mechanism unknown. HbA$_{1c}$ reduction: 0.5-1%

<u>Advantages</u>: No hypoglycemia; ↓ LDL

<u>Disadvantages</u>: Constipation; ↑ triglycerides; Interferes with absorption of other medications

Cost: High

## Bile acid sequestrants *(Colesevelam)*
<u>Mechanism & action</u>: Binds bile acids and cholesterol; hypoglycemic mechanism unknown

<u>Advantages</u>: No hypoglycemia; ↓ LDL

<u>Disadvantages</u>: Constipation; ↑ triglycerides; Interferes with absorption of other medications
<u>Cost</u>: High

## Dopamine-2 agonists *(Bromocriptine)*
<u>Mechanism & action</u>: Activates DA receptors; Alters hypothalamic metabolism regulation, ↑ insulin sensitivity
<u>Advantages</u>: No hypoglycemia
<u>Disadvantages</u>: Dizziness, nausea, fatigue, rhinitis, unknown long-term safety
<u>Cost</u>: Medium

## Insulin
<u>Action & kinetics</u>: Anabolic hormone maintains glucose homeostasis via glucose translocation, inhibition of glycogenolysis and gluconeogenesis, and stimulation of glycogen synthesis. Suppresses lipolysis and ketogenesis. Drives potassium into cells. Used in hyperglycemia, diabetic ketoacidosis, acute hyperkalemia. Intensive insulin targeting blood glucose 80-110mg/dL probably increases mortality; a higher target glucose range (ICU 140-180 mg/dL) is now preferred[49].
<u>Kinetics</u>: Renal excretion. Plasma $T_{1/2}$ 5-15 min.
<u>IV (regular only)</u>: Mix 100 units in 100 mL NS or D5W; flush first 10 mL through tubing and waste.
<u>Ketoacidosis</u>: Bolus 0.1 units/kg, then 0.1 units/kg/h. Rebolus and increase infusion rate if glucose does not fall 50-75 mg/dL/hr. Halve rate when glucose is < 250 mg/dL. See DKA on page 87 for alternative Joslin dosing. <u>Severe hyperkalemia</u>: Onset 15-30 min. Give 10 units along with 50 g dextrose 50% during first hour. May re-bolus or infuse 20 units insulin in 1 liter 10% dextrose at 50 mL/h. <u>Severe β-adrenergic blocker or calcium-channel-blocker overdose ("insulin-euglycemic therapy")[50]</u>: 1 unit/kg bolus + 0.5

---

[49] Finfer S, *et al.* Intensive versus conventional glucose control in critically ill patients. *N Engl J Med* 2009; 360: 1283-1297.
[50] Kerns W. Insulin-Euglycemia Therapy. In: Nelson LS, *et al.*, editors. Goldfrank's Toxicologic Emergencies, 9/e. 2010.

unit/kg/h. Titrate upwards by 2 unit/kg if no improvement in 30 min. Add dextrose 0.5g/kg if glucose < 400 mg/dL and monitor glucose q 15-30 min, maintaining glucose 100-250 mg/dL.

<u>Renal failure:</u>  $T_{\frac{1}{2}}$ ↑. Give 75% dose if CrCl 10-50 mL/min; 50% if CrCL <10 mL/min.

## Insulin preparations:

| Formulation | Onset | Peak | Effectiveness |
|---|---|---|---|
| Short-acting = prandial insulin | | | |
| Aspart (*Novolog*) | 5-15 min | 30-90 min | 2-4 |
| Lispro (*Humalog*) | 5-15 min | 30-90 min | 2-4 |
| Glulisine (*Apidra*) | 5-15 min | 30-90 min | 2-4 |
| Regular | 30-60 min | 2-3 h | 3-6 hr |
| Long-acting = basal insulin | | | |
| NPH | 2-4 h | 4-10 h | 10-16 hr |
| Glargine (*Lantus*) | 2-4 h | Minimal | 20-24 hr |
| Detemir (*Levemir*) | 3-8 h | None | 12-24 hr |

## Dosing regimens
*See* Inpatient Hyperglycemia on *page 84.*

## Sliding Scale Insulin (units regular)
Not generally acceptable as sole form of insulin therapy

| Glucose mg/dL | With Meals | | | At Bedtime |
|---|---|---|---|---|
| | Highly insulin sensitive | Normal insulin sensitivity | Highly insulin resistant | |
| < 150 | 0 | 0 | 0 | |
| 150–199 | 1 | 2 | 3 | |
| 200-249 | 2 | 4 | 6 | |
| 250-299 | 3 | 6 | 9 | 0-2 |
| 300-349 | 4 | 8 | 12 | 2-4 |
| > 350 | 5 | 10 | 15 | 4-6 |

## Joslin ICU Insulin Infusion Algorithm (Target 140-180mg/dL)[51]

| Current Blood Glucose | Previous Blood Glucose (mg/dL) | | | | | | | |
|---|---|---|---|---|---|---|---|---|
| | < 100 | 100-140 | 141-180 | 181-200 | 201-250 | 251-300 | 301-400 | >400 |
| < 100 | Stop insulin, give glucose until BG > 140, then restart at ½ previous infusion | | | | | | | |
| 101-140 | ↓1 unit/ hr | ↓ 25% or 0.5 unit/hr* | | ↓ 50% or 2 unit/hr* | | | ↓ 75% or 2 unit/hr* | |
| 141-180 | — | | | ↓ 50% or 2 unit/hr* | | | | |
| 181-200 | ↑1 unit /hr | ↑0.5 unit/hr | ↑ 25% or 1 unit /hr* | — | ↓ 25% or 2 unit/hr* | | | |
| 201-250 | ↑ 25% or 2 unit/hr* | | ↑ 25% or 1 unit/hr* | | ↑1 unit/hr | — | | |
| 251-300 | ↑ 33% or 2.5 unit/hr* | | ↑ 25% or 1.5 unit /hr | ↑ 25% or 1 unit/hr* | ↑ 1 unit /hr | ↑1.5 unit /hr | ↑ 25% or 2 unit/hr* | — |
| 301-400 | ↑ 40% or 3 unit/hr | | | | | | | |
| >400 | ↑ 50% or 4 unit/hr | | | | | | | |

*= whichever is greater.  Check blood glucose hourly until stable, then less frequently.*

## Ibutilide[52] *(Convert)*

<u>Action</u>: Short-acting class III antiarrhythmic used to convert atrial fibrillation (AF) or flutter to sinus rhythm. Dose-related QT prolongation associated with antiarrhythmic activity. Ibutilide treatment prior to electrical cardioversion reduces energy threshold and increases success rate.[53]

<u>Kinetics</u>: Rapid redistribution terminates drug effect. Hepatic metabolism. Elimination $T_{\frac{1}{2}}$ ~6 hr (range 2-12).

<u>IV</u>: AF or flutter < 48 hr duration: 1 mg infused over 10 min (0.01 mg/kg if < 60kg). Repeat once if

[51] Gonda O. Joslin Clinical Guideline for Inpatient Management of Surgical and ICU Patients with Diabetes. *http://www.joslin.org/ joslin_clinical_guidelines.html. 2015.*

[52] Stambler BS, *et al.* Efficacy and safety of repeated intravenous doses of ibutilide for rapid conversion of atrial flutter or fibrillation. *Circulation 1996; 94:* 1613-1621.

[53] Oral H, *et al.* Facilitating transthoracic cardioversion of atrial fibrillation with ibutilide pretreatment. *N Engl J Med 1999; 340:* 1849-1854.

arrhythmia persists 20 min after start of infusion. Continue ECG monitoring ≥ 4-6 hr post-infusion (longer if hepatic dysfunction), with immediate access to defibrillator, pacing, antiarrhythmic capability. Consider initiation of long-term oral anti-arrhythmic if cardioversion successful. Start IV heparin prior to infusion and continue anticoagulation for 4 wk afterward. AF of unclear duration or lasting > 48 hr: Anticoagulate > 3 wks before cardioversion and 4 wk afterwards.

<u>Renal & hepatic failure</u>: Dose adjustment may not be necessary.

<u>Caution</u>: Avoid other antiarrhythmics (especially class I or III agents) before and within 4 hr of administering drug. Do not give if decompensated CHF, EF < 30% or recent MI. Avoid in hypokalemia, hypomagnesemia, $QT_c$ > 440ms or hemodynamic instability. Unsuitable for chronic atrial fibrillarion.

<u>Warning</u>: Can cause lethal polymorphic ventricular tachycardia (*torsades de pointes*). VT generally begins during or shortly after infusion, and is more common in women, CHF, reduced EF and those with slower heart rates. Low incidence (< 2%) of self-limited high-grade AV block and bundle-branch block.

<u>Interactions</u>: Excess risk of *torsades* if co-administered with drugs that prolong QT (antiarrhythmics, tricyclic antidepressants, phenothiazines, $H_1$-antagonists).

<u>Pregnancy</u>: Category C.

## Idarucizumab (*Praxbind*)
## reversal of Dabigatran[54]

<u>Action</u>: Reversal of Dabigatran anticoagulation. Humanized Fab. Binds free and thrombin-bound Dabigatran. No procoagulant effect.

<u>Kinetics</u>: Normalizes coagulation tests (aPTT, dilute thrombin time, or ecarin clotting time) within minutes. Initial $T_{1/2}$ 47 min, terminal $T_{1/2}$ 10.3 hr. Re-

---

54 Pollack CV, Jr., *et al.* Idarucizumab for Dabigatran Reversal. *N Engl J Med* 2015; 373: 511-520.

nal elimination and protein catabolism.

<u>IV</u>: 5 g as two consecutive bolus injections or infusions. A second 5 g dose may be administered 12-24 hr after 1st dose for persistent bleeding and elevating coagulation tests, or additional invasive procedures needed.

<u>Renal failure</u>: No dose adjustment necessary.

<u>Warning</u>: Dabigatran $T_{1/2}$ 12-17 hr and 80% renal excreted. Dabigatran can be restarted after 24 hr. No activity on anticoagulants other than dabigatran.

# Iron intravenous[55]

## Ferumoxytol, ferric gluconate, ferric carboxymaltose, iron sucrose

<u>Action</u>: Rapid repletion of iron stores when oral fails including malabsorption, gastroduodenal bypass, inflammatory bowel (oral may exacerbate) or celiac disease, hereditary telangiectasia, chronic kidney disease, failed erythropoiesis stimulators esp cancer. MRI contrast agent (off-label). Lower molecular weight agents may have fewer adverse effects. Compared with maximum oral iron absorbed ~25 mg/d. FDA indication in CKD typically dialysis with or without erythropoietin.

<u>IV Dose (mL)</u>: body weight (kg) x 2.3 x (target – patient Hb g/dL) ÷ [Elemental iron mg/mL in specific drug] + supplement 500 mg to replenish iron stores. Maximum dose 1000 mg.

<u>Warning</u>: Observed anaphylaxis rate is low apart from iron dextran, which is not listed below. Iron dextran had highest anaphylaxis rate and is not listed here. Observe for 30 min afterwards. May cause hypotension during infusion. Alters MRI contrast for days-weeks.

---

[55] Auerbach M, *et al*. Clinical use of intravenous iron: administration, efficacy, and safety. *Hematology Am Soc Hematol Educ Program 2010; 2010*: 338-347; Avni T, *et al*. The safety of intravenous iron preparations. *Mayo Clin Proc 2015; 90*: 12-23.

IV: Start at 2 mcg/min, titrate up to 10 mcg/min.
Contraindication: Digitalis induced bradycardia, angina
Side effects: Hypotension from vasodilatation; tachycardia; ischemia and increased infarct size during MI; malignant ventricular arrhythmias.

## Ferumoxytol (*Feraheme*)

Formulation: 30 mg/mL elemental iron as polyglucose sorbitol carboxymethylether. 750 kDa.
Maximum: 510 mg per session. Separate doses by 3-8 d.
Kinetics: $T_{\frac{1}{2}} \sim$ 15 hr
IV: 510mg diluted in 50-200mL infused over 15 min. Off-label infuse over as little as 1min, especially as MRA contrast agent.
Warning: **Black box warning** risk of anaphylaxis (estimated 0.1%).

## Ferric gluconate (*Ferrlecit*)

Formulation: 12.5 mg/mL elemental iron. 289-440 kDa.
Maximum: 125mg. (Off-label:) 250mg. Maximum 187.5mg at one time.
Kinetics: $T_{\frac{1}{2}} \sim$ 1-1.5 hr
IV: May be diluted and infused over 20-30 min. Slow injection up to 12.5mg/min.
Warning: No black box warning. No test dose suggested. Risk of hypersensitivity.

## Ferric carboxymaltose (*Injectafer*)

Formulation: 50 mg/mL elemental iron. 150 kDa.
Maximum: 750 mg per session, may repeat in 7 d.
Kinetics: $T_{\frac{1}{2}} \sim$ 7-12 hr
IV: Slow push or diluted 100 mg/min.
Warning: No black box warning. Risk of hypersensitivity.

## Iron sucrose (*Venofer*)

Concentration: 20 mg/mL elemental iron.
Maximum: 300mg per session.
Kinetics: $T_{\frac{1}{2}}$ 6 hr

<u>IV</u>: 100-200 mg per session as slow injection over 2-5 min.

<u>Warning</u>: No black box warning. Risk of hypersensitivity.

# Isoproterenol *(Isuprel)*

<u>Action</u>: Nonspecific β-adrenergic agonist. Potent inotrope and chronotrope. Hepatic metabolism. 3$^{rd}$ line agent (after dopamine, epinephrine) for bradycardia unresponsive to atropine if transcutaneous or transvenous spacing is unavailable; temporizing measure prior to overdrive pacing for *torsades de pointes*.

<u>Kinetics</u>: Plasma T$_{1/2}$ < 5 min. Onset < 5 min, duration <1 hr.

<u>IV</u>: Start at 2 mcg/min, titrate up to 10 mcg/min.

<u>Contraindication</u>: Digitalis-induced bradycardia, angina

<u>Side Effects</u>: hypotension from vasodilation; tachycardia; ischemia and increased infarct size during MI; malignant ventricular arrhythmias.

## Kayexalate

*See sodium polystyrene sulfonate, page 351*

# Ketamine *(Ketalar)*

<u>Action</u>: Rapid-acting non-barbiturate "dissociative" anesthetic, related to phencyclidine. Causes marked analgesia, amnesia, normal tone and reflexes, cardiovascular and respiratory stimulation. Mild bronchodilator. Increases HR and BP and myocardial oxygen demand. Side effects attenuated by benzodiazepines or clonidine.

<u>Kinetics</u>: Onset 1-2 min, duration 5-15 min. Alpha T$_{1/2}$ 10-15 min; Beta T$_{1/2}$ 2.5 hr. Alpha redistribution to peripheral tissues. Hepatic elimination.

<u>Renal failure</u>: No dose reduction.

<u>Liver failure</u>: Consider dose reduction.

<u>IV</u>: <u>Induction</u> 1-4.5 mg/kg IV. Typical dose 2 mg/kg can cause surgical anesthesia for 5-10 min.

<u>Combination</u> 1-2mg/kg IV at 0.5mg/kg/min with diazepam 2-5mg IV via separate route over 1 min

(typical 10-15 mg diazepam). <u>Maintenance</u> repeat half- or full-induction dose as needed, or 0.1-0.5 mg/kg/min combined with diazepam 2-5 mg IV as needed.

<u>Caution:</u> Emergence dysphoria (hallucinations, delirium, agitation) ~ 12%. Combination with benzodiazepine may reduce emergence reactions. Cardiovascular stimulation may be marked and cause hypertension ischemia or arrhythmia. Although considered respiratory stimulant, watch for transient apnea. Increases intracranial pressure.

<u>Warning:</u> Do not admix with diazepam.

# Labetalol

<u>Action:</u> Selective α-1 antagonist, nonselective β-antagonist. α:β 1:3 oral, 1:7 IV. No β-1 agonism but may be partial β-2 agonist. Dose-related antihypertensive effect without reflex brady/tachycardia. Tachyphylaxis uncommon. Predominant β-effect makes it a 2$^{nd}$ line agent for sympathomimetic crises[56] (e.g. cocaine overdose, pheochromocytoma), for which pure α-antagonists are preferred, e.g. phentolamine.

<u>Kinetics:</u> T$_½$ 5-8 hr. IV onset 3-5 min. Liver clearance with extensive first-pass metabolism; reduce dose in liver disease.

<u>Renal failure:</u> T$_½$ unchanged. No dosage adjustment. Not dialyzed.

<u>IV:</u> 20-80 mg IV bolus (over 2 min) q 10 min to max 300 mg for rapid BP control. Infuse 0.5-2 mg/min to maximum of 2400 mg/day. Stop infusion after satisfactory BP. Change to PO by abruptly stopping infusion and waiting for BP to rise.

<u>PO:</u> 1:1 PO-IV conversion (total daily dose divided in two intervals). Usual dose 200-400 mg bid, max 1200 mg bid. Titrate to **standing** BP.

---

56 Hollander JE. The management of cocaine-associated myocardial ischemia. N Engl J Med 1995; 333: 1267-1272; McCord J, et al. Management of cocaine-associated chest pain and myocardial infarction. Circulation 2008; 117: 1897-1907.

Caution: Postural hypotension. Abrupt discontinuation may precipitate angina, hypertension, myocardial ischemia like all β-blockers. β-predominance may precipitate paradoxical hypertension in sympathomimetic crisis.

Side effects: Bradycardia, 3° AVB (all less than in pure β-blockers). Postural hypotension, paresthesias, hepatocellular damage, tremor, low-titer insignificant (+) antinuclear antibody, halothane hypotension.

Pregnancy: Category C although may be useful.

# Levetiracetem (*Keppra*)

Action: Parenteral anticonvulsant with unknown mechanism of action, possibly synaptic vesicle protein 2A antagonism. Attractive pharmacokinetic profile and high therapeutic index. Neither inducer nor substrate of CYP enzymes. High oral bioavailability. Compared with lorazepam for seizures, comparable efficacy, less respiratory depression and hypotension[57]. Off-label for status-epilepticus.

IV: Initiate 500 mg IV over 15 min, bid. Advance q 2 wk to 1500 mg bid.

PO: Same dose and interval as IV. Complete bioavailability.

Kinetics: Peak corresponds to infusion time. $T_{\frac{1}{2}}$ 6-8 hr, ESRD 24 hr. Enzymatic hydrolysis, renal excretion.

Renal insufficiency: Reduce dose in proportion to GFR. GFR > 80 mL/min: 500-1500 mg q 12 hr; GFR 50-80: 500-1000 mg q 12 hr; GFR 30-50: 250-750 mg q 12 hr; GFR < 30: 250-500 mg q 12. ESRD hemodialysis: 500-1000 mg q 24 hr + 250-500 mg supplement after every dialysis.

Liver impairment: No dosage adjustment.

Side effects: Behavior disorder, irritability, aggression, mood disorder.

---

[57] Prasad M, *et al.* Anticonvulsant therapy for status epilepticus. *Cochrane Database Syst Rev* 2014; 9: CD003723.

# Levothyroxine (T4)

*See* Liothyronine, page 314. *See* myxedema coma on *page 80*.

<u>Action:</u> Thyroid hormone. Must undergo peripheral conversion to T3 for biological activity. Conversion blocked by severe non-thyroid illness.

<u>Kinetics:</u> Onset of action 6-12 hr. $T_{1/2}$ one week.

<u>IV:</u> <u>Myxedema coma:</u> Bolus 300-500 mcg IV then 50-100 next day. Lower dose in cardiovascular disease. Consider combination with liothyronine (T3). **Maintenance:** half of regular dose or 50-100 mcg IV qd.

<u>PO:</u> Oral bioavailability 50-80%. **Maintenance:** Average dose 1.6 mcg/kg. Start at 12.5-50 mcg in elderly or cardiac disease and titrate upwards every 2-3 weeks. **Non-adherent patients (off-label):** Long $T_{1/2}$ allows "directly observed therapy" in form of weekly dosing (7 x usual daily dose).

<u>Caution:</u> Cardiovascular effects (ischemia, arrhythmia especially atrial fibrillation, high output CHF).

<u>Drug interactions:</u> Estrogens bind T4, higher doses may be needed. Decreased oral absorption with iron, antacids, bile resins, calcium. Thyroid replacement increases clotting factor metabolism, thereby increasing warfarin effect and potential for bleeding.

# Lidocaine

<u>Action:</u> Class IB antiarrhythmic depresses automaticity. Used to suppress ventricular arrhythmias, especially associated with acute ischemia. Not warranted as routine prophylaxis in acute MI. Second line agent in cardiac arrest.

<u>Kinetics:</u> $T_{1/2}$ 1.5-2 hr initially lengthens to 3h with infusions > 1day. $T_{1/2}$ increases with CHF, age, liver disease. Extensive hepatic metabolism; metabolites accumulate in renal failure and may cause CNS toxicity. Rapid redistribution of initial load ($T_{1/2}$ ~ 4-8 min) requires re-bolus. Amenable to emergency re-distribution by fat emulsion.

<u>IV</u>: <u>Ventricular tachycardia or fibrillation</u>:  Load 1-1.5 mg/kg over 1-2 min then 0.5-0.75 mg/kg q 5-10 min to max 3 mg/kg. May give initial bolus via ETT at 2-4 mg/kg. **Maintenance**: 30-50 mcg/kg/min (1-4mg/min). Re-bolus 0.5 mg/kg and increase infusion for breakthrough arrhythmias. Reduce infusion after 1 day. No need to taper before discontinuing.

<u>Renal failure</u>: Minimal $T_{1/2}$ change: no dose change, not dialyzed. However, active metabolite accumulates in renal failure and may contribute to neurological side effects.

<u>Side-effects</u>: Neurologic, including drowsiness, slurred speech, paresthesias, confusion (seen almost universally > 7 mcg/mL). Severe: seizures.

<u>Interactions</u>: $T_{1/2}$ prolonged by beta-blockers (which decrease hepatic blood flow) and by cimetidine (reduces hepatic metabolism). Lidocaine potentiates action of neuromuscular blocking agents.

<u>Levels</u>: Therapeutic: 1.5-5.0 mcg/mL. Seizures seen at levels > 5 mcg/mL.

# Liothyronine (T3; *Triostat IV*)

*See* levothyroxine, *page 313*. *See* myxedema coma on *page 80*.

<u>Action</u>:  Biologically active form of thyroid hormone (converted from T4 in periphery).

<u>Kinetics</u>:  Onset 2-4 hr. Elimination $T_{1/2}$ ~ 2.5d , compared with ~ 7 d for T4.

<u>Indication</u>: T3 is generally avoided except in severe hypothyroidism (myxedema coma) in which **(1)** T4 monotherapy would pose unacceptable delay in recovery or **(2)** concurrent severe non-thyroid illness inhibits peripheral conversion from T4 to T3.

<u>Dose</u>: No data or consensus on optimal dosing.

<u>Myxedema coma</u>: 10-20 mcg IV, then 10 mcg q 4-6 hr based on clinical response. In known cardiovascular disease, halve dose.  FDA dose is higher.  Often combined with T4 (levothyroxine).

<u>Adverse effects</u>:  Cardiovascular (ischemia, hypertension, CHF, cardiac arrest). Not indicated for weight loss.

# Lipid or fat emulsion[58] (*Intralipid*)

<u>Action</u>: Off-label emergency treatment for cardiac arrest induced by lipid-soluble agents: quaternary amine anesthetics (lidocaine, bupivacaine), tricyclic antidepressants, verapamil, lipophilic beta-adrenergic blockers, chlorpromazine. May act as "lipid-sink" or may have other electrophysiological properties. Benefit is anecdotal.

<u>IV</u>: 20% fat emulsion 1.5 mg/kg bolus then 0.25 mL/kg/min x 30-60 min. Repeat bolus q 3-5 min up to 10mL/kg until circulation restored. Increase infusion to 0.5 mL/kg/min if BP declines. Maximum total dose 8 mL/kg.

<u>Warning</u>: Use is off-label and anecdotal. Note propofol and clevidipine are dissolved in fat emulsion.

# Magnesium

<u>Action</u>: Hypomagnesemia common with diuretics, alcohol, nephrotoxic agents (aminoglycosides, amphotericin). Shortens QT interval and may suppress polymorphic VT associated with hypomagnesemia. Correction of deficit facilitates correction of hypocalcemia, hypokalemia. Anticonvulsant in eclampsia. No benefit to supplementation in acute MI. Third-line agent in acute asthma. **Note:** In severe hypomagnesemia deficit is 1-2 mEq/kg; half of administered Mg is excreted renally. Replace half in first day and remainder in 2-3 d. Serum levels correlate poorly with body stores.

<u>IV</u>: 1-2 g IV as 10% solution in 50-100 mL D5W or NS over > 20-30 min. 1 g $MgSO_4$ = 8.12 mEq. <u>Torsades de Pointes</u>: 1-2 g IV over 5 min. <u>Eclampsia</u>: 2-4 g IV push over 2-4 min then 1-4 g/hr titrated to respiratory drive, loss of patellar reflexes, levels. Levels of 4-7 mg/dL therapeutic in eclampsia and seizures. Levels > 7 mg/dL toxic. <u>Asthma</u>: 1.2-2 g IV

---

[58] Bania TC. Intravenous fat emulsions. In: Nelson LS, *et al.*, editors. Goldfrank's Toxicologic Emergencies, 9/e. 2010; Rothschild L, *et al.* Intravenous lipid emulsion in clinical toxicology. *Scand J Trauma Resusc Emerg Med* 2010; 18: 51; Soar J, *et al.* Advanced life support. *Resuscitation* 2015; 95: e71-e120.

over 15-30 min in addition to β-blockers, oxygen, glucocorticoids, may reduce hospital admission[59].

<u>IM</u>: IV dose given as 1 g of 25% solution q 4-6 hr.

<u>Side effects</u>: Hypotension, hypothermia, CNS depression, respiratory paralysis. Atropine-responsive bradycardia. Extreme caution in renal failure.

## Mannitol[60]

<u>Action</u>: Osmotic diuretic sugar alcohol causing dehydration to achieve hyperosmolarity. Indicated as osmotic diuretic and to reduce intracranial pressure. Used in traumatic brain injury to lower intracranial pressure.

<u>Kinetics</u>: $T_{\frac{1}{2}}$ ~ 100 min. Acts within 10-15 min, and halves intracranial pressure within 20-60 min.

<u>IV</u>: 0.25-1.0g/kg of 20% solution q 2-4 hr. Target intracranial pressure <20 mmHg and osmolarity 300-320 mOsm/L; verify serum osmolar gap (*see page 2*) is low 20 min after infusion to assure fidelity.

<u>Caution</u>: Causes acute renal failure especially > 200g/d. Avoid excessive hypernatremia.

## Methylene Blue

<u>Action</u>: Reduces methemoglobin from ferric to ferrous state via NADPH-dehydrogenase. Requires NADPH generated by pentose phosphate pathway, itself requiring G6PD. Used to treat methemoglobinemia; *see page 251*.

<u>Indication</u>: Symptomatic methemoglobinemia > 40%. Note: remove toxins as warranted with charcoal, catharsis, hemodialysis. Exchange transfusion or hemodialysis indicated if > 50% MetHb.

<u>IV</u>: 1-2 mg/kg of 1% solution over 5 min, repeat in 1 hr if cyanosis persists.

<u>Kinetics</u>: Partially reduced in tissue. Slow renal excretion over days.

---

[59] Kew KM, *et al*. Intravenous magnesium sulfate for treating adults with acute asthma in the emergency department. *Cochrane Database Syst Rev* 2014; 5: CD010909.

[60] Ropper AH. Hyperosmolar therapy for raised intracranial pressure. *N Engl J Med* 2012; 367: 746-752.

<u>Warning</u>: High doses oxidize reduced hemoglobin iron to ferric, which produces methemoglobin. Therefore infuse slowly. Do not use in cyanide toxicity because of superior efficacy of nitrate + thiosulfate.

<u>Contraindication</u>: G6PD deficiency (causes hemolysis). Consider alternative treatment with ascorbic acid 100-500 mg po or IV.

<u>Adverse reactions</u>: Colors urine bright blue-green. Irritates bladder. Cumulative doses > 7 mg/kg can cause dyspnea, chest pain, tremor, cyanosis, hemolysis. Can contribute to serotonin syndrome.

## Methylnaltrexone[61] *(Relistor)*

<u>Action</u>: Peripherally-acting μ-opioid antagonist unable to cross blood-brain barrier, used to treat opioid-induced constipation during palliative care.

<u>Dose</u>: 38-62 kg: 8 mg SQ; 62-114 kg: 12 mg SQ; otherwise 0.15 mg/kg. Typically every other day, but no more than daily.

<u>Kinetics</u>: Peak concentration 30 min, elimination $T_{1/2}$ ~ 8 hr, eliminated unchanged in urine & feces.

<u>Renal failure</u>: Reduce dose by half if CrCl < 30 mL/min.

<u>Hepatic impairment</u>: No adjustment if mild.

<u>Contraindication</u>: Bowel obstruction.

<u>Adverse reactions</u>: Abdominal pain, flatulence, diarrhea, nausea, dizziness. Risk of GI perforation in disorders of intestinal wall integrity.

## Midazolam[62] *(Versed)*

<u>Action</u>: Benzodiazepine used for sedation and as anticonvulsant. Also has amnestic, anxiolytic, and muscle relaxant properties. High risk for respiratory depression. Individualize dose using hemodynamic and oximetric monitoring.

---

[61] Becker G, *et al.* Novel opioid antagonists for opioid-induced bowel dysfunction and postoperative ileus. *Lancet 2009; 373:* 1198-1206.

[62] Jacobi J, et al. Clinical practice guidelines for the sustained use of sedatives and analgesics in the critically ill adult. *Crit Care Med. 2002; 30:*119.

<u>Kinetics</u>: Onset 2-5 min, $T_{1/2}$ 3 -11 hr. Liver metabolism, renal excretion.

<u>IV</u>: <u>Procedural sedation</u>: 0.01-0.05 mg/kg IV over 2 min repeated prn Q10-15 min or 0.07-0.08 mg/kg IM. Observe for 2 min before re-bolusing; > 3.5-5 mg usually unnecessary. Use 0.25-0.5 mg as initial IV dose in elderly. Reduce dose by 30% if used with narcotic. <u>Continuous infusion for ventilated patient</u>: Bolus 0.02 - 0.08 mg/kg, then infuse 0.04 - 0.2 mg/kg/hr. <u>Status epilepticus (off-label)</u>[62]: Bolus 0.2 mg/kg IV, then infuse 0.05-0.4 mcg/kg/min (titrated to EEG burst suppression). Therapeutic levels may require intubation and blood pressure support. <u>Intranasal (off-label)</u>[63]: similar kinetics, 80% bioavailability, but mucosal burning from excipient. 10 mg IN for seizures. Use atomizer.

<u>Renal failure</u>: $T_{1/2}$ unchanged, distribution different. Use 50% for CrCl < 10mL/min.

<u>Warning</u>: Be prepared to support respiration.

<u>Contraindications</u>: Narrow-angle glaucoma.

<u>Adverse reactions</u>: Respiratory depression, hypotension.

<u>Pregnancy</u>: Teratogenic.

## Milrinone *(Primacor)*

<u>Action</u>: Phosphodiesterase-III inhibitor used as inotrope-vasodilator in acute CHF and low cardiac output state after cardiac surgery. No reduction in mortality, length of stay, readmission in RCT; ↑ mortality with chronic oral therapy. May work additively with dobutamine. May counteract β-blockers.

<u>IV</u>: Load 50 mcg/kg over 10 min, then infuse 0.375 (minimum), 0.50 (standard), or 0.75 mcg/kg/min. Duration typically less than 72 hr.

<u>Kinetics</u>: Onset 5-15 min. Terminal elimination $T_{1/2}$ 2.4 hr. 70% protein-bound, 80% urine elimination, remainder glucuronide.

---

[62] Meierkord H, *et al.* EFNS guideline on the management of status epilepticus in adults. *Eur J Neurol* 2010; 17: 348-355.

[63] Veldhorst-Janssen NM, *et al.* Pharmacokinetics and tolerability of nasal versus intravenous midazolam in healthy Dutch volunteers. *Clin Ther* 2011; 33: 2022-2028.

<u>Renal Failure:</u> Adjustments in bolus may be necessary. Infusion adjusted based on CrCl (mL/min): for 50 mL/min give 0.43 mcg/kg/min, decrease infusion by 0.05 mcg/kg/min for every additional 10 mL/min decrease in CrCl (to 10 mL/min). For CrCl 5 mL/min, rate is 0.2 mcg/kg/min.

<u>Incompatibility:</u> Precipitates IV furosemide.

<u>Side Effects:</u> Hypotension, tachycardia, aggravates ventricular arrhythmia, accelerates ventricular response to atrial fibrillation.

# Naloxone *(Narcan)*[64]

<u>Action:</u> Direct opiate competitive antagonist, no agonist properties. Indicated in opiate overdose, reversal of opiate sedation/hypotension

<u>Kinetics:</u> Initial response 2-3 min. Elimination $T_{1/2}$ 30-80 min. IM more prolonged than IV. Liver metabolism.

<u>IV/IM/SQ/nasal:</u> <u>Opiate intoxication:</u> Initial dose 0.04 mg, escalate rapidly q 2-3 min → 0.5mg → 2 mg → 4 mg → 10 mg → 15 mg. If no response at highest dose, doubtful opiate intoxication. <u>Postop:</u> 0.1-0.2 mg IV q 2-3 min. **Infusion:** 0.4-0.8 mg/hr titrated to effect, or give 2/3 dose that caused reversal hourly.

<u>Renal failure:</u> No dosage adjustment.

<u>Caution:</u> Reversal of opiate toxicity is often transient because opiate $T_{1/2}$ may exceed that of naloxone. Abrupt reversal of narcotic depression can cause HTN, tachycardia, N/V, tremulousness, seizures (especially with meperidine), pulmonary edema, cardiac arrest. Large doses needed for pentazocine or propoxyphene.

<u>Incompatibility:</u> polyanions (heparin, albumin), alkali, bisulfite.

# Neostigmine
*See* Anticholinesterases on *page 262*

---

[64] Boyer EW. Management of opioid analgesic overdose. *N Engl J Med* 2012; 367: 146-155.

# Neuromuscular blockers[65]

<u>Warning</u>: **In patients not already intubated, neuromuscular blockers should be used only by physicians skilled in advanced airway management including endotracheal intubation.**

<u>Action</u>:    Quaternary ammonium compounds that block motor response at neuromuscular junction (nicotinic acetylcholine receptor).    Most are non-depolarizing, and block acetylcholine without altering resting electrical potential.    Succinylcholine is a depolarizing agent and has biphasic response: phase I produces tetany and twitching from depolarization and electrolyte shifts; phase II resembles non-depolarizing block.    Sequentially affect eyes, face, neck THEN limbs, abdomen, chest THEN diaphragm. Ideally, ongoing blockade should be monitored by twitch response from an electrical nerve stimulator in addition to clinical assessment of voluntary muscle movements.    Adequate tidal volumes with T-piece breathing may **not** predict ability to maintain airway if extubated. Used in ICU to facilitate ventilation and reduce ventilator dyssynchrony, reduce intracranial pressure, treat muscle spasm, reduce oxygen consumption.    Brief systematic application may improve outcomes in ARDS[66].

<u>Side-effects</u>: **Histamine release:** Most with succinyl-choline; less with vecuronium, rocuronium, and cisatracurium. **Cardiovascular:** Hypotension, tachycardia, bronchospasm, conduction abnormalities; seen to some degree in all agents, but least with vecuronium and newer agents (rocuronium, cisatracurium, and mivacurium). **Malignant hyperthermia:** Treat with dantrolene (*see page 274*). **Muscarinic side effects**: Bradycardia, hypotension, salivation; blocked by

[65] Murray MJ, *et al.* Clinical practice guidelines for sustained neuromuscular blockade in the adult critically ill patient. *Crit Care Med* 2002; 30: 142-156.

[66] Papazian L, *et al.* Neuromuscular blockers in early acute respiratory distress syndrome. *N Engl J Med* 2010; 363: 1107-1116.

pre-treatment with atropine-like drugs.

Reversal: Nondepolarizing agents with cholinesterase inhibitors (neostigmine or pyridostigmine) plus atropine; IV calcium.

Caution/Interactions: Hyperkalemia, especially with succinylcholine (exacerbated by digoxin). Neuromuscular blockade accentuated in presence of myasthenia gravis or myasthenic syndromes, hypothyroidism, dehydration, aminoglycosides; effects also potentiated by hypokalemia, hypocalcemia, hypermagnesemia, respiratory acidosis, metabolic alkalosis, hypothermia, and liver failure. Extended infusion may result in prolonged neuromuscular blockade, especially with steroidal agents (pancuronium, vecuronium, rocuronium); risk factors include renal failure and high-dose steroid use for associated asthma.[67] Syndrome often but not always associated with elevated CK levels. All chemically paralyzed patients should receive adequate sedation and analgesia, as well as <u>eye protection</u> and proper positioning to prevent pressure sores, nerve palsies, etc.

## Atracurium (Tracrium)

Indication: Paralysis in mechanically ventilated patient.

Dose: 0.4-0.5 mg/kg IV bolus followed by infusion 4-12 mcg/kg/min. Typical infusion 11-13 mcg/kg/min.

Kinetics: Onset 2-8 min, duration 25-35 min.

Advantages: Safe in renal dysfunction.

Disadvantages: Metabolite (laudanosine) accumulates in liver failure and may cause possible CNS effects. Histamine release at higher doses.

## Cisatracurium (Nimbex)

Indication: Paralysis in mechanically ventilated patient.

Dose: 0.15- 0.2 mg/kg IV bolus or 2.5-3 mcg/kg/min continuous infusion.

Kinetics: Onset 2-8 min, duration 45-60 min.

---

[67] Segredo V, et al. Persistent paralysis in critically ill patients after long-term administration of vecuronium. *N Engl J Med* 1992; 327: 524-528.

<u>Advantages</u>: No cardiovascular effects or histamine release. Can be used with liver and renal dysfunction. Pregnancy category B.
<u>Disadvantages</u>: May cause prolonged neuromuscular blockade.

## Pancuronium *(Pavulon)*
<u>Indication</u>: Paralysis in mechanically ventilated patient.
<u>Dose</u>: Bolus 0.06-0.1 mg/kg; repeat incremental doses of 0.01 mg/kg q 25-60 min or infuse 1-2 mcg/kg/min.
<u>Kinetics</u>: Onset 2-3 min, duration 90-100 min.
<u>Disadvantage</u>: Caution in renal failure because of reduced plasma clearance and doubling of $T_{\frac{1}{2}}$. Recovery of blockade may be slower in renal failure. Vagolytic causes tachycardia, increased myocardial demand.
<u>Advantage</u>: Inexpensive.

## Rocuronium *(Zemuron)*
<u>Indications</u>: May be used for intubation as well as paralysis in ventilated patient. <u>Dose</u>: Intubation: 0.6-1.0 mg/kg IV. Maintenance: 0.1-0.2 mg/kg as bolus or 10 - 12 mcg/kg/min continuous infusion.
<u>Kinetics</u>: Onset 45-60 sec, duration 45-70 min.
<u>Advantages</u>: No histamine release or cardiovascular effects. Safe in renal failure and liver disease. Pregnancy Category B. Non-depolarizing alternative to succinylcholine for intubation. Similar to vecuronium.

## Succinylcholine
<u>Indications</u>: Intubation; sub-optimal for long-term paralysis of ventilated patient.
<u>Dose</u>: Intubation: 0.6-1.5 mg/kg IV. No maintenance bolus; infusion 0.5-10 mg/min (1 mg/mL).
<u>Kinetics</u>: Onset 30-60 sec, duration 5-15 min. Rapidly hydrolyzed in plasma & liver.
<u>Advantages</u>: Rapid onset; doesn't cross placenta. Kidney-independent.
<u>Disadvantages</u>: Depolarization causes hyperkalemia (usual increase 0.5 mEq/L); avoid in predisposed patients, *e.g.* renal insufficiency, burns, crush

injury. Prolonged paralysis with decreased hepatic production of cholinesterase. Vasopressor action may increase intracranial pressure. Avoid in stroke, 48 hr - 6 mo after head or spinal cord injury (proliferation of postjunctional receptors may cause denervation hypersensitivity). Bradyarrhythmia (rare in adults; prophylax with atropine).

## Vecuronium (Norcuron)

<u>Indications:</u> Primarily used for paralysis of ventilated patient. May be used for intubation although onset slower compared to other agents.

<u>Dose:</u> Intubation: 0.08-0.10 mg/kg IV. Maintenance: 0.8-1.2 mcg/kg/min infusion.

<u>Kinetics:</u> Onset 60-90 sec, duration 25-30 min.

<u>Advantages:</u> No histamine release or related adverse hemodynamic effects

<u>Disadvantages:</u> May cause prolonged neuromuscular blockade, especially in ESRD.

## Comparison summary of neuromuscular blockers

|  | Atra curium | Cisatra curium | Pancuro nium | Rocuro nium | Succinyl choline | Vecuroni um |
|---|---|---|---|---|---|---|
| Onset | Intermed | Intermed | Intermed | Rapid | Ultrarapid | Rapid |
| Duration | Intermed | Intermed | Long | Intermed | Ultrashort | Intermed |
| Renal failure* | Yes | Yes | No | Yes | Yes | No |
| Liver failure* | Yes | Yes | No | Yes | No | No |
| Histamine release | Yes | No | No | No | Yes | No |
| Cardio-vascular effects | Yes | No | Yes | No | Yes | No |

*\* May be used without dosage adjustment in these conditions*

## Nicardipine IV (Cardene)

*See also* clevidipine on *page 272.*

<u>Action:</u> Dihydropyridine calcium-channel blocker relaxes vascular smooth muscle. Used as parenteral antihypertensive as alternative to nitroprusside.

<u>Kinetics:</u> $\alpha$ T½ 2.7 min, $\beta$ T½ 45 min. Onset 5-15 min, duration 3 hr. Rapid hepatic clearance.

<u>IV:</u> Infuse 5 mg/hr, increase by 2.5 mg/hr q 5-15

min until desired BP or maximum 15 mg/hr. After achieving blood pressure goal, reduce to 3 mg/hr.

Transition to oral: Give PO nicardipine 1 hr before discontinuing infusion. 20 mg PO q 8 $\cong$ 0.5 mg/hr; 30 mg PO q 8 $\cong$ 1.2 mg/hr; 40 mg PO q 8 $\cong$ 2.2 mg/hr.

Renal failure: No dosage adjustment.

Liver failure: Delayed clearance. May exacerbate portal hypertension.

Contraindication: Critical aortic valvular stenosis.

Caution: Causes reflex tachycardia, which may provoke/exacerbate myocardial ischemia. Negative inotrope in severe left ventricular dysfunction. Decreases GFR in renal dysfunction. Incompatible with bicarbonate or lactate Ringers coinfusion.

Interactions: Beta and calcium channel blockers have additive hypotensive effects. Levels increased by cimetidine. Increases cyclosporine levels.

Pregnancy: Category C. Embryocidal in certain animals.

## Nimodipine

Action: Dihydropyridine calcium-channel blocker, highly lipophilic, affects cerebral arteries preferentially. Used to relieve cerebral vasospasm (which causes secondary ischemia and poor outcome) after subarachnoid hemorrhage (SAH).

Kinetics: Peak onset 1 hr, elimination $T_{1/2}$ 1-2 hr, terminal $T_{1/2}$ 8-9 hr. Hepatic metabolism, renal excretion.

Dose oral: 60 mg po q 4 hr for 21 days. Start within 4 d of SAH.

Black Box Warning: Do not administer IV or parenterally, which may cause lethal hypotension.

Caution: CYP3A4 metabolism; activity enhanced by macrolides, azoles, HIV protease inhibitors, cimetidine, valproate, etc. Avoid grapefruit juice. Hypotension most common effect.

## Nitric Oxide (Inomax)

See Pulmonary Vasodilators page 346.

**Nitrite**
*See* cyanide poisoning *page 249.*

# Nitroglycerin

<u>Action</u>: Dose-dependent arterial and venous vasodilator via stimulation of guanylate cyclase. Increases coronary perfusion, decreases $MVO_2$, LV filling pressure, pulmonary and systemic vascular resistance. Used to control ongoing ischemic discomfort, hypertension especially related to ischemia, or management of pulmonary congestion.

<u>Kinetics</u>: Plasma $T_{1/2}$ 1-4 min.

<u>IV</u>: Begin 5-20 mcg/min, titrate 10-20 mcg/min increments q 3-5 min. Predominantly hypotensive (arteriolar dilator) effect > 200 mcg/min.

<u>Ointment 2%</u>: Antianginal onset 30 min. Begin 0.5 inch q 6 hr until desired effects achieved using a 10-12 hr nitrate-free interval. 1" corresponds to ~ 10-40 mcg/min IV; 2" ~ 80 mcg/min IV. **Explosive** during cardioversion.

<u>Renal failure</u>: $T_{1/2}$ unchanged. No dosage adjustment.

<u>Contraindication</u>: Avoid in hypotension. Life-threatening hypotension used with sildenafil, tadalafil, vardenafil, or related PDE-5 inhibitors. ↑ intracranial pressure or ↓ cerebral perfusion; narrow-angle glaucoma; preload dependent states (pericardial tamponade or constriction, right ventricular infarct, hypertrophic cardiomyopathy).

<u>Side effects</u>: Headache, dizziness, dermatitis.

<u>Note</u>: Absorbed by plastic/PVC; usually mixed in glass bottle. Use non-absorbtive tubing. Tachyphylaxis after prolonged infusion/exposure without nitrate-free interval. Propylene glycol excipient.

# Nitroprusside *(Nipride)*

<u>Action</u>: Arterial and venous vasodilator. Used for afterload reduction in acute heart failure, mitral regurgitation, aortic insufficiency, ventricular septal defect. Antihypertensive for most causes of severe hypertension including pheochromocytoma. Useful

in aortic stenosis with decompensated heart failure despite prior adverse reports[68]. Free NO relaxes vascular, not visceral, smooth muscle. Reacts with hemoglobin to yield methemoglobin and unstable compound releasing cyanide. Cyanide converted (using thiosulfate) in liver and kidney to thiocyanate.

Kinetics: $T_{1/2}$ < 10 min.

IV: Initial 0.3-0.5 mcg/kg/min. Titrate upwards to desired BP incrementally q 3-15 min, do not exceed 10 mcg/kg/min rate for > 10 min. **Withdraw slowly** to avoid rebound vasoconstriction. Use concurrent hypotensive to lower nitroprusside dose and limit toxicity.

Renal failure and liver failure: $T_{1/2}$ unchanged. No dosage adjustment. However, risk of thiocyanate much higher (removed by dialysis).

Levels: Blood cyanide levels not predictive of tissue levels or of toxicity. Follow **thiocyanate** daily after 48-72 hr infusion, especially if abnormal CNS function at baseline. Symptoms at 60 mcg/mL; "toxicity" at 100 mcg/mL. Toxicity unlikely when infused < 72 hr at less than 2 mcg/kg/min (normal kidneys) or less than 1 mcg/kg/min (anuric). Thiocyanate elimination $T_{1/2}$ of 3 d (normals), 9 d (renal dysfunction). Keep **methemoglobin** < 10%.

Toxicity: Manifested clinically by tinnitus, blurred vision, confusion, psychosis, seizure, delirium, lactic acidosis, marrow suppression, pink color, electromechanical dissociation. Metabolic acidosis or failure to respond to adequate infusion may represent increased free cyanide. Infusion of **hydroxycobalamin** (not cyanocobalamin) 25 mg/h may reduce cyanide toxicity[69]. Cyanide accumulates in liver disease; thiocyanate accumulates in renal dysfunction.

Contraindications: Severe liver disease (rhodanase

---

[68] Khot UN, *et al.* Nitroprusside in critically ill patients with left ventricular dysfunction and aortic stenosis. *N Engl J Med* 2003; 348: 1756-1763.

[69] Cottrell JE, *et al.* Prevention of nitroprusside-induced cyanide toxicity with hydroxocobalamin. *N Engl J Med* 1978; 298: 809-811.

deficiency), vitamin B12 deficiency, hypothyroidism (exacerbated by thiocyanate), aortic dissection, aortic coarctation, Leber congenital optic atrophy or tobacco amblyopia (absent rhodanase).

Caution: Hypovolemia, renal or liver disease, cerebrovascular disease, elevated intracranial pressure. Protect from light to reduce cyanide release.

Overdose: *See cyanide poisoning page 249.*

Pregnancy: Category C.

## Norepinephrine *(Levophed)*

Action: Potent β-1 and α-agonist. No β-2 action (unlike epinephrine). β-1 prominent at low doses; α-1 predominates at higher doses. Vasoconstriction increases afterload and $MVO_2$, decreases splanchnic perfusion and exacerbates peripheral ischemia, but spares cerebral and coronary circulation. Baroreceptor stimulation → no net change in heart rate or cardiac output. Chronic use causes decreased circulatory volume related to vasoconstriction. Compared with epinephrine: half as potent chronotrope and inotrope, equipotent vasoconstrictor, no vasodilator properties, less demand on $MVO_2$, less arrhythmogenic. May exacerbate mitral and aortic regurgitation. Used for hypotension due to peripheral artery vasodilation, sepsis, myocardial dysfunction, cardiac arrest. Also used for hepatorenal syndrome in combination with albumin, *etc.*

Kinetics: Rapid onset, duration 1-2 min.

IV: Mix 4, 6, 8 mg in 250 mL dextrose not saline = 16, 24, 32 mcg/mL. Typical starting dose 0.1-0.5 mcg/kg/min. Incompatible with alkali.

Cautions: Avoid extravasation; use long peripheral IV or central lines. Suspect volume depletion if hypotension develops, especially with chronic use. MAO inhibitors and tricyclics dramatically potentiate activity.

Extravasation: *See phentolamine page 335.*

# Novel Oral Anticoagulants (NOACs)[70]

<u>Common indication:</u> Direct factor Xa inhibitors indicated for nonvalvular atrial fibrillation, DVT prophylaxis after hip/knee surgery, DVT or PE treatment. No coagulation monitoring required.

<u>Common risks:</u> Risk of thrombotic events after premature discontinuation. Risk of life-threatening bleeding. Avoid in mechanical heart valve. Risk of spinal/epidural anesthesia causing hematoma.

## Apixaban *(Eliquis)*

<u>Action:</u> Direct factor Xa inhibitor.

<u>Kinetics:</u> $T_{1/2}$ ~ 12 hr. No dosage adjustment for renal or impairment except atrial fibrillation below. Avoid in moderate+ hepatic impairment.

<u>Coagulation test:</u> Anti-Xa activity, PT, aPTT are elevated.

<u>PO:</u> <u>Stroke reduction in non-valvular atrial fibrillation:</u> 5mg po bid. Reduce dose to 2.5 mg bid if two of (age ≥ 80 yr, weight ≤ 60kg, serum creatinine ≥ 1.5 mg/dL). <u>DVT prophylaxis after orthopedic surgery:</u> 2.5 mg bid. <u>DVT or PE therapy:</u> 10 mg bid x 7 d, then 5 mg bid. <u>Prevent recurrent DVT or PE:</u> 2.5 mg bid.

<u>Interruption for surgery:</u> 24 hr before low-bleeding-risk procedures, 48 hr before moderate-high bleeding risk procedures. Bridging probably harmful.

<u>Conversion:</u> From warfarin: Start after INR < 2.0; To warfarin: start parenteral anticoagulant and warfarin at time of next apixaban dose, then follow INR. To/from other NOAC: switch when next dose is due.

<u>Missed dose:</u> Take as soon as possible on same day and resume bid; do not double-dose.

<u>Interaction:</u> Reduce dose 50% when coadministered with CYP3A4 + PGp dual inhibitors (ketoconazole, itraconazole, ritonavir, clarithromycin).

---

[70] Kovacs RJ, *et al.* Practical management of anticoagulation in patients with atrial fibrillation. *J Am Coll Cardiol* 2015; 65: 1340-1360.

**Reversal:** There is no antidote. Utility of 4-factor PCC unclear.

**Pregnancy:** Category B.

## Dabigatran *(Pradaxa)*

Action: Direct thrombin inhibitor.

Kinetics: $T_{1/2}$ 12-17 hr. Renal elimination. Kinetics unchanged in moderate hepatic impairment. Not suitable for mechanical heart valves.

Coagulation test: Elevates TT, aPTT or ECT, not INR unless above therapeutic.

PO: Swallow whole. Stroke reduction in non-valvular atrial fibrillation 150 mg po bid for CrCL > 30 mL/min; 75 mg po bid for CrCL 15-30 mL/min. Reduce dose to 75 bid if CrCL 30-50 mL/min and co-administration of dronadarone or systemic keto-conazole. DVT or PE therapy: CrCL > 30 mL/min: 150 mg bid; CrCL < 30 mL/min: no recommendation. Avoid co-administration of PGp inhibitor if CrCL < 50 mL/min. DVT prophylaxis after joint replacement: CrCL > 30 mL/min: 110 mg day 1, then 220mg qd. CrCL < 30 mL/min: no recommendation. Avoid co-administration of PGp inhibitor if CrCL < 50 mL/min.

Interruption for surgery: Stop 1-2 d (CrCL > 50 ml/min) or 3-5 d (CrCL < 50 mL/min) before procedures with high bleeding risk.

Conversion: From warfarin: Start after INR < 2.0; To warfarin: CrCL > 50 ml/min: start warfarin 3 d before stopping dabigatran; CrCL 31-50: start warfarin 2 d before; CrCL 15-30: start warfarin 1 d before; CrCL < 15 no recommendation. To/from parenteral: start dabigatran 0-2 hr before next scheduled dose is due or when UFH discontinued.

Missed dose: Skip dose if cannot be taken > 6 hr before next dose. Do not double to compensate for missed doses.

Interactions: Renal impairment and PGp coadministration ↑ exposure to dabigatran (see PO above). Avoid with PGp inducers (rifampin).

Reversal: *See idarucizumab on page 307.* May be dialyzable.

Pregnancy: Category C.

## Rivaroxaban *(Xarelto)*

Action: Direct factor Xa inhibitor.

Kinetics: $T_{1/2}$ 5-9 hr young, 11-13 hr elderly. Avoid in moderate+ hepatic impairment.

Coagulation test: Anti-Xa activity, PT, aPTT are elevated.

PO: Stroke reduction in non-valvular atrial fibrillation: CrCL > 50 mL/min: 20 qd with evening meal; CrCL 15 - 50 mL/min: 15mg qd with evening meal. DVT prophylaxis after joint replacement: Hip: 10 mg qd x 35 d. Knee: 10 mg qd x 12 d. DVT or PE therapy: 15 mg bid with food x 21 d, then 20 mg qd with food. Prevent recurrent DVT or PE: 20mg qd with food.

Interruption for surgery: Stop at least 24 hr before procedure.

Conversion: From warfarin: Start after INR < 3.0; To warfarin: start parenteral anticoagulant and warfarin at time of next rivaroxaban dose, then follow INR. To other NOAC or parenteral: switch when next dose is due. From other NOAC or parenteral: start rivoroxaban 0 - 2 hr before next scheduled evening dose and omit other drug.

Missed dose: If receiving 15 bid, take missed dose even if 30 mg total. If receiving daily, take missed dose immediately without doubling.

Interaction: Avoid use along with CYP3A4/ PGp dual inhibitors (ketoconazole, itraconazole, ritonavir, clarithromycin), and along with strong CYP3A4/ PGp dual inducers (rifampin, phenytoin, carbamazepine).

Reversal: There is no antidote. Utility of 4-factor PCC unclear.

Pregnancy: Category C.

# Octreotide (Sandostatin)

<u>Action:</u> Cyclic octapeptide somatostatin analogue. Suppresses release of GI peptides including gastrin, VIP, insulin, glucagon, secretin, motilin, and decreases splanchnic blood flow. Indicated for acromegaly, carcinoid tumor, VIPoma. Also used IV to control bleeding esophageal varices, intractable secretory diarrhea (AIDS) & fistulae.

<u>Kinetics:</u> $T_{1/2}$ 1.7-1.9 hr; GFR < 10: 3.1 hr. Hepatic metabolism and renal excretion.

<u>IV:</u> <u>Variceal esophageal hemorrhage (off-label):</u> 50 mcg bolus, then 50 mcg/h x 5 d[71]. <u>Sulfonylurea overdose (off-label):</u> 50-100 mcg SQ or IV plus dextrose 10%, then q 6-8 hr until spontaneous euglycemia[72]. <u>Hepatorenal syndrome (off-label):</u> 100-200 µg SC tid combined with midodrine po and albumin IV.

<u>SQ:</u> Begin 50 mcg SQ qd, advance prn up to 600 mcg/day divided bid-qid.

<u>Renal insufficiency:</u> Reduce maintenance dose.

<u>Interactions:</u> Reduces insulin requirements. Incompatible with insulin in TPN.

<u>Adverse effects:</u> Biliary sludge & stones, pancreatitis. Injection site pain. Nausea, vomiting, abdominal pain. Hypoglycemia in Type I DM. Torsades de Pointes.

# Ondansetron (Zofran)

<u>Action:</u> Serotonin 5-HT3 receptor antagonist, used as anti-emetic.

<u>Kinetics:</u> Elimination $T_{1/2}$ 3.5-5.5 hr, hepatic metabolism.

<u>IV:</u> <u>Postoperative nausea</u> 4 mg IV over 0.5-5 min before induction or immediately after surgery.

<u>Chemotherapy nausea:</u> 0.15 mg/kg over 15 min beginning ½ hr before chemotherapy, repeat q 4 hr x 2. Alternatively 32 mg IV over 15 min once.

---

[71] Chan MM, et al. Octreotide. Chest 2013; 144: 1937-1945.

[72] Dougherty PP, et al. Octreotide's role in the management of sulfonylurea-induced hypoglycemia. J Med Toxicol 2010; 6: 199-206.

<u>PO</u>: 8 mg po 30 min before highly emetogenic chemotherapy, then q 12 hr for 1-2 d. Alternatively 24 mg po once. Not superior to dexamethasone 4 mg bid

<u>Renal failure</u>: No dose adjustment.

<u>Liver disease</u>: Do not exceed 8 mg daily.

<u>Cautions</u>: May prolong ECG QT interval. May mask ileus or gastric distention. Serotonin syndrome especially in combination with serotonergic drugs. See page 242.

<u>Pregnancy</u>: Category B.

## Opiate analgesics[73]

<u>Caution</u>: there is wide variability and limited data to support these equivalences. When converting or rotating opiate analgesics, switch to 50-67% of the oral equi-analgesic dose, consider the total daily dose.

| Drug | Equi-analgesic dose (mg) | | Typical first dose | |
|------|------|------|------|------|
| | Oral | Parenteral | Oral | Parenteral |
| Codeine | 180-200 | 120 | 30 mg q 3-4 hr | 10 mg q 3-4 hr |
| Fentanyl Patch (Duragesic) | — | — | — | 25 mcg/h q 72 h [a] |
| Fentanyl | — | 0.1 | — | — |
| Hydrocodone (Vicodin) | 30 | — | 5-10 mg q 4-6 hr | — |
| Hydromorphone (Dilaudid) | 7.5 | 1.5 | 2-4 mg q 3-4h | 1.5 mg q 3-4 hr |
| Levorphanol (Levo-Dromoran) | 4 | 2 | 4 mg q 6-8 hr | 2 mg q 6-8 hr |
| Meperidine (Demerol)[b e] | 300 | 100 | 100 mg q 3 hr | 100 mg q 3 hr |
| Methadone (Dolophine)[c] | 2-4 | 10-20 (acute), 2-4 (chronic) | 5 mg q 8-12 hr | 5 mg q 8-12 hr |

[73] Veterans Administration and Department of Defense. Clinical Practice Guideline for the Management of Opioid Therapy for Chronic Pain 2/e. 2010; Ballantyne JC, et al. Opioid therapy for chronic pain. N Engl J Med 2003; 349: 1943-1953. See also Knotkova H, et al. Opioid rotation. J Pain Symptom Manage 2009; 38: 426-439. Shaheen PE, et al. Opioid equianalgesic tables. J Pain Symptom Manage 2009; 38: 409-417.

| Drug | Equi-analgesic dose (mg) | | Typical first dose | |
|---|---|---|---|---|
| | Oral | Parenteral | Oral | Parenteral |
| Morphine | 30 | 10 | 15 mg q 3-4 hr | 10 mg q 3-4 hr |
| Oxycodone (Percodan) | 30 | — | 5 mg q 6 hr | — |
| Remifentanil | — | 0.05 | — | — |
| Tramodol[d][e] | 100 | — | 25 mg q AM | — |

Comments: (a) Do not use fentanyl patch in opiate naive. Use only for unremitting pain. The lowest dose 25 mcg/h x 72 hr may compare with 50-75 mg oral morphine/d; (b) meperidine is contraindicated for sustained use because of toxic metabolites; (c) equi-analgesic dose to morphine is often lower-than-expected; (d) Associated with suicide in addiction-prone; Note risk of seizure and anaphylaxis. (e) Avoid with monoamine oxidase or selective serotonin reuptake inhibitors.

## Pamidronate *(Aredia)*

See zoledronate on *page 357*. See hypercalcemia on *page 220*.

<u>Action</u>: Bisphosphonate inhibits osteoclastic bone resorption for treatment of malignancy-related hypercalcemia and Paget disease.

<u>Kinetics</u>: Onset 1-2 d, peak action 6 d in malignancy. Excreted unchanged by kidney $T_{\frac{1}{2}}$ 28 hr. Bone terminal elimination $T_{\frac{1}{2}}$ estimated 1 yr.

<u>IV</u>: <u>Hypercalcemia of malignancy</u>: Dose based on serum calcium: for $[Ca^{++}]$ 12-13.5 mg/dL give 60-90 mg; for $[Ca^{++}] > 13.5$ mg/dL give 90 mg. Infuse each over 2-24 hr. Assure vigorous prehydration. May retreat after 7 d after complete or partial response.
<u>Moderate-severe Paget disease</u>: 30 mg IV over 4 hr x 3 consecutive days.

<u>Renal insufficiency</u>: Not recommended in Cr >3.0 mg/dL or GFR < 30 mL/min.

<u>Hepatic insufficiency</u>: No dosage adjustment.

<u>Toxicity</u>: Fever in 20%; hypertension, thrombophlebitis, nausea, jaw osteonecrosis, severe late musculoskeletal pain.

<u>Caution</u>: "Overshoot" hypocalcemia (also low Mg, $PO_4$, $K^+$); may exacerbate pre-existing myelosuppression. Risk of dose-dependant renal failure: do not exceed single doses > 90 mg. Avoid concurrent

nephrotoxic drugs and diuretics. Reports of jaw osteonecrosis confounded by frequent concurrent glucocorticoids, chemotherapy, infection, but assure adequate dental hygiene before treatment, avoid invasive dental procedures after treatment.
<u>Pregnancy:</u>  Category D.

## Pancuronium
*See* Neuromuscular blockers on *page 320*

## Pentobarbital *(Nembutal)*
<u>Action:</u> Short-acting parenteral barbiturate anesthetic used mainly in refractory convulsive status epilepticus. Controlled substance.
<u>Kinetics:</u> Immediate onset. Elimination $T_{1/2}$ 15-48 hr. Hepatic metabolism.
<u>IV:</u> Load 15mg/kg over 60 min, then 0.5-3 mg/kg/hr to achieve EEG burst-suppression. Follow levels (range 15-40 mcg/mL). Patients should be intubated with continuous arterial pressure and EEG monitoring.
<u>Renal failure:</u> No dosage adjustment. Not dialyzed.
<u>Caution:</u> CYP3A4 inducer
<u>Adverse Effects:</u> Profound hypotension, respiratory depression. Direct myocardial suppressant. Often requires concurrent vasopressor support.

## Phenobarbital sodium
<u>Action:</u> Barbiturate used in generalized and partial seizures.
<u>Kinetics:</u> Peak onset 30-60 min. Elimination 25% renal unchanged, 75% liver metabolites via urine. $T_{1/2}$ 53-118 hr.
<u>IV:</u> 15-20 mg/kg load at 50-100 (ideally < 60) mg/minute; if seizures persist may re-bolus 5-10 mg/kg to maximum of 30 mg/kg.
<u>Maintenance:</u> 60-250 mg/day PO (bioavailability 70-90%) divided bid-tid.
<u>Levels:</u> Therapeutic: 10-25 mcg/mL; acute therapy: 15-40 mcg/mL; coma: > 65 mcg/mL.
<u>Renal failure:</u> Give q 12-16 hr for CrCl < 10 mL/min.

Supplement full dose after hemodialysis or hemofiltration; ½ dose after peritoneal dialysis.

Side effects: Respiratory depression, marked hypotension. Sedation, nystagmus and ataxia at toxic levels. Agitation and confusion in elderly and those with cognitive impairment. Maculopapular, morbilliform, scarlatiniform rashes 1-3%; erythema multiforme or Stevens-Johnson syndrome rarely. Chronic: folate and vit. D deficiency.

Drug interactions: Induces hepatic microsome oxidase. Decreases levels of phenytoin, warfarin, beta blockers, corticosteroids, contraceptives, quinidine, doxycycline, vitamin D. Increases levels of tricyclics. Displaces thyroxine from albumin. Causes production of toxic metabolites of chlorocarbon anesthetics and carbon tetrachloride.

Pregnancy: Category D.

## Phentolamine *(Regitine)*

Action: Nonspecific $\alpha$-adrenergic antagonist used in excess adrenergic states, *e.g.* pheochromocytoma, clonidine withdrawal, MAO inhibitor drug interactions, cocaine toxicity. Also used to limit skin necrosis from extravasation of catecholamines.

Kinetics: Liver metabolism. Elimination $T_{\frac{1}{2}}$ 19 min.

IV: Pheochromocytoma: 5 mg IV/IM given 1-2 hr preoperatively, titrate for effect. Sympathomimetic hypertensive crisis (Off-Label): 5-10 mg IV q 5 min to total of 20-30 mg. Administer prior to $\beta$-blocker to prevent unopposed $\alpha$-mediated vasoconstriction. Possible utility in cocaine coronary artery spasm and myocardial ischemia[74]. Extravasation of catecholamines: Infiltrate area liberally with 5-10 mg/10-mL NS via 25 g needle (should cause conspicuous hyperemia if used within 12 hr). Pralidoxime-induced hypertension (off-label): 5 mg IV.

Overdose: Fluids, norepinephrine (**not** epinephrine).

Pregnancy: Category C.

---

[74] McCord J, *et al.* Management of cocaine-associated chest pain and myocardial infarction. *Circulation 2008; 117: 1897-1907.*

## Phenylephrine *(Neo-Synephrine)*

<u>Action</u>: Postsynaptic α-adrenergic agonist with virtually no β activity, used as a vasoconstrictor. Less demand on $MVO_2$ compared to epinephrine or dopamine. Causes marked reflex bradycardia (prevented by atropine). Less arrhythmogenic than other catecholamines. Constricts cerebral, pulmonary, and splanchnic vessels but may relax coronaries. Exacerbates mitral and aortic regurgitation. Reduces dynamic left ventricular outflow obstruction in hypertrophic cardiomyopathy. Used in hypotension or shock, as a vasoconstrictor in spinal or regional anesthesia, or drug-related hypotension.

<u>Dose</u>: Bolus: 0.1-0.5 mg IV q 15 min. Continuous infusion: 100-180 mcg/min. Titrate down to maintenance dose, usually 40-60 mcg/min. Maximum infusion rate not specified by manufacturer (add 10 mg increments to infusion bag to maintain acceptable infusion rate).

<u>Kinetics</u>: Effects sustained compared with epinephrine, ~ 20 min after IV.

<u>Caution</u>: MAO inhibitors, tricyclics, and oxytocic agents potentiate pressor effect; use vastly reduced doses of phenylephrine.

Pregnancy: Category C.

## Phenytoin *(Dilantin)*

<u>Indications</u>: First-line anticonvulsant for generalized, partial complex, or simple partial seizures. Not used in absence, myoclonic, or atonic seizures. Ability to enhance AV node conduction used (rarely) in digitalis-induced arrhythmia and after Tetralogy of Fallot repair.

<u>Kinetics</u>: Maximal therapeutic effect within 20-25 min of IV infusion. $T_{\frac{1}{2}}$ 6-24 hr initially, 20-60 hr at therapeutic levels.

<u>IV</u>: Load 10-15 mg/kg (off-label but recommended 15-20 mg/kg) not faster than 50 mg/min; if refractory seizures may give additional 5-10 mg/kg doses to total of 30 mg/kg. Maintenance 100 mg IV or po q 6-8 hr. Observe for hypotension (28-50% of patients)

and arrhythmia (2%), especially with rapid infusion. **Fosphenytoin** (a water-soluble prodrug) is measured in phenytoin equivalents (PEs) but dosing is the same (15-20 mg/kg); may be administered more rapidly at 100-150 PEs mg/min and may cause less hypotension. However, no apparent difference in time to onset of clinical effect. May be given IM.

<u>PO</u>: Load 400 mg, then 300 mg q 2 hr x 2; then initial maintenance dose of 100 mg PO tid. Once stable may switch to once-daily dosing if no adverse symptoms. Increase doses in increments of 30-50 mg. Steady-state levels not reached until 7-10 d after dose change.

<u>Levels</u>: Therapeutic 10-20 mcg/mL, may use up to 30-40 mcg/mL in comatose patient with status epilepticus. Obtain level 2 hr after IV load. Measure **free** phenytoin levels (therapeutic 1-2 mcg/mL) in renal or liver failure, albumin < 2.8, warfarin, sulfonamides, salicylates, valproate.

<u>Renal failure</u>: $T_{1/2}$ unchanged. No adjustment; however, the active drug (free phenytoin) is completely dialyzed, such that patients may seize with "normal" total phenytoin levels during or after dialysis. *See "levels" above.*

<u>Side effects</u>: Hypotension given IV (due to propylene glycol excipient); folate, vitamin D and vitamin K antagonism; inhibition of insulin release, interstitial nephritis.

<u>Toxicity</u>: Ataxia, diplopia, slurred speech, stupor. May cause venous irritation, distal limb discoloration, edema ("purple glove syndrome"), and skin necrosis related to infusion or extravasation. <u>Hypersensitivity</u>: Fever, lymphadenopathy, eosinophilia, blood dyscrasias, polyarteritis, Stevens-Johnson syndrome. Propylene glycol excipient

<u>Interactions</u>: CYP2C9 and CYP2C19 metabolism. **Decrease phenytoin levels**: anticancer drugs in combination (cisplatin, doxorubicin, methotrexate), barbiturates, carbamazepine, diazepam, ritonavir,

sucralfate, chronic ethanol, calcium antacids, folic acid. **Increase phenytoin levels**: amiodarone, antiepileptics, azoles, chloramphenicol, chlordiazepoxide, cimetidine, disulfiram, estrogens, acute ethanol ingestion, isoniazid, metronidazole, omeprazole, phenothiazines, salicylates, sulfonamides, trimethoprim, trazodone, valproate. Free phenytoin increased in hyperbilirubinemia, hypoalbuminemia, uremia. Tricyclics lower seizure threshold. **Levels reduced by phenytoin**[75]: Cardiac: amiodarone, propranolol, metoprolol, nifedipine, felodipine, nimodipine, digoxin, lovastatin, simvastatin, warfarin, quinidine; Psychiatric: diazepam, alprazolam, amitriptyline, nortriptyline, imipramine, desipramine, clomipramine, citalopram, paroxetine, buproprion, haloperidol, chlorpromazine, clozapine, olanzapine, risperidone, quetiapine; Antineoplastic: Cyclophosphamide, busulfan, etoposide, methotrexate, teniposide, vinca alkaloids; Antiinfective: doxycycline, nevirapine, efavirenz, delavirdine, indinavir, ritonavir, saquinavir, praziquantel, azoles; Other: prednisone, oral contraceptives, theophylline, cyclosporine, tacrolimus, methadone.
Pregnancy: Fetal hydantoin syndrome, neonatal coagulopathy; however, short-term use probably safe.

## Phosphorus[76]

PO: 1-2 g daily in 3 divided doses, increment as tolerated. Milk (skim 1 L = 1 g P). Neutra-Phos 4 x 1250 mg tabs = 1 g P + 28.5mEq Na + 28.5mEq K; Neutra-Phos-K 4 x 1450 mg tabs = 1 g P + 57mEq K.
IV: Reserve for patients who are symptomatic or unable to tolerate PO. Dispensed as 94 mg = 3 mmol phosphorus + 4.4 mEq Na or K per mL. Give 0.08-0.16mmol/kg in 50-500mL fluid over 6 hr. The following simplified weight-based surgical ICU regimen

[75] French JA, *et al*. Initial management of epilepsy. *N Engl J Med* 2008; 359: 166-176.
[76] Brunelli SM, *et al*. Hypophosphatemia: clinical consequences and management. *J Am Soc Nephrol* 2007; 18: 1999-2003.

was effective and well-tolerated, IV over 6 hr[77]:

| Serum PO₄ | Serum PO₄ | Weight 40-60 kg | Weight 61-80 kg | Weight 81-120 kg |
|---|---|---|---|---|
| 0.58 - 0.70 mM | 1.8 - 2.2 mg/dL | 10 mmol | 15 mmol | 20 mmol |
| 0.32 - 0.54 mM | 1.0 - 1.7 mg/dL | 20 mmol | 30 mmol | 40 mmol |
| < 0.32 mM | < 1.0 mg/dL | 30 mmol | 40 mmol | 50 mmol |

If serum [K] < 4.0 mEq/L use K-phosphate; if [K] > 4.0 mEq/L use Na- phosphate. **Warning** 1 mmol K-PO₄ contains ~ 1.5 mEq K.

Conversion: 1 mg phosphorus = 0.032 mmol phosphate
Caution: Rapid IV infusion may cause hypocalcemic tetany, renal failure, tissue calcification, and hyperkalemia. Large oral (doses > 3-5 mg/kg phosphorus) doses may cause diarrhea. Avoid in severe renal impairment.
Interactions: Precipitates in fluids with calcium gluconate > 9.6 mEq/L.

## Physostigmine
See "Anticholinesterases" on *page 262*

## Platelet P2Y₁₂ Inhibitors
### Clopidogrel, ticagrelor, prasugrel
Actions: Potent inhibitors of platelet P2Y₁₂ ADP receptor. Used to prevent thrombotic events after myocardial infarction, after coronary stent.
Caution: Avoid lapses and premature discontinuation after coronary stent, generally 30 d after bare metal stent and 12 mo after drug-eluting stent.

### Clopidogrel
Kinetics: T₁/₂ ~ 6 hr. Irreversible P2Y₁₂ blocker. Requires metabolic conversion for action.
PO: 300-600 mg load then 75 mg qd
Stop before surgery: 5 d;

---

[77] Taylor BE, *et al.* Treatment of hypophosphatemia using a protocol based on patient weight and serum phosphorus level in a surgical intensive care unit. *J Am Coll Surg* 2004; 198: 198-204.

Notes: Possible reduced effect in CYP2C19 poor metabolizers; consider alternative treatment. Possible reduced effect with CYP2C19-inhibiting PPIs (omeprazole, esomeprazole); consider alternative PPI.

## Ticagrelor

Kinetics: $T_{1/2} \sim 12$ hr. Reversible $P2Y_{12}$ blocker. No renal adjustment. Avoid in severe hepatic failure
PO: 180 mg load + 90 mg bid
Stop before surgery: 5 d
  Warning: Do not use with ASA > 100 mg which ↑bleeding risk
Adverse effects: Dyspnea 15%; Bradycardia;
  Switching from alternative: Begin 24 hr after last clopidogrel. May use loading dose if clopidogrel-unresponsive.

## Prasugrel

Kinetics: $T_{1/2} \sim 7$ hr. Onset < 30 min; Biological effect 5-9 d. Irreversible $P2Y_{12}$ blocker. No renal/hepatic adjustment. Requires metabolic conversion for action.
PO: 60 mg load then 10 mg qd
Stop before surgery: 7 d
  Caution: Bleeding ↑ compared with clopidogrel; Net harm in age > 75 yr, weight < 60 kg.
  Not recommended 'upfront' NSTEMI.

## Pralidoxime (2-PAM, *Protopam*)[78]

Action: Quaternary ammonium reactivates acetylcholinesterase rendered inactive by organophosphate insecticides, slows irreversible "aging" of anticholinesterase. Also directly detoxifies certain organophosphates. Used to reverse (respiratory) muscle paralysis. Possible role in tetanus. Effectively reverses nicotinic toxicity (skeletal muscle, sympathetic ganglia); less effective against muscarinic (including

---

[78] Newmark J. Therapy for nerve agent poisoning. *Arch Neurol* 2004; 61: 649-652.

central respiratory) effects but synergistic with atropine. Most effective given within 48 hr of exposure, indicated in all symptomatic exposures and those with RBC cholinesterase < 50% normal.

<u>Kinetics:</u> Onset 5-15 min IV, $T_{\frac{1}{2}}$ 7-77 min. Renal excretion.

<u>IV:</u> <u>Organophosphate antidote:</u> 2 g over 30 min, then 1 g/hr for 48hr, then 1 g/4hr until weaned from ventilator[79]. Pre-treat with atropine 2-4 mg IV. Reduce dose for renal insufficiency, elderly or frail.

<u>Carbamate anticholinesterase toxicity:</u> After atropine as above, 1-2 g IV over 5-30 min then 250 mg IV q 5 min until reversal. Max infusion rate 200 mg/min. Follow with benzodiazepine anticonvulsant. *See* Nerve Agents *page 252.*

<u>Caution:</u> May precipitate myasthenic crisis. Reduce in renal failure.

<u>Interactions:</u> Theophylline, aminophylline, succinylcholine, respiratory depressants.

<u>Adverse effects:</u> Rapid infusion may cause tachycardia, laryngospasm, neuromuscular blockade, hypertension (difficult to distinguish from organophosphate toxicity).

## Procainamide

<u>Indications:</u> **(1)** Treatment of persistent, recurrent or intermittent ventricular fibrillation. **(2)** Treatment of wide-complex tachycardias of unclear etiology (in presence of normal ventricular function). **(3)** Pharmacologic conversion or suppression of supraventricular tachycardias (particularly atrial fibrillation or flutter) **(4)** Control of rapid ventricular rate via accessory pathway conduction in pre-excitation syndromes

<u>Action:</u> Class IA antiarrhythmic. Depresses conduction velocity and automaticity, prolongs refractoriness of atrial and ventricular myocardium and of accessory pathways while shortening refractoriness (via

[79] Pawar KS, *et al.* Continuous pralidoxime infusion versus repeated bolus injection to treat organophosphorus pesticide poisoning: a randomised controlled trial. *Lancet 2006; 368: 2136-2141.*

anticholinergic activity) of AV node. Mild anticholinergic without α-adrenergic blockade of quinidine. Negative inotropy in severe heart failure. Prolongs P-R and Q-T intervals.

**Metabolism:** Acetylated to NAPA in liver (20% of dose in slow and 30% of dose in fast-acetylators). NAPA excreted in urine; accumulates in renal failure. PCA associated with lupus-like syndrome; infrequent in rapid-acetylators, in whom procainamide levels are lower. Plasma $T_\frac{1}{2}$ 3-4 hr.

**IV:** **Loading dose:** 15-18 mg/min over 25-30 min. Alternatively 100 mg bolus over 2 min, repeat q 5 min as needed to total dose 1 g. **Emergency** 20 mg/min until arrhythmia stops **or** adverse effect (QRS prolonged 50%, QT prolonged > 35%, or hypotension) **or** maximum total dose of 17 mg/kg. Infuse up to 50 mg/min as tolerated during emergencies. **Maintenance:** 2 mg/min, range 1-4 mg/min.

**PO:** Total 2-6 g/d, begin at 50 mg/kg/d. First dose one renal $T_\frac{1}{2}$ (3-4 hr) after last IV dose. Regular formulation q 3-4 hr; sustained release q 6 hr. If CrCl 10-50 mL/min give q 6-12 hr; CrCl < 10mL/h give q 8-24 hr, following levels. Peak levels at 90 min after oral dose.

**Therapeutic levels:** Procainamide 3-10 mcg/mL, sometimes higher. NAPA 10-30 mcg/mL.

**Renal failure:** Procainamide $T_\frac{1}{2}$ 5-6 hr; NAPA $T_\frac{1}{2}$ 42-70 hr (normal 6-8 hr). Adjust per levels. Pending levels, reduce maintenance infusion by one third for moderate renal or cardiac dysfunction and by two-thirds for severe cardiac or renal dysfunction.

**Contraindications:** Complete AV block (may produce asystole), *torsades* or long QT.

**Interactions:** Increased levels with cimetidine, β-blockers, amiodarone.

**Caution:** Myasthenia gravis, renal insufficiency, atrial fibrillation or flutter (may accelerate ventricular response), negative inotrope in high-doses (esp. severe LV dysfunction). Prolongs sinus node recovery time in sick-sinus syndrome, unpredictable effects in digitalis toxicity, prolongs QT (may predispose to *torsades*). Rarely causes agranulocytosis or lupus-like syndromes. Hypotension at supratherapeutic concentrations, especially during IV load.

## Propofol[80] *(Diprivan)*

Action: Water-insoluble sedative-hypnotic produces rapid unconsciousness with short duration of action. Crosses blood-brain barrier rapidly, then redistributed and eliminated. Formulated as lipid emulsion.

Indications: **(1)** Rapid IV sedation for procedures **(2)** Maintenance sedation of mechanically ventilated patient **(3)** Alternative (off-label) agent for status epilepticus.

Kinetics: Onset 1-2 min, duration 3-10 min. $V_d = 60L/kg$ reflects water-insolubility and extensive tissue redistribution. Plasma $T_{1/2}$ 5 min after 1 hr infusion, 7 min after 10 hr infusion. Eliminated by hepatic conjugation then renal excretion.

IV: Monitored anesthesia care for procedures: Slow injection of 0.5 mg/kg over 3-5 min, or begin infusion of 100-150 mcg/kg/min (6 - 9 mg/kg/hr). Follow with maintenance infusion of 25-75 mcg/kg/min. Sedation for mechanical ventilation: 5 mcg/kg/min x 5 min then increase 5 - 10 mcg/kg/min q 5 - 10 min until desired sedation; max ~ 80 mcg/kg/min. Status epilepticus (off-label)[81]: 2 - 3 mg/kg initially, then boluses 1-2 mg/kg until seizure control, then 4-10 mg/kg/min (titrated to EEG). Withdraw slowly.

Renal failure/liver disease: No dose adjustment necessary.

Adverse effects: Dose-related myocardial depression, hypotension (often severe), respiratory depression or apnea, bradycardia. Injection pain reduced with lidocaine or large vein. Lipid emulsion supports

---

[80] Barr J, *et al.* Clinical practice guidelines for the management of pain, agitation, and delirium in adult patients in ICU. *Crit Care Med* 2013; 41: 263-306.

[81] Meierkord H, *et al.* EFNS guideline on the management of status epilepticus in adults. *Eur J Neurol* 2010; 17: 348-355.

microbial overgrowth[82]; use sterile technique and replace drug and tubing q 12 hr.  Long infusions (days) slow time to awakening. "Propofol infusion syndrome[83]" of lactic acidosis, rhabdomyolysis, renal and circulatory failure, Brugada-pattern ECG, brady-asystole associated with prolonged infusions.
Caution: Use aseptic technique.  Consider lipid emulsion calories (1.1 fat kcal/mL) in nutritional calculations.  Avoid prolonged > 48 hr infusions.
Interactions:  Concurrent opioids potentiate cardio-pulmonary depression.

# Propylene Glycol Diluent[84]

Action and adverse effects: Not a drug and not groovy. Diluent (excipient) for intravenous diazepam, loraze-pam, esmolol, nitroglycerin, phenytoin. Estimated safe up to 1 g/kg/d. Consider as an iatrogenic cause of unexplained anion gap metabolic acidosis, and hy-perosmolarity.  $T_{1/2}$ ~ 5hrs. Renal and hepatic metabo-lism incl to D-lactic acid.

# Protamine[85]

Action: Polycation from salmon sperm forms inactive complex with heparin, thereafter probably metabo-lized and fibrinolysed with release of some heparin. Weak anticoagulant via platelet and fibrinogen action. Neutralizes heparin instantly, but protamine effect often shorter duration than heparin.   Neutralizes anti-thrombin activity completely but anti-factor-Xa activity incompletely.

IV: 1 mg neutralizes ~ 100 units estimated circulating

[82] Bennett SN, *et al.* Postoperative infections traced to contamina-tion of an intravenous anesthetic, propofol. *N Engl J Med* 1995; 333: 147-154.
[83] Kam PC, *et al.* Propofol infusion syndrome. *Anaesthesia* 2007; 62: 690-701.
[84] Wilson KC, *et al.* Propylene glycol toxicity: a severe iatrogenic ill-ness in ICU patients receiving IV benzodiazepines. *Chest* 2005; 128: 1674-1681.
[85] Garcia DA, *et al.* Parenteral anticoagulants: ACCP Guidelines. *Chest* 2012; 141: e24S-43S.

heparin (assume heparin $T_\frac{1}{2}$ of 60 min). Give IV over 10 min not more than 50 mg/10 min. If 30 - 60 min have elapsed since heparin dose, reduce 25 - 50%; if > 2 hr since heparin reduce 75%. Subcutaneous heparin may require protamine continuous infusion to neutralize. Less effective in LMW heparin overdose but: 1 mg protamine per 100 anti-Xa units (~ 1 mg enoxaparin) within previous 8 hr. Repeat 0.5 mg protamine per 100 anti-Xa units enoxaparin if aPTT prolonged 2-4 hr after first infusion. Excessive protamine probably causes mild anticoagulation.

Kinetics: Elimination $T_\frac{1}{2}$ 7.5 min, which is shorter than heparin.

Warning: Prior sensitization may occur from NPH insulin, protamine, vasectomy; predisposes to possible anaphylactoid reactions. Corticosteroid & antihistamine pretreatment may be helpful in risk of allergic reaction. Rebound heparin effect and bleeding may occur 0.5-18 hr after protamine administration. Too-rapid administration causes hypotension and anaphylactoid reaction.

Incompatibility: Penicillins and cephalosporins.

# Prothrombin complex concentrate (4-factor PCC; *Kcentra*)

Action: Rapid reversal warfarin anticoagulation associated with bleeding, using all four factors (II, VII, IX, X) inhibited by vitamin K antagonists. Low volume allows rapid infusion compared with fresh frozen plasma, without risk of transfusion associated lung injury.

Kinetics: $T_\frac{1}{2}$ 4-60 hr depending on factor.

IV: For INR 2-4: 25 units/kg of Factor IX maximum 2500; For INR 4-5: 35 units/kg maximum 3500; For INR > 6: 50 units/kg maximum 5000 units. Infuse at 0.12 mL/kg/min (~ 3 units/kg/min) up to maximum 8.4 mL/min. Expect INR to fall to ~ 2.5 within 30 min. Administer vitamin K concurrently in order to reconstitute clotting factors after PCC metabolized.

<u>Caution</u>: Contains heparin; avoid in HIT. Associated with serious thromboembolism risk possibly related to underlying thrombotic tendency.

# Pulmonary Vasodilators[86]
Nitric oxide, calcium blockers, ambrisentan, bosentan, macicentan, sildenafil, tadalafil, riociguat, epoprostenol, iloprost, trepostinil

## Nitric Oxide (Inomax)[87]
<u>Indications</u>:   Pulmonary vasodilator selective for ventilated alveoli. Indicated for newborn hypoxic respiratory failure with pulmonary artery hypertension. All adult usage is off-label. Diagnostic test for reversibility of pulmonary artery hypertension and responsiveness to vasodilators. May improve ventilation:perfusion matching.
<u>Kinetics</u>: $T_{1/2}$ < 10 sec. Primarily renal excretion as nitrate.
<u>Dose</u>: <u>Pediatric inhalation</u>: 20 ppm. **Off-label** acute pulmonary vasodilator, ARDS, acute right ventricular dysfunction complicating cardiac surgery, sickle acute chest syndrome: 10-80 ppm via nasal cannula, face mask, or ventilator.
<u>Toxicity</u>:    Methemoglobinemia, especially with doses > 20 ppm.
<u>Caution</u>: Administered in an adequately ventilated room. Consider monitoring methemoglobin and $NO_2$ up to every 6 hr.   Do not discontinue abruptly. May cause acute pulmonary edema in left ventricular dysfunction.   Contraindicated in patients dependent on R → L blood shunting.

## Calcium Channel Blockers
<u>Indication</u>:   PAH and positive vasoreactivity study. Not evidently helpful in connective tissue dz, HIV,

---

[86] Galie N, *et al.* 2015 ESC/ERS Guidelines for the diagnosis and treatment of pulmonary hypertension. *Eur Respir J* 2015; 46: 903-975.
[87] Griffiths MJ, *et al.* Inhaled nitric oxide therapy in adults. *N Engl J Med* 2005; 353: 2683-2695.

porto-pulmonary hypertension, and pulmonary venoocclusive dz.

<u>PO</u>: <u>Nifedipine</u> long-acting 120-240 mg; <u>Diltiazem</u> 240-720 mg; <u>Amlodipine</u> 20 mg. Begin at quarter dose and escalate cautiously to maximum tolerated dose.

<u>Adverse effects</u>: Limiting symptomatic hypotension and peripheral edema.

<u>Monitoring</u>: Reassess by RHC at 3-4 mo.

## Ambrisentan *(Letairis)*

<u>Action</u>: Endothelin receptor antagonist, binds receptor type A. Effective in PAH, connective tissue disease, HIV infection. Abnormal liver function tests up to 3%. Indicated for WHO group 1 FCII-IV symptoms.

<u>Kinetics</u>: $T_{\frac{1}{2}}$ ~ 9 hr.

<u>PO</u>: 5 mg daily with or without tadalafil 20 mg qd. Increment either drug at 4 wk intervals to ambrisentan 10 mg qd or tadalafil 40 mg qd.

<u>Warning</u>: Test for and avoid use in pregnancy because of embryo-fetal toxicity.

<u>Pregnancy</u>: Category X.

## Bosentan *(Tracleer)*

<u>Action</u>: Endothelin receptor antagonist, blocks type A and B receptors. Effective in PAH, connective tissue disease, Eisenmenger. Indicated for WHO group 1 FCII-IV symptoms.

<u>Kinetics</u>: $T_{\frac{1}{2}}$ ~ 5 hr. Avoid liver impairment. No adjustment for renal impairment.

<u>PO</u>: 62.5 bid for 4 wk then increase to 125 mg bid.

<u>Interactions</u>: Ritonavir requires dosing qod.

<u>Warning</u>: Test for and avoid use in pregnancy because of embryo-fetal toxicity. Hepatotoxicity 10% requires monthly liver function test checks.

<u>Pregnancy</u>: Category X.

## Macitentan *(Opsumit)*

<u>Action</u>: Endothelin receptor antagonist, blocks type A and B receptors. Effective in PAH. Indicated for WHO group 1 FCII-III symptoms.

<u>Kinetics</u>: $T_{1/2}$ ~ 16 hr; active metabolite 48 hr. No adjustment renal or hepatic impairment.

<u>PO</u>: 10 mg daily.

<u>Interactions</u>: Potentiated by ritonavir, ketoconazole, strong CYP3A4 inhibitors.

<u>Warning</u>: Test for and avoid use in pregnancy because of embryo-fetal toxicity.

<u>Pregnancy</u>: Category X.

## Sildenafil *(Revatio)*

<u>Action</u>: Phosphodiesterase Type 5 (PDE5) inhibitor. Indicated for WHO group 1 FCII-III symptoms.

<u>Kinetics</u>: $T_{1/2}$ ~ 4 hr whether PO or IV. Clearance reduced in hepatic and renal impairment.

<u>PO</u>: 20 mg tid.

<u>IV</u>: 10 mg tid is equivalent to 20 mg tid.

<u>Interactions</u>: Riociguat effect potentiated. Ritonavir not recommended. No incremental value to added bosentan.

<u>Contraindicated</u>: Concomitant organic nitrate.

<u>Pregnancy</u>: Category B.

## Tadalafil *(Adcirca)*

<u>Action</u>: PDE5 inhibitor. Indicated for WHO group 1 FCII-III symptoms.

<u>Kinetics</u>: $T_{1/2}$ ~ 35 hr. Renal impairment halve dose. Hepatic impairment no data.

<u>PO</u>: 40 mg once daily. ESC recommends 2.5 mg as lowest dose.

<u>Interactions</u>: Ritonavir, organic nitrates.

<u>Contraindicated</u>: Concomitant organic nitrate.

<u>Pregnancy</u>: Category B.

### Riociguat *(Adempas)*

<u>Action:</u> Cyclic GMP inhibitor. Indicated in chronic thromboembolic pulmonary hypertension (CTEPH); also WHO group 1 FCII-III symptoms.

<u>Kinetics:</u> $T_{1/2}$ ~ 12 hr. Avoid in severe hepatic impairment and in CL-Cr < 15 mL/min or dialysis.

<u>PO:</u> Start 0.5-1.0 mg tid, uptitrate ≥ q 2 wk if SBP > 95, to maximum 2.5 mg tid on background endothelin antagonist or prostanoids.

<u>Contraindicated:</u> Concomitant PDE5 inhibitor or nitrate or nitric oxide donor. Pregnancy.

<u>Warning:</u> Test for and avoid use in pregnancy because of embryo-fetal toxicity.

<u>Pregnancy:</u> Category X.

### Epoprostenol (Flolan, Prostacyclin, PGI2)

<u>Action:</u> Short-acting pulmonary and systemic vasodilator and inhibitor of platelet aggregation. Improves exercise and survival in pulmonary arterial hypertension WHO group 1 FCIII-IV symptoms. Use in functional class IV and rapidly progressive disease.

<u>Kinetics:</u> Rapid hydrolysis in blood, $T_{1/2}$ 6 min.

<u>IV:</u> Initiate 2 ng/kg/min, then ↑ 2 ng/kg/min increments q ≥ 15 min until dose-limiting effects (hypotension, nausea, headache, abdominal pain), then reduce 2 ng/kg/min to establish infusion rate. Expect subsequent adjustments 1-2 ng/kg/min q ≥ 15 min based on symptoms. Optimal chronic monotherapy as high as 150 ng/kg/min in adults.

<u>Contraindication:</u> Severe left ventricular dysfunction.

<u>Side-effects:</u> Hypotension, nausea, vomiting, headache, flushing, lightheadedness, restlessness, anxiety, abdominal pain, dyspnea, tachycardia, bradycardia, platelet dysfunction.

<u>Caution:</u> Exacerbates R → L shunt (hypoxemia), *e.g.* across atrial septal defect. Consider paradoxical shunt complications of indwelling infusion device. Avoid abrupt discontinuation.

<u>Pregnancy:</u> Category B.

## Iloprost *(Ventavis)*

<u>Action</u>: Prostanoid. Indicated for WHO group 1 FCIII-IV symptoms

<u>Inhaled</u>: 2.5 mcg via dedicated nebulizer 6-9 times daily, maximum q 2 hr. Increase to 5 mcg per dose as tolerated.

<u>Kinetics</u>: $T_{1/2}$ 20-30 min . Increase dosing interval to q3-4 hr in hepatic impairment. No adjustment for renal impairment.

<u>Pregnancy</u>: Category C.

## Treprostinil
### *(Orenitram po, Remodulin IV, Tyvaso inhaled)*

<u>Action</u>: Prostanoid. Indicated for WHO group 1 FCII-IV symptoms.

<u>Kinetics</u>: $T_{1/2}$ 4 hr. Hepatic elimination. Adverse effects may be increased in hepatic and renal impairment.

<u>SQ</u> or <u>IV</u>: 1.25 ng/kg/min, increment weekly for first four weeks, then 2.5 ng/kg/min per week thereafter. Dose interruptions should not last more than a few hours and otherwise may require dose reduction.

<u>Inhaled</u>: 6 mcg breaths x 3 per session, qid. Reduce as needed to 1-2 breaths if not tolerated. Escalate by 3 breaths per session q 1-2 wk to target 9 breaths per session.

<u>PO</u>: 0.25 mg q 12 hr or q 8 hr. Increment every 3-4 d. Maximum dose 12-21 mg bid. Take with food. Do not crush.

<u>Warning</u>: Inhibits platelet aggregation and may increase bleeding.

<u>Pregnancy</u>: Category B.

## Pyridostigmine
*See* Anticholinesterases on *page 262*

## Rasburicase *(Elitek)*

<u>Action</u>: Recombinant urate oxidase. Degrades uric acid to allantoin and peroxide, in contrast to allopurinol which generates stone-forming xanthine. Effective

against preformed uric acid, unlike allopurinol and febuxostat; therefore treats hyperuricemia despite acute renal failure.

<u>Kinetics</u>: Terminal $T_{1/2}$ 15-23 hr.

<u>IV</u>: 0.2 mg/kg over 30 min, daily for 5 d (7 d in EU)

<u>Contraindicated</u>: G6PD deficiency.  Prior anaphylaxis from rasburicase.

<u>Adverse effects</u>: Anaphlyaxis especially subsequent treatment cycles.  Causes methemoglobinemia. Degrades uric acid in test tubes, yielding spuriously low lab values; ice specimens for measurement.

## Reteplase (rPA; *Retavase*)

*See* Fibrinolytic Agents on *page 284*

## Remifentanil *(Ultiva)*

<u>Action</u>: Rapid-acting μ-opioid agonist indicated for general anesthesia and perioperative pain. Used as ICU sedative.

<u>Kinetics</u>: Rapid-distribution $T_{1/2}$ 1 min, slower distribution $T_{1/2}$ 6 min, terminal elimination $T_{1/2}$ 10-20 min. Unaffected by renal or hepatic function. Hydrolyzed by blood and tissue esterases.

<u>IV</u>: <u>ICU sedation</u> (off-label): Load 0.4-0.8 mcg/kg, then 0.5-2 mcg/kg/min.  <u>Postoperative analgesia</u>: 0.1mcg/kg/min, range 0.025-0.2mcg/kg/min.

<u>Adverse effects</u>: Bradycardia, hypotension, constipation, respiratory depression.

<u>Caution</u>: Analgesia ends 5-10 min after discontinuing remifentanil.

<u>Pregnancy</u>: Category C.

## Rivaraoxaban *(Xarelto)*

*See* Novel Oral Anticoagulants on *page 328*

## Rocuronium *(Zemuron)*

*See* Neuromuscular Blockers on *page 320*

## Sodium polystyrene sulfonate *(Kayexalate)*

<u>Action</u>: Cation-exchange resin exchanges $K^+$ for $Na^+$ in the gut.  Treats severe hyperkalemia by removing K

from body, along with other cations. Binds ~ 1 mEq K$^+$ per gram sodium polystyrene sulfonate. Onset 2-12 hr PO; 30-90 min per rectum. 15 g = 4 level teaspoons. <u>PO</u>: 15-60 g Kayexalate + 20-100 mL water or syrup q 2-6 hr.

<u>PR</u>: 30-50 g Kayexalate + 100 mL warm water as retention enema (for several hours) q 6 hr followed by voluminous (up to 2L) cleansing enema.

<u>Adverse effects</u>: Hypomagnesemia, hypocalcemia, alkalosis, overshoot hypokalemia. Sodium load may precipitate heart failure. May cause constipation or impaction if used without laxative. <u>Black box warning</u>: Rare reports colonic necrosis when administered PR in uremic patients, attributed to sorbitol. Admixture with sorbitol not recommended.

**Succinylcholine**
*See* Neuromuscular blockers on *page 320*

**Tenecteplase (TNK-tPA; *TNKase*)**
*See* Fibrinolytic Agents on *page 284*

**Thiosulfate**
*See* "Cyanide Poisoning" on *page 249*

**Thrombolytics**
*See* Fibrinolytic Agents on *page 284*

**Triiodothyronine (T3)**
*See* Liothyronine on *page 314*

**Tirofiban (Aggrastat)**
*See* Glycoprotein II$_b$III$_a$ inhibitors on *page 293*

**Torsemide (Demadex)**
*See* Loop diuretics on *page 279*

# Vasopressin
*See also* Desmopressin on *page 274*
<u>Action</u>: Antidiuretic hormone; potent direct vasoconstrictor via V1 receptor on vascular smooth muscles independent of adrenergic mechanisms; procoagulant. Adjunctive with epinephrine in cardiac arrest,

probably does not improve outcome[88]. Adjunct norepinephrine-sparing agent in vasodilatory shock, no mortality benefit[89]. Used in esophageal variceal hemorrhage to reduce portal pressure, hepatic flow, and as procoagulant. Used also in diabetes insipidus (DI) and as GI promotility agent.

<u>Kinetics:</u>    Hepatic and renal metabolism. Renal excretion. $T_{1/2}$ 10-20 min.

<u>IV:</u> All off-label except DI. <u>Cardiac arrest</u>[90]: 20 units IV push with each cycle of epinephrine combined with methylprednisolone 40mg and stress dose steroids after ROSC. <u>Upper GI hemorrhage</u>[91]: 0.2-0.4 units/min to maximum 0.6 units/min until bleeding controlled for 24 hr. Combine with nitroglycerin 40-400 mcg/min keeping SBP > 90 mmHg. <u>Diabetes insipidus:</u> 5-10 units SQ/IM q 6-12 h. <u>Adjunct to NE in shock</u> 0.01-0.03 units/min IV.r

<u>Adverse effects:</u> Myocardial ischemia via coronary vasoconstriction; water intoxication; skin necrosis if extravasated; abdominal cramps, sweating.

<u>Interactions:</u>    Ganglionic blocking agents markedly increase vasopressor effects. Antidiuretic effect potentiated by carbamazepine, tricyclics, clofibrate, fludrocortisone, chlorpropamide. Antidiuretic effect antagonized by norepinephrine, lithium, alcohol, demeclocycline.

## Vecuronium

*See* Neuromuscular blockers on *page 320*

---

[88] Wenzel V, *et al.* A comparison of vasopressin and epinephrine for out-of-hospital cardiopulmonary resuscitation. *N Engl J Med* 2004; 350: 105-113; Gueugniaud PY, *et al.* Vasopressin and epinephrine vs. epinephrine alone in cardiopulmonary resuscitation. *N Engl J Med* 2008; 359: 21-30.

[89] Russell JA, *et al.* Vasopressin versus norepinephrine infusion in patients with septic shock. *N Engl J Med* 2008; 358: 877-887.

[90] Mentzelopoulos SD, *et al.* Vasopressin, steroids, and epinephrine and neurologically favorable survival after in-hospital cardiac arrest: a randomized clinical trial. *JAMA* 2013; 310: 270-279.

[91] Garcia-Tsao G, *et al.* Management of varices and variceal hemorrhage in cirrhosis. *N Engl J Med* 2010; 362: 823-832.

# Verapamil

*See diltiazem on page 278.*

<u>Action</u>: Slow calcium channel antagonist. Depresses SA node, slows AV node conduction (but not AV bypass tracts). Reduces myocardial contractility. Antihypertensive via cardiac and vascular smooth muscle relaxation. Used IV to interrupt reentrant rhythms involving AV node and to slow ventricular response to atrial fibrillation and flutter. Used PO to lower BP, suppress angina and supraventricular tachycardias.

<u>Kinetics</u>: Onset 3-5 min. Liver metabolism. Terminal $T_{1/2}$ 2 hr acute, 4-12 hr chronic, extended in hepatic disease.

<u>IV</u>: <u>Narrow complex tachycardia</u>: 2.5-10 mg (38-150 mcg/kg) over 2-3 min. May repeat 5-10 mg (75-150 mcg/kg) after 15-30 min.

<u>Renal failure</u>: No adjustment.

<u>Liver failure</u>: Reduce dose by up to 50%.

<u>Contraindications</u>: Undiagnosed wide-complex tachycardia; Wolff-Parkinson-White syndrome; severe left ventricular dysfunction, sinus node dysfunction.

<u>Adverse reactions</u>: Hypotension; bradycardia or asystole when given IV, especially with concurrent β-blockers, digoxin, hypokalemia, or in sinus node dysfunction. May exacerbate heart failure.

<u>Interactions</u>: Many. Digoxin clearance halved (reduce digoxin dose by 50%). Neuromuscular blockers potentiated; reports of vascular collapse with dantrolene.

<u>Pregnancy</u>: Category C.

# Warfarin[92] *(Coumadin)*

<u>Action</u>: Oral anticoagulant. Blocks vitamin-K-dependent factors II, VII, IX, X, proteins C & S. Heterogeneous half-lives of clotting factors causes transient hypercoagulability upon starting therapy, especially in partial factor C & S deficiency. Use concomitant anticoagulation until INR is therapeutic to overcome this phenomenon, especially in high thrombotic risk. Genotyping CYP2C9 or VKORC1 does not reduce

---

[92] Holbrook A, *et al.* Evidence-based management of anticoagulant therapy. Chest 2012; 141: e152S-184S.

complications.

**Kinetics:** Complete bioavailability, highly albumin-bound, hepatic metabolism, enterohepatic circulation. $T_{1/2}$ 1-2 d, biological effect 2-7 d.

**Renal failure:** No adjustment.

**PO:** Start 5 mg qd x 3-4 d (consider 2.5 mg in elderly, malnourished, liver disease, or high bleeding risk); adjust subsequent doses to achieve target INR. Check

$$INR = \left[\frac{Patient\ PT}{Control\ PT}\right]^{ISI}$$

INR qd after day 2 until INR range achieved x 2 d, then 2-3 times weekly for 1-2 ws, followed by less frequent monitoring until INR stable. ACCP 2012 recommends starting 10 mg d.

**Monitoring:** International Normalized Ratio (INR). "ISI" (international sensitivity index) varies with reagent batch. INR may overestimate *in vivo* anti-coagulation during first few days of therapy.

**Adverse effects:** Major hemorrhage; risk increased if age > 65, stroke or GI bleeding history, renal insufficiency or anemia. Hypercoagulant during initiation of therapy. Skin necrosis via thrombosis of venules and capillaries of SQ fat (usually seen in protein C and S deficiency on therapy d 3-8), atheroembolism or purple toe syndrome.

**Pregnancy**[93]**:** Category X, especially gestation weeks 6-12. In mechanical valves & planned or actual pregnancy, LMWH recommended despite ↑ valve thrombosis risk. Warfarin may be substituted after wk13 until close to delivery. ASA 75-100 mg may be added if high risk of thromboembolism. Safe to nurse.

---

[93] Bates SM, *et al.* VTE, thrombophilia, antithrombotic therapy, and pregnancy: ACCP Guidelines. *Chest* 2012; *141: e691S-736S.*

## INR targets

| Indication, Duration | INR (range) |
|---|---|
| • Prosthetic heart valve: • Mechanical heart valve in mitral position; • Cage-ball valve in any position | 3.0 (2.5-3.5) |
| • Prosthetic heart valve: • Mechanical heart valve in aortic position; • Bioprosthetic heart valve in mitral position; • DVT or PE whether provoked or related to coagulopathy • Atrial fibrillation | 2.5 (2.0-3.0) |

## High INR

No bleeding: • INR > 10: Give vitamin K 2 mg po and withhold warfarin; • INR 4.5-10: No evident benefit to vitamin K beyond withholding warfarin

Bleeding: Give four-factor plasma complex concentrate (*see PCC on page 345*)

## Thrombotic risk of perioperative warfarin interruption[94]

| Risk | Mechanical Heart Valve | Atrial fibrillation | Venous thromboembolism (VTE) |
|---|---|---|---|
| High > 10% | Any mitral prosthesis Any caged-ball or tilting-disc aortic Stroke or TIA < 6 mo | $CHADS_2 \geq 5$ Stroke or TIA < 3 mo Rheumatic valve dz | VTE within 3 mo Clotting disorder (Prot C or S deficiency, APL, etc) |
| Medium 5-10% | Bileaflet aortic valve prosthesis and: afib, prior stroke/TIA, HTN, DM, CHF, age > 75 | $CHADS_2 = 3-4$ | VTE < 3-12 mo Recurrent VTE Active cancer treated < 6 mo or palliation Non-severe thrombophilia" |
| Low < 5% | Bileaflet aortic valve prosthesis without risks above | $CHADS_2 = 0-2$ and no prior stroke/TIA | Single VTE ≥ 12 mo ago without |

# non-severe thrombophilia: Factor V Leiden or prothrombin mutation

## Managing warfarin before surgery

High bleeding risk surgery: • Urology (TURP, bladder resection, tumor ablation, nephrectomy, renal biopsy); • Cardiac device: (ICD, pacemaker implant); • Colon polypectomy (esp > 1-2 cm); • General

---

[94] Douketis JD, *et al*. Perioperative management of antithrombotic therapy: ACCP Guidelines. *Chest* 2012; 141: e326S-350S.

<u>surgery</u>: Vascular organs, Bowel resection, Any major surgery with extensive tissue injury; • <u>Cardiac</u> surgery; • <u>Brain</u> surgery; • <u>Spinal</u> surgery

<u>Stop warfarin</u> 5d before surgery, restart 12-24 h after surgery

<u>Bridge anticoagulation:</u> • recommended in high ACCP thrombosis risk; • consider in moderate ACCP thrombosis risk. • Initiate bridging when INR is sub-therapeutic. • Bridge using LMWH or UFH. • No benefit and ↑ bleeding in RCT[95] of bridging for elective surgery in atrial fibrillation, mostly postoperative, using LMWH bridging.

<u>Selected drug interactions that increase risk of bleeding</u>

• <u>NSAIDs</u>; <u>Antiplatelet agents</u> including ASA, clopidogrel, other P2Y12 inhibitors; • <u>Antibiotics</u>: cephalosporins esp cefradine; amoxicillin; doxycycline; metronidazole; cotrimoxazole; ciprofloxacin; levofloxacin; norfloxacin; fluconazole; • <u>SSRIs</u>; • Tramadol; • CoenzymeQ; • Ginger

# Zoledronic acid (*Zometa*)

*See* pamidronate on *page 333. See* hypercalcemia on *page 220*.

<u>Action</u>: Bisphosphonate inhibits osteoclast activity. Indicated in hypercalcemia of malignancy.

<u>Kinetics</u>: Primarily eliminated via kidney; $T_{1/2}$ = 167 hr. 56% bound to plasma proteins

<u>IV</u>: 4 mg IV single dose IV infusion over > 15 min. Assure adequate hydration prior to drug administration. May repeat (4 mg) after 7 d if calcium does not return to normal.

<u>Renal dysfunction</u>: eGFR 50-60 mL/min: 3.5 mg; 40-49: 3.3 mg; 30-39: 3.0 mg.

<u>Interactions</u>: Additive renal toxicity when given with aminoglycosides and other nephrotoxic drugs. Risk of renal dysfunction increased in multiple myeloma, particularly when given with thalidomide

[95] Douketis JD, *et al.* Perioperative Bridging Anticoagulation in Patients with Atrial Fibrillation. *N Engl J Med 2015; 373: 823-833*

<u>Adverse effects</u>: Nephrotoxicity (including acute renal failure), fever, flu-like symptoms, nausea/vomiting, rash, chest pain. Reports of jaw osteonecrosis confounded by frequent concurrent glucocorticoids, chemotherapy, infection, but assure adequate dental hygiene before treatment, avoid invasive dental procedures after treatment. Hypocalcemia, especially used with loop diuretics.

<u>Incompatibility</u>: Calcium-containing infusion solutions (*i.e.* lactated Ringers)

<u>Pregnancy</u>:  Category D

# INDEX

ABCD2 score, 158
Abciximab, 294
Acarbose, 302
Acebutolol, 267
Acetaminophen toxicity, 245, 258
Acetazolamide, 208
Acetylcysteine, 246, 258
Acid-base map, 1
Acidosis, 268
    Lactic, 201, 204
    Metabolic, 1, 168, 201, 203, 243, 245, 247, 268, 344
    Renal tubular, 206
    Respiratory, 1
ACLS, 13
ACTH, 89
    Stimulation test, 89
Activated partial thromboplastin time, 128
Acute coronary syndrome, 17, 296
Acute coronary syndromes, 43, 48, 49, 291, 293, 294, 297, 298, 300
Adenosine, 15, 33, 258, 259
Adrenal insufficiency, 81, 88
    in sepsis, 89
Airway, 10
Airway obstruction, 188
Alcohol, 2
Alcohol ketoacidosis, 168
Alcohol withdrawal, 166
Alkalosis
    Metabolic, 1, 207
    Respiratory, 1, 248
Allopurinol, 224
Alteplase, 287
Ambrisentan, 347
American Society of Anesthesia (ASA) classification, 44, 198
Aminophylline, 259
Amiodarone, 12, 15, 33, 260
Amyl nitrite, 21, 250
Amylase, 105
Analgesics, 332, 351

Anaphylaxis, 62, 281, 293
Anatomy
    Bronchoscopic, 185
    Chest, 181
    Coronary, 24
    Cross-sectional, 184
    Heart, 23
    Peripheral nerves, 172
Anemia, 113
    Chronic disease, 118
    Iron-deficiency, 116
    Microcytic, 118
    Pernicious, 120
Anesthetic, 310
Aneurysm, intracranial, 149
Angina
    Unstable, 43, 49, 297, 300, 325
Angioplasty, coronary, 264, 291, 293, 294, 299
Anion gap, 201, 202
Antianginal, 325
Antiarrhythmic, 261, 265, 266, 278, 306, 313, 315, 341, 354
Anticholinergic syndromes, 237, 262
Anticholinesterases, 262
    Toxicity, 265, 341
Anticoagulants, 51, 53, 122, 124, 193, 291, 296, 298, 299, 328, 344, 354, 357
    reversal, 307, 344, 345, 355
Anticonvulsant, 165, 312, 315, 317, 336, 343
Antidiuretic hormone, 352
Antidotes, 236
Anti-emetic, 331
Anti-Factor-$X_a$ Activity, 129, 300, 328
Antihypertensives, 42, 43, 272, 300, 311, 323, 325, 335
Antinuclear antibody, 225
Antiphospholipid antibody, 130
Antipsychotic, 295
Antithrombin, 264, 291, 296

Aortic
  stenosis, 20, 22, 54, 326
  valve area, 54
  valve regurgitation, 56
  valve stenosis, 55
Aortic dissection, 43, 151, 282
APACHE II score, 64
Apixaban, 328
ARDS, xiv, 61, 66, 70, 109, 111, 125, 127, 320, 346
Argatroban, 124, 264
Arthritis, 232
Ascites, 100
Aspirin, 50
Asthma, 189
Asystole, 13
Atenolol, 267
ATN, 223, 224
Atracurium, 321
Atrial fibrillation, 35, 276, 278, 306, 328, 354, 356
Atrial flutter, 306
Atropine, 14, 254, 265
Autoantibody, 225
Autonomic instability, 241, 242
Azotemia, 223, 224
B12 deficiency, 118
Balloon pump, 40
Barbiturate, 334
Barotrauma, 70
Benzodiazepines, 164, 167, 289
  Overdose, 289
Beta-Adrenergic Blockers, 43, 50, 266, 282, 293, 310, 311
  Overdose, 305
  Toxicity, 240, 292
Betamethasone, 273
Betaxolol, 267
Bicarbonate, 204, 239, 240, 244, 249, 268
  Deficit, 204
BiPAP, 73
Bisoprolol, 267
Bisphosphonate, 333, 357
Bivalirudin, 124, 269
Blatchford score, 91
Bleeding, 91
Blood transfusion, 125, 134
Body surface area, 4

Bosentan, 347
Bradycardia, 14, 39, 265, 293, 310
Brain Abscess, 169
Brain Death, 178
Bromocriptine, 304
Bronchodilator, 187, 281
Bronchospasm, 281
Brugada, 27, 34
Brugada criteria, 31
Bumetanide, 279
Bundle branch block, 29, See LBBB or RBBB
C. difficile, 95
Calcitonin, 222
Calcitriol, 220
Calcium, 3, 219, 220, 240, 270
Calcium channel blockers, 270, 272, 278, 323, 324, 347, 354
  Toxicity, 240, 292
  Overdose, 304
Calcium gluconate, 220
Calculators, 9
Carbon dioxide, 5, 12
Cardiac arrest, 313, 353
Cardiac cycle, 19
Cardiac index, 6
Cardiac output, 4, 6
Cardiopulmonary resuscitation, 10
Cardioselective, 282
Carteolol, 267
Carvedilol, 267
Catecholamine extravasation, 335
Catecholamines, 279, 280, 281
Central pontine myelinolysis, 211
Cerebral vasospasm, 324
Cerebrospinal fluid, 140, 168
CHADS₂, 35
Charcoal, 235, 246, 249, 271
Chest anatomy
  CT, 184
  Radiographs, 181
Child-Pugh score, 101
Chlordiazepoxide, 167
Chloride
  Urine, 208
Chlorothiazide, 271
Cholinergic syndromes, 237

Chronic thromboembolic pulmonary hypertension, 349
Cirrhosis, 100, 101
Cisatracurium, 321
Clearance, renal, 3
Clevidipine, 272, 315
Clonidine, 272
Clopidogrel, 339
Clostrodium difficile colitis, 97
Coagulation, 128
Cocaine, 43
Codeine, 332
Cold agglutinins, 113, 115
Colesevelam, 303
Colonic pseudo-obstruction, 262
Coma, 159, 178
Compliance, 70
  Lung, 5
Constipation, 317
Conversion, Units, 6
Coombs, 115
Cornell criteria LVH, 28
Coronary artery anatomy, 24
Coronary artery disease, 36
Coronary interventions, percutaneous (PCI), 264, 291, 293, 294, 299
Coronary stent, 92, 339
Corticosteroids, 273
Cortisol, 89
Cosyntropin, 89
Creatinine clearance, 2
Crystalloid, 60
CT scan, 184
CURB-65 Score, 141
Cyanide, 249, 301, 326
Cyproheptadine, 243
Cytochrome P450, 256
Cytomegalovirus, 134
Dabigatran, 307, 329
Dantrolene, 241, 274
Dead space, 5
Deep venous thrombosis, 190, 291, 296, 298, 327, 355
Delirium tremens, 166
Delta-delta gap, 202
Demyelination, osmotic, 211
Dermatomes, 172

Desmopressin, 103, 213, 274
Dexamethasone, 141, 273
Dexmedotomidine, 275
Diabetes insipidus, 212, 275, 353
Diabetic ketoacidosis (DKA), 84, 86
Diarrhea, 95, 96, 132
Diazepam, 164, 167, 244, 254, 344
Digoxin, 276
  Toxicity, 277, 336
Digoxin Immune Fab, 277
Diltiazem, 278
Dipyridamole, 259
Diuretic, 271, 316
Diuretics
  Loop, 279
  Thiazide, 271
DL$_{CO}$, 188
Dobutamine, 60, 192, 279
Dopamine, 14, 16, 280
Duke criteria, 135
Duke treadmill prognostic score, 38
DVT, 190
ECG, 25, 37
  Acute MI, 29, 30
  Bundle branch block, 29
  Fascicle block, 30
  Hypercalcemia, 221
  Hyperkalemia, 216
  Hypertrophy, 28
  Hypokalemia, 215
  Hypomagnesemia, 218
  Myxedema, 81
Eclampsia, 43, 315
Effusion
  Pleural, 194
eGFR, 2
Embolectomy, 192
Empyema, 194
Encephalopathy
  Hepatic, 102
  Hypertensive, 42
  Wernicke, 167
Endocarditis, 135, 136
  Prophylaxis, 136

Endothelin receptor antagonists, 197, 347
Enoxaparin, 298
Epilepticus, 166, 343
Epinephrine, 12, 14, 16, 60, 62, 63, 281
Epoprostenol, 349
Eptifibatide, 294
Esmolol, 267, 282, 344
Esophageal varices, 331, 353
Ethanol, 166, 283
Ethylene glycol, 2, 202, 243, 283, 290
Etomidate, 284
Euthyroid sick, 79
Exenatide, 303
Exercise tests, 37
Exudate, 194
Fascicular block, 30
FEMg, 218
FENa, 3, 223
Fentanyl, 332
Ferric carboxymaltose, 309
Ferric gluconate, 309
Ferritin receptor, 117
Ferumoxytol, 309
FE-Urea, 224
Fever, 82, 88, 127, 131, 135, 138, 148, 190, 227, 232
postoperative, 133
Fibrinolytics, 53, 155, 192, 287, 297
Fidaxomicin, 98
Fludrocortisone, 273
Fluid
Ascitic, 100
Cerebrospinal, 140, 168
Pleural, 193
Synovial, 231
Flumazenil, 234, 289
Folate deficiency, 119
Fomepizole, 245, 290
Fondaparinux, 124, 291
Formaldehyde, 202
Fosphenytoin, 164, 165, 337
Free water deficit, 213
Furosemide, 279
G6PD deficiency, 115, 251
Gallium nitrate, 222

Gap
Anion, 2
Osmolal, 2
Gastrointestinal hemorrhage, 90, 101, 353
Geneva Score, 191
Glasgow coma scale, 65, 176
Gliclazide, 302
Glimepiride, 302
Glipizide, 302
Glomerular filtration rate, 2
Glucagon, 236, 240, 292
Glucocorticoids, 61
Glyburide, 302
Glycoprotein II$_b$III$_a$ Inhibitors, 51, 293
Gout, 231
Gradient
Alveolar oxygen, 6
Grave's disease, 82
Haloperidol, 295
Haptoglobin, 115
Harris-Benedict Equation, 107
HAS-BLED, 35
Heart failure, 43, 271, 276, 279, 325, 326
Heart murmurs, 20, 22
Hemodialysis, 248
Hemodynamics, 6, 19
Hemolytic Anemia, 113
Hemolytic-Uremic Syndrome, 114
Hemorrhage, 90, 274, 331, 353
Heparin, 296
Low-Molecular Weight, 298
Overdose, 344
Heparin-induced thrombocytopenia, 264, 269, 291
Hepatorenal syndrome, 104, 331
Homocysteine, 119
Hydralazine, 300
Hydrochloric acid, 208
Hydrocodone, 332
Hydromorphone, 332
Hydroxocobalamin, 301
Hypercalcemia, 220, 333, 357
Hyperglycemia, 84, 305
Hyperkalemia, 27, 216, 268, 270, 304, 351

Hypernatremia, 212
Hyperosmolar hyperglycemic state, 84, 86
Hyperparathyroidism, 220
Hypertension, 42, 272, 278, 311, 323, 325, 326
Hyperthyroidism, 82
Hypertrophic cardiomyopathy, 20
Hypocalcemia, 219, 270
Hypoglycemia, 86, 292
Hypoglycemic agents, 301
Hypoglycorrhachia, 168
Hypokalemia, 214
Hypomagnesemia, 217, 315
Hyponatremia, 82, 209
Hypophosphatemia, 222
Hyporeninemic Hypoaldosteronism, 206, 207, 216
Hypothermia, 80
Hypothyroidism, 80, 314
Hypoxemia, 70, 71
Ibutilide, 306
Idarucizumab, 330
Ideal body weight, 4
Iloprost, 350
Immune thrombocytopenia, 120
Innervation, 169
Inotropes, 279, 280, 281, 292, 310, 318
Insulin, 85, 217, 304
International Normalized Ratio, 355
Intra-aortic balloon pump, 40
Intracerebral hemorrhage, 42
Intracranial hemorrhage, 150
Intralipid, 315
Iodine, 83
Iron, 117
Iron deficiency, 117
Iron Intravenous, 308
Iron sucrose, 309
Iron supplementation, 117
Iron-Deficiency Anemia, 116
Isopropanol, 2
Isoproterenol, 310
Joslin, 87, 306
Jugular venous pulsations, 20
Kayexalate, 217, 351, 352

Ketamine, 310
Ketoacidosis, 201, 304
    Diabetic, 202
Korsakoff's psychosis, 167
Labetalol, 267, 311
Lactic acidosis, 201, 204
LBBB, 29, 31, 285
Left bundle branch block, 29
Left ventricular hypertrophy (LVH), 27, 28
Lepirudin, 124
Levetiracetem, 312
Levorphanol, 332
Levothyroxine, 81, 313
Lidocaine, 251, 313
Liothyronine, 81, 314
Lipase, 105
Lipid or fat emulsion, 239, 240, 315, 343
Liraglutide, 303
Loading dose, 3
Long QT, 33
Lorazepam, 164, 165, 167, 244, 254, 344
Lower GI bleeding, 94
Lugol's solution, 83
Lumbar puncture, 139
Lung cancer resection, 199
Lung volumes, 186
Macitentan, 348
Macrocytic Anemia, 118
Magnesium, 13, 217, 218, 220, 315
Malignant hyperthermia, 134, 274, 320
Mannitol, 202, 316
Mechanical ventilation, 61, 68
Megaloblastic, 118
MELD Score, 102
Melena, 90
Meningitis, 139, 168
    TB, 169
    Tranplant patients, 148
Meningococcemia, 138
Meperidine, 332
Metabolic acidosis. See Acidosis: Metabolic
Metformin, 205, 301
Methadone, 332

Methanol, 2, 202, 283, 290
    Toxicity, 243
Methemoglobin, 236, 251, 316, 326
Methimazole, 83
Methylene blue, 250, 251, 316
Methylmalonic acid, 119
Methylnaltrexone, 110, 317
Methylprednisolone, 273
Metoprolol, 267
Metronidazole, 98
Microangiopathic hemolytic anemia, 121
Midazolam, 165, 317
Midodrine, 104
Miglitol, 302
Milrinone, 318
Mini-Mental State, 175
Minute ventilation, 5
Mitral valve stenosis, 54, 56
Mitral valve regurgitation, 20, 22, 57, 67
Mixing study, 130
Molarity, 2
Morphine, 333
Müller maneuver, 20
Murmurs, 20
Muscarinic, 237, 265
Muscles, 169
Myasthenia gravis, 262
Myeloma, 220
Myocardial infarction, 27, 43, 49, 50, 285, 297, 299, 300, 339
Myocardial ischemia, 325
Myxedema, 80, 313, 314
N-acetylcysteine. See Acetylcysteine
Nadolol, 267
Naloxone, 10, 13, 110, 234, 319
Nateglinide, 302
Nausea, 331
Nebivolol, 267
Neostigmine, 262, 340
Nerve agents, 252, 265, 341
Nerves, 169, 170
Neuroleptic malignant syndrome, 134, 241, 274
Neurologic Prognosis, 177

Neuromuscular blockers, 72, 73, 262, 320
    Reversal, 262
Nicardipine, 323
Nicotinic, 238
NIH stroke scale, 152
Nimodipine, 324
Nitric Oxide, 346
Nitrite, 250, 326
Nitrogen balance, 108
Nitroglycerin, 43, 50, 325, 344
Nitroprusside (Nipride), 43, 325
Norepinephrine, 16, 60, 105, 327
Novel Oral Anticoagulants, 328
NSTEMI, 48
Nutrition, 107
Octreotide, 104, 331
Omeprazole, 340
Ondansetron, 331
Opiate, 237, 332
    Toxicity, 319
Organ donation, 180
Organophosphate toxicity, Organophosphates, 340
    Toxicity, 265, 341
Orogastric lavage, 235
Osmolal gap, 201
Osmolality, 201
Osmolarity, 2, 201, 209
Oxazepam, 167
Oxygen, 5, 16, 69
Oxygen content, 6
$P2Y_{12}$ platelet inhibitor, 51, 52
Pacemaker, 39
Pamidronate, 222, 333
Pancreatitis, 105, 111
Pancuronium, 322
Paralyzing agents. See Neuromuscular blockers
Parathyroid, 220
Parenteral nutrition, 107
Paroxysmal cold hemoglobinuria, 114, 115
PCWP, 58, 66, 325, 326
PDE5 inhibitors, 197
Peak flow, 189
Pediatric vital signs, 9
PEEP, 70, 71
    Auto-, 71

Penbutalol, 268
Pentobarbital, 334
Pericardial tamponade, 67
Pericarditis, 27
Perioperative, 44, 101, 126, 197, 356
Phenobarbital, 165, 334
Phentolamine, 335
Phenylephrine, 336
Phenytoin, 164, 165, 336, 344
Pheochromocytoma, 43, 282, 325, 335
Phosphorus, 222, 338
Physical Examination, 20
Physostigmine, 262, 263
Pindolol, 268
Pioglitazone, 302
Plateau pressure, 74
Platelet P2Y$_{12}$ Inhibitors, 339
Platelet transfusion, 121, 126
Pleural effusion, 193
Pneumonia, 141
Pneumonia Severity Index/PORT Score, 142
Poison control hotline, 234
Poisoning, 289
  Acetaminophen, 245
  Anticholinergic, 237
  Anticholinesterase, 265, 341
  Cholinergic, 237
  Cyanide, 236, 326
  Ethylene glycol, 236, 243
  General management, 234
  Methanol, 236, 243
  Nerve agents, 252
  Opiate, 237, 319
  Organophosphate, 341
  Salicylate, 247
  Sedative, 237
  Sulfonylurea, 331
  Sympathomimetic, 237
Polydipsia, 210
Portal hypertension, 100
Positive End Expiratory pressure (PEEP), 70
Potassium, 3, 27, 214, 216
Pralidoxime, 254, 340
Prasugrel, 340

Prednisolone, 273
Prednisone, 273
Pre-operative risk assessment
  Liver disease, 101
Procainamide, 15, 33, 341
Procalcitonin assay, 134
Propanolol, 267
Propofol, 165, 315, 343
Propranolol, 83, 268
Propylene Glycol Diluent, 337, 344
Propylthiouracil, 83
Prostacyclin, 349
Prostanoids, 197
Prosthetic heart valve, 356
Protamine, 344
Prothrombin complex concentrate, 345
Prothrombin time, 128
Pulmonary artery catheters, 65
Pulmonary edema, 65
Pulmonary function testing, 186
Pulmonary hypertension, 195, 346, 347, 349
Pulmonary infiltrates, 148
Pulmonary mass, 186
Pulmonary thromboembolism, 190, 291, 296, 297, 298, 299, 328
  Thrombolytic therapy, 287
Pulmonary vasodilators, 318, 346
Pulseless electrical activity, 12
Purpura fulminans, 138
Pyridostigmine, 262, 263
Radiocontrast nephropathy, 258
Rankin Score, 153
Rasburicase, 224, 350
Rashes, 138
RBBB, 29
Red blood cell transfusion, 125
Regadenoson, 260
Remifentanil, 333, 351
Renal failure, 223
  Acute, 43, 223
Renal tubular acidosis, 206, 216
Repaglinide, 302
Reptilase time, 129

Resistance
Pulmonary vascular, 5, 6
Systemic vascular, 6
Restrictive lung disease, 72
Reteplase, 288
Reticulocyte production index, 113
Right bundle branch block, 29
Right ventricular dysfunction, 191, 319, 346
Right Ventricular Hypertrophy, 28
Riociguat, 197, 349
Risk score, 9, 35, 38, 45, 49, 90, 101, 109, 122, 158, 186, 197
Rivaroxaban, 330
Rockall score, 91
Rocky mountain spotted fever, 138
Rocuronium, 322
Romhilt-Estes criteria LVH, 28
Rosiglitazone, 302
rPA, 288
RVH, 28
SAAG, 100
Salicylate toxicity, 204, 247, 268
Sarin, 252
Schilling test, 120
Sedation, 72, 77, 275, 284, 295, 317, 343, 351
reversal, 289, 319
Seizures, 163, 166, 336
Sensitivity, statistical, 7
Sensivity, 8
Sepsis, 60
Serotonin syndrome, 134, 242
Shock, 58, 65, 281, 353
Cardiogenic, 40, 54, 58, 204
Septic, 58
Shunt, 6
SIADH, 210, 211
Sildenafil, 348
Sitagliptin, 303
SLE, 225
Sodium, 3, 209, 212, 223
Urinary, 209
Sodium polystyrene sulfonate, 351
Soman, 252
Sotalol, 15
Specificity, statistical, 7, 8

Spirometry, 187, 200
Spontaneous bacterial peritonitis, 100
Staphylococcal toxic shock syndrome, 139
Statistics, 7
Status epilepticus, 163, 318, 334, 336
Streptococci, 135, 139
Stress tests, 37
Stroke, 35, 42, 149, 151, 154, 286, 298, 300
Stroke Risk, 158
Subarachnoid hemorrhage, 43, 324
Succinylcholine, 322
Sulfonylurea overdose, 331
Sympathomimetic syndromes, 43, 237
Synovial Fluid Analysis, 231
Systemic Lupus Erythematosus, 229
Tabun, 252
Tachycardia, 15, 31, 261, 354
Supraventricular, 341
Ventricular, 15, 31, 261, 313
Wide-QRS, 259, 261, 341
Tadalafil, 348
Tamponade
Pericardial, 67
Targeted temperature management, 17, 77
Tenecteplase, 288
Tetany, 270
Therapeutic hypothermia, 77
Thiamine, 234
Thiocyanate, 326
Thiosulfate, 250, 326
Thrombocytopenia, 120
Heparin-induced, 121, 264
Thromboembolism
Venous, 287, 296, 300
Thrombolytics, 284
Thrombotic thrombocytopenia purpura, 114
Thyroid, 79, 80, 82, 313, 314
Storm, 82
Thyroid function tests, 79
Thyrotoxicosis, 82

Thyroxine, 81, 313
TIA, 158
Ticagrelor, 340
Tidal volume, 5
TIMI-Risk score, 49
Timolol, 268
Tirofiban, 295
TNK-tPA, 288
Torsades de pointes, 33, 218, 240, 307, 310, 315, 341, 343
Torsemide, 279
Toxic shock syndrome, 139
Toxic syndromes, 237
tPA, 287
Tramodol, 333
Transferrin, 117
Transfusion, 61, 125
    Lung injury, 127
    Reactions, 126
Transplantation
    Infections, 146
Transudate, 100, 194
Treprostinil, 350
Tricyclic antidepressant toxicity, 204, 238, 315
TTKG, 214
Tuberculosis, 169
Tumor lysis syndrome, 224, 350
Upper GI hemorrhage, 353
Urate oxidase, 350
Urea, 224
    Fractional excretion, 224
Urinary alkalinization, 269
Urinary anion gap, 203
Urinary tract infection, 132
Urine chloride, 208

Valsalva, 21
Valvuloplasty, 56
Vancomycin, 98
Varices, 331
    Bleeding, 93
    Hemorrhage, 353
Vasculitis, 227
Vasodilator, 266, 272, 282, 300, 311, 324, 325, 349, 354
Vasopressin, 60, 213, 352
Vasopressor, 60, 280, 281, 327, 336, 352
Vecuronium, 323
Ventilator, 68
    Emergencies, 74
    Non-invasive, 73
Ventilator Emergencies, 74
Ventricular Septal Defect, 67
Ventricular tachycardia, 314
Verapamil, 354
Vildagliptin, 303
Visual acuity, 174
Von Willebrand factor, 274
VX Gas, 252
Warfarin, 328, 329, 345, 354
Weaning, ventilator, 75
Wedge pressure. See PCWP
Weight, Ideal, 4
Well's Score, 190
Wernicke encephalopathy, 150, 167
Whole bowel irrigation, 235
Wide-complex tachycardia, 31
Zoledronate, 222, 357

# GROOVY DRUGS BY CATEGORY

**Cardiovascular & Pulmonary Drugs**
Abciximab (ReoPro), 258, 293
Adenosine (Adenocard), 258
Ambrisentan (Letairis), 347
Aminophylline, 259
Amiodarone (Cordarone), 260
Apixaban (Eliquis), 328
Argatroban, 264
Atropine, 265
Beta-Adrenergic Blockers, 266
Bosentan (Tracleer), 347
Calcium Blockers, 270, 272, 278,
   323, 324, 354, 346
Chlorothiazide (Diuril), 271
Clevidipine (Cleviprex), 272
Clonidine (Catapres), 272
Dabigatran (Pradaxa), 278, 328
Digoxin, 276
Diltiazem IV, 278
Diuretics, Loop, 279
Dobutamine, 279
Dopamine, 280
Epinephrine (Adrenalin), 281
Epoprostenol (Prostacyclin), 282,
   349
Esmolol (Brevibloc), 282
Fibrinolytic Agents, 284
Fondaparinux (Arixtra), 291
Glycoprotein II$_b$III$_a$ Inhibitors, 293
Heparin Unfractionated, 296
Heparin, LMWH, 298
Hydralazine (Apresoline), 300
Ibutilide (Corvert), 306
Idarucizumab (Praxbind), 307
Iloprost, 350
Isoproterenol (Isuprel), 310
Labetalol, 311
Macitentan (Opsumit), 348
Milrinone (Primacor), 318
Nicardipine IV (Cardene), 323
Nimodipine, 324
Nitric Oxide (Inomax), 346
Nitroglycerin, 325
Nitroprusside (Nipride), 325

Norepinephrine (Levophed), 327
Novel oral anticoagulants (NOACS),
   328
Phentolamine (Regitine), 335
Phenylephrine, 336
Procainamide, 341
Protamine, 344
Riociguat (Adempas), 349
Rivaroxaban (Xarelto), 330
Sildenafil (Revatio), 348
Tadalafil (Adcirca), 348
Treprostinil, 350
Vasopressin, 352
Verapamil, 354
Warfarin (Coumadin), 354

**Cardiac Rhythm Drugs**
Adenosine (Adenocard), 258
Amiodarone (Cordarone), 360
Atropine, 265
Digoxin, 276
Ibutilide (Corvert), 306
Lidocaine, 313
Procainamide, 341

**Coagulation and Hematology
Drugs**
Abciximab (ReoPro), 258, 293
Alteplase, 259, 284
Apixaban (Eliquis), 328
Argatroban, 264
Bivalirudin (Angiomax), 269
Clopidogrel, 339
Dabigatran (Pradaxa), 278, 328
Desmopressin (ddAVP), 274
Fibrinolytic Agents, 284
Fondaparinux (Arixtra), 291
Glycoprotein II$_b$III$_a$ Inhibitors, 293
Heparin Unfractionated, 296
Heparin, LMWH, 298
Idarucizumab (Praxbind), 307
Iron intravenous, 308
Novel oral anticoagulants (NOACS),
   328

Prasugrel, 340
Protamine, 344
Prothrombin complex concentrate (4-factor PCC; Kcentra), 345
Reteplase, 351, 284
Rivaroxaban (Xarelto), 351, 328
Tenecteplase, 352, 284
Thrombolytics, 352, 284
Ticagrelor, 340
Tirofiban (Aggrastat), 295
Vasopressin, 352
Warfarin (Coumadin), 354

**Endocrine Drugs**
Corticosteroids, 273
Glucagon, 292
Hypoglycemics other than insulin, 301
Insulin, 304
Levothyroxine (T4), 313
Liothyronine (T3), 314
Octreotide (Sandostatin), 331
Pamidronate (Aredia), 333
Triiodothyronine, 352, 314
Zoledronic acid (Zometa), 357

**Gastrointestinal Drugs**
Desmopressin (ddAVP), 274
Ethanol, 283
Methylnaltrexone (Relistor), 317
Octreotide (Sandostatin), 331

**Neurology Drugs**
Levetiracetem (Keppra), 312
Mannitol, 316
Nimodipine, 324
Pentobarbital, 334
Phenobarbital, 334
Physostigmine, 339, 262
Propofol (Diprivan), 343

**Renal Drugs**
Acetylcysteine (Mucomyst), 258
Bicarbonate, 268
Calcium, 270
Diuretics, Loop, 279

Iron intravenous, 308
Magnesium, 315
Mannitol, 316
Phosphorus, 338
Rasburicase (Elitek), 350
Sodium Polystyrene (Kayexalate), 310, 351
Torsemide, 352, 279

**Sedation, Anesthesia, and Reversal Drugs**
Anticholinesterases, 262
Atracurium, 265, 320
Cisatracurium (Nimbex), 321
Dexmedotomidine (Precedex), 275
Etomidate (Amidate), 284
Flumazenil (Romazicon), 289
Haloperidol (Haldol), 295
Ketamine (Ketalar), 310
Methylnaltrexone (Relistor), 317
Midazolam (Versed), 317
Naloxone (Narcan), 319
Neostigmine, 319, 262
Neuromuscular blockers, 320
Ondansetron (Zofran), 331
Opiate analgesics, 332
Pancuronium, 334, 320
Phenytoin (Dilantin), 336
Physostigmine, 339, 262
Pralidoxime (2-PAM), 340
Propofol (Diprivan), 343
Propylene glycol diluent, 344
Pyridostigmine, 263
Remifentanil, 351
Rocuronium, 351, 320
Succinylcholine, 352, 320
Vecuronium, 353, 320

**Toxicology Drugs**
Acetylcysteine (Mucomyst), 258
Charcoal, activated, 271
Cytochrome P450 (CYP) interactions, 256
Dantrolene, 274
Digoxin Immune Fab (Digifab), 277
Ethanol, 283

Fomepizole (Antizol), 290

Hydroxocobalamin (Cyanokit), 301

Lipid or fat emulsion (Intralipid), 315

Methylene Blue, 316

Naloxone (Narcan), 319

Phentolamine (Regitine), 335

Phenytoin (Dilantin), 336

Pralidoxime (2-PAM), 340

Pyridostigmine, 263

Thiosulfate, 352, 249

Glucagon, 292

# Notes

# Notes

# Notes

# Notes

# Notes

# Notes

# Notes

# Notes